T0213365

Clinical Cases in
Periodontics

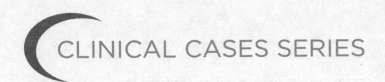

CLINICAL CASES SERIES

Clinical Cases in
Periodontics

Nadeem Karimbux, DMD, MMSc

Associate Professor
Department of Oral Medicine, Infection, and Immunity
Assistant Dean
Office of Dental Education
Harvard School of Dental Medicine
Harvard University
Boston, MA
USA

WILEY-BLACKWELL
A John Wiley & Sons, Inc., Publication

This edition first published 2012 © 2012 by John Wiley & Sons, Inc.

Wiley-Blackwell is an imprint of John Wiley & Sons, formed by the merger of Wiley's global Scientific, Technical and Medical business with Blackwell Publishing.

Registered office: John Wiley & Sons Ltd, The Atrium, Southern Gate, Chichester, West Sussex, PO19 8SQ UK

Editorial offices: 2121 State Avenue, Ames, Iowa 50014-8300, USA
                     The Atrium, Southern Gate, Chichester, West Sussex, PO19 8SQ UK
                     9600 Garsington Road, Oxford, OX4 2DQ UK

For details of our global editorial offices, for customer services and for information about how to apply for permission to reuse the copyright material in this book please see our website at www.wiley.com/wiley-blackwell.

Authorization to photocopy items for internal or personal use, or the internal or personal use of specific clients, is granted by Blackwell Publishing, provided that the base fee is paid directly to the Copyright Clearance Center, 222 Rosewood Drive, Danvers, MA 01923. For those organizations that have been granted a photocopy license by CCC, a separate system of payments has been arranged. The fee codes for users of the Transactional Reporting Service are ISBN-13: 978-0-8138-0794-2/2012.

Designations used by companies to distinguish their products are often claimed as trademarks. All brand names and product names used in this book are trade names, service marks, trademarks or registered trademarks of their respective owners. The publisher is not associated with any product or vendor mentioned in this book. This publication is designed to provide accurate and authoritative information in regard to the subject matter covered. It is sold on the understanding that the publisher is not engaged in rendering professional services. If professional advice or other expert assistance is required, the services of a competent professional should be sought.

Cover artwork: Top, center image created by Exan using axiUm Electronic Health Record.

Library of Congress Cataloging-in-Publication Data
Karimbux, Nadeem.
   Clinical cases in periodontics / Nadeem Karimbux.
      p. ; cm. – (Clinical cases)
   Includes bibliographical references and index.
   ISBN 978-0-8138-0794-2 (pbk. : alk. paper)
   I. Title. II. Series: Clinical cases (Ames, Iowa)
   [DNLM: 1. Periodontal Diseases–therapy–Case Reports. 2. Periodontics–methods–Case Reports. WU 240]
   617.632–dc23

                              2011036319

A catalogue record for this book is available from the British Library.

This book is published in the following electronic formats: ePDF 9780470962923; ePub 9780470962954; Mobi 9780470962985

Set in 10/13 pt Univers Light by Toppan Best-set Premedia Limited

1   2012

DEDICATION

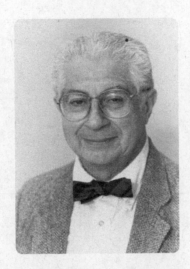

Henry David Epstein, 1914–2011
(Courtesy of the Epstein family.)

Founding member of the Department of Periodontology at the Harvard School of Dental Medicine and an inspiring role model, educator, mentor, and friend.

CONTENTS

CONTRIBUTORS

Veerasathpurush Allareddy, BDS, MBA, MMSc, MHA, PhD
Instructor
Department of Developmental Biology
Director of Pre-Doctoral Orthodontics
Harvard School of Dental Medicine
Harvard University
Boston, MA
USA

Athbi Alqareer, BDM
Advanced Graduate Resident
Department of Developmental Biology
Division of Orthodontics
Harvard School of Dental Medicine
Harvard University
Boston, MA
USA

Emilio I. Arguello, DDS, MSc
Board Diplomate
Clinical Instructor
Department of Oral Medicine, Infection, and Immunity
Division of Periodontics
Harvard School of Dental Medicine
Harvard University
Boston, MA
USA

Kasumi Kuse Barouch, DDS, PhD
Clinical Assistant Professor
Department of Periodontology and Oral Biology
Goldman School of Dental Medicine
Boston University
Boston, MA
USA
Instructor
Department of Oral Medicine, Infection, and Immunity
Division of Periodontology
Harvard School of Dental Medicine
Harvard University
Boston, MA
USA

Ryan D. Blissett, DMD, MMedSc
Private Practice, Brookline, MA
Clinical Instructor and Lecturer
Department of Restorative Dentistry and Biomaterials Sciences
Harvard School of Dental Medicine
Boston, MA
USA

Guillaume Campard, DDS, MMSc
Advanced Graduate Resident
Department of Oral Medicine, Infection, and Immunity
Division of Periodontology
Harvard School of Dental Medicine
Harvard University
Boston, MA
USA

Maria Dona, DDS, MSD
Advanced Graduate Resident, DMSc Candidate
Department of Oral Medicine, Infection, and Immunity
Division of Periodontology
Harvard School of Dental Medicine
Harvard University
Boston, MA
USA

Satheesh Elangovan, BDS, DSc, DMSc
Assistant Professor
Department of Periodontics
University of Iowa College of Dentistry
Iowa City, IA
USA

Ronald M. Fried, DMD, MMSc
Assistant Clinical Professor
Department of Oral Medicine, Infection, and Immunity
Division of Periodontology
Harvard School of Dental Medicine
Harvard University
Boston, MA
USA

Martin Ming-Jen Fu, BDS, MS
Advanced Graduate Resident
Department of Oral Medicine, Infection, and Immunity
Division of Periodontology
Harvard School of Dental Medicine
Harvard University
Boston, MA
USA

Luca Gobbato, DDS, MS
Clinical Instructor
Department of Oral Medicine, Infection, and Immunity
Harvard School of Dental Medicine
Harvard University
Boston, MA
USA

Kevin Guze, DMD, DMSc
Instructor
Department of Oral Medicine, Infection, and Immunity
Division of Periodontology
Harvard School of Dental Medicine
Harvard University
Boston, MA
USA

Mohamed H. Hassan, BDS, DMD, MS, FICD
TMD Fellowship
Diplomate, American Board of Periodontology
Clinical Instructor
Department of Oral Medicine, Infection, and Immunity
Division of Periodontology
Harvard School of Dental Medicine
Harvard University
Boston, MA
USA

Daniel Kuan-te Ho, DMD, MSc
Advanced Graduate Resident
Department of Oral Medicine, Infection, and Immunity
Division of Periodontology
Harvard School of Dental Medicine
Harvard University
Boston, MA
USA

T. Howard Howell, DDS
A. Lee Loomis Professor of Periodontology
Department of Oral Medicine, Infection, and Immunity
Division of Periodontology
Harvard School of Dental Medicine
Harvard University
Boston, MA
USA

Giuseppe Intini, DDS, MS, PhD
Instructor
Department of Development Biology
Clinical Instructor
Department of Oral Medicine, Infection, and Immunity
Harvard School of Dental Medicine
Harvard University
Boston, MA
USA

Alice Y. Kim-Bundy, DMD
Private Practice
West Hollywood, CA

David M. Kim, DDS, DMSc
Assistant Professor
Director of Pre-doctoral Periodontology
Department of Oral Medicine, Infection, and Immunity
Division of Periodontology
Harvard School of Dental Medicine
Harvard University
Boston, MA
USA

Soo-Woo Kim, DMD, MS
Advanced Graduate Resident
Department of Oral Medicine, Infection, and Immunity
Division of Periodontology
Harvard School of Dental Medicine
Harvard University
Boston, MA
USA

Samuel Koo, DDS, MS
Advanced Graduate Resident
Department of Oral Medicine, Infection, and Immunity
Harvard School of Dental Medicine
Harvard University
Boston, MA
USA

Walter S. Krawczyk, DDS
Assistant Clinical Professor
Department of Oral Medicine, Infection,, and Immunity
Harvard School of Dental Medicine
Harvard University
Boston, MA
USA

N. Joseph Laborde III, DDS
Advanced Graduate Resident
Department of Oral Medicine, Infection, and Immunity
Division of Periodontology
Harvard School of Dental Medicine
Harvard University
Boston, MA
USA

Samuel Soonho Lee, DDS
Advanced Graduate Resident, DMSc Candidate
Harvard School of Dental Medicine
Harvard University
Boston, MA
USA

Mark A. Lerman, DMD
Instructor
Department of Oral Medicine, Infection, and Immunity
Harvard School of Dental Medicine
Harvard University
Boston, MA
USA

Paul A. Levi, Jr., DMD
Associate Clinical Professor
Department of Periodontology
School of Dental Medicine
Tufts University
Boston, MA
USA
Universitat Internacional de Catalunya
Hospital General
Sant Cougat, Barcelona
Spain

Helen Livson, DMD, MMSc
Advanced Graduate Resident
Department of Oral Medicine, Infection, and Immunity
Division of Periodontology
Harvard School of Dental Medicine
Harvard University
Boston, MA
USA

Mohamed A. Maksoud, DMD
Clinical Instructor
Department of Oral Medicine, Infection, and Immunity
Division of Periodontology
Harvard School of Dental Medicine
Harvard University
Boston, MA
USA

Howard L. Needleman, DMD
Senior Associate in Dentistry
Children's Hospital Boston
Boston, MA
USA
Clinical Professor of Developmental Biology (Pediatric Dentistry)
Harvard School of Dental Medicine
Boston, MA
USA

Myron Nevins, DDS
Assistant Clinical Professor
Department of Oral Medicine, Infection, and Immunity
Harvard School of Dental Medicine
Harvard University
Boston, MA
USA

Campo E. Perez, Jr., DDS
Post-Doctoral Resident
Department of Periodontology
School of Dental Medicine
Tufts University
Boston, MA
USA
Assistant Clinical Professor
Department of Oral Pathology
Dental School
Zulia University
Maracaibo, Venezuela

Vinicius Souza Rodrigues, DDS
Advanced Graduate Resident, DMSc Candidate
Department of Oral Medicine, Infection, and Immunity
Division of Periodontology
Harvard School of Dental Medicine
Harvard University
Boston, MA
USA

Sarah D. Shih, DDS, MS, DMSc
Clinical Instructor
Department of Oral Medicine, Infection, and Immunity
Division of Periodontology
Harvard School of Dental Medicine
Harvard University
Boston, MA
USA

Jennifer F. Taschner, DDS, MMSc
Private Practice
Fort Myers, FL
USA

Ronny S. Taschner, DDS
Private Practice
Fort Myers, FL
USA

Ricardo Teles, DDS, DMSc
Associate Director
Center for Clinical and Translational Research
Associate Member of the Staff
Department of Periodontology
Clinical Instructor
The Forsyth Institute
Cambridge, MA
USA
Clinical Instructor
Department of Oral Medicine, Infection, and Immunity
Division of Periodontology
Harvard School of Dental Medicine
Harvard University
Boston, MA
USA

Anisha K. Thondukolam, DDS
Advanced Graduate Resident
Department of Oral Medicine, Infection, and Immunity
Division of Periodontology
Harvard School of Dental Medicine
Harvard University
Boston, MA
USA

Philip M. Walton, DDS
Advanced Graduate Resident
Department Oral Medicine, Infection, and Immunity
Division of Periodontology
Harvard School of Dental Medicine
Harvard University
Boston, MA
USA

Robert F. Wright, DDS, FACP
Associate Professor, Department of Restorative
Dentistry and Biomaterials Sciences
Director, Advanced Graduate Prosthodontics
Diplomate, American Board of Prosthodontics
Harvard School of Dental Medicine
Harvard University
Boston, MA
USA

Clinical Cases in
Periodontics

1

Examination and Diagnosis

Clinical Cases in Periodontics, First Edition. Nadeem Karimbux.
© 2012 John Wiley & Sons, Inc. Published 2012 by John Wiley & Sons, Inc.

Case 1

Examination and Documentation

CASE STORY

A 40-year-old African-American male (LD) in no apparent distress presented with a chief complaint of: "My dentist told me I have gum disease and I should see a periodontist." Figures 1–5 are the patient's intraoral photographs.

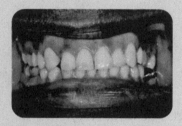

Figure 1: Frontal view.

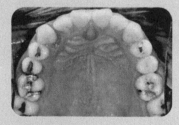

Figure 2: Maxillary view.

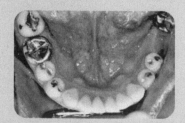

Figure 3: Mandibular view.

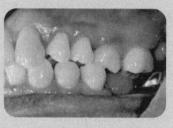

Figure 4: Right occlusal view.

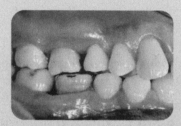

Figure 5: Left occlusal view.

LEARNING GOALS AND OBJECTIVES

- The patient's chief complaint
- Medical and dental history
- Soft tissue and gingival examination
- Periodontal charting
- Radiographic interpretation and diagnosis of periodontal condition

Past Dental History

This patient denied having bleeding gums during brushing or flossing, he had no loose teeth, and he was not in pain. The patient claimed to brush twice a day and flossed sporadically. His last dental visit was a year ago for a cleaning.

This particular patient presented with a blood pressure of 140/90, a pulse of 70 beats per minute, and a respiration rate of 14 breaths per minute. The patient denied having any significant health problems, had no known allergies, and denied taking any medications.

Soft Tissue and Gingival Examination

The patient had no pathologic masses or lesions upon extraoral and intraoral examination (Figures 1–5). He presented with generalized coral pink gingiva with normal pigmentation, scalloped gingival contour with knife-edged margins, pyramidal papillae with localized areas of blunted papilla, stippling, localized areas of recession, and firm consistency with localized edematous areas. There was mild plaque, with no significant supra/subgingival calculus. There was some normal pigmentation associated with the attached gingiva (Figures 1, 4, and 5).

Periodontal Charting

A thorough periodontal examination was completed. The periodontal chart (Figures 6 and 7) shows that the patient had generalized bleeding on probing, minimal plaque, pocket depths ranging from 2 to 15 mm with the more severe probing depths in the posterior teeth, class 1–2 furcations, class 1–3 mobility, and localized recession.

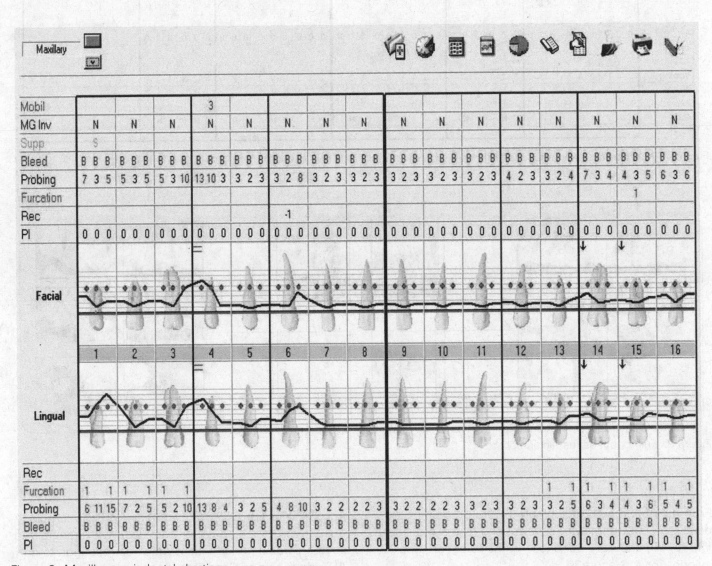

Figure 6: Maxillary periodontal charting.

Mandibular

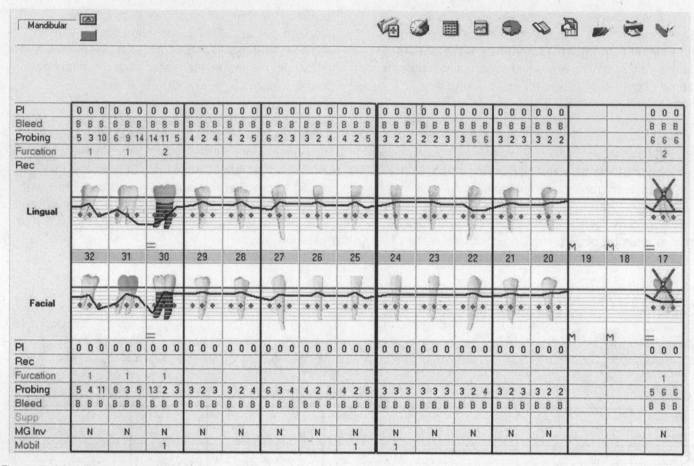

Lingual / Facial charting (teeth 32–17)

	32	31	30	29	28	27	26	25	24	23	22	21	20	19	18	17
PI	0 0 0	0 0 0	0 0 0	0 0 0	0 0 0	0 0 0	0 0 0	0 0 0	0 0 0	0 0 0	0 0 0	0 0 0	0 0 0			0 0 0
Bleed	B B B	B B B	B B B	B B B	B B B	B B B	B B B	B B B	B B B	B B B	B B B	B B B	B B B			B B B
Probing	5 3 10	6 9 14	14 11 5	4 2 4	4 2 5	6 2 3	3 2 4	4 2 5	3 2 2	2 2 3	3 6 6	3 2 3	3 2 2			6 6 6
Furcation	1		1	2												2
Rec																
Lingual																
Facial														M	M	
PI	0 0 0	0 0 0	0 0 0	0 0 0	0 0 0	0 0 0	0 0 0	0 0 0	0 0 0	0 0 0	0 0 0	0 0 0	0 0 0			0 0 0
Rec																
Furcation	1		1	1												1
Probing	5 4 11	8 3 5	13 2 3	3 2 3	3 2 4	6 3 4	4 2 4	4 2 5	3 3 3	3 3 3	3 2 4	3 2 3	3 2 2			5 6 6
Bleed	B B B	B B B	B B B	B B B	B B B	B B B	B B B	B B B	B B B	B B B	B B B	B B B	B B B			B B B
Supp																
MG Inv	N	N	N	N	N	N	N	N	N	N	N	N	N			N
Mobil			1					1	1							

Figure 7: Mandibular periodontal charting.

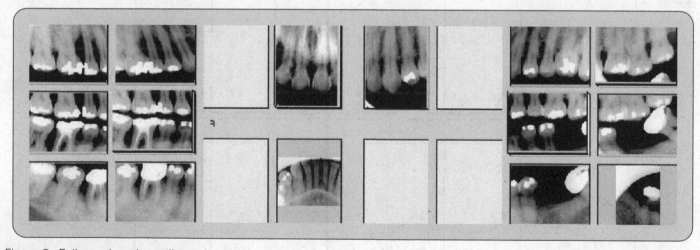

Figure 8: Full mouth series radiographs.

Radiographic Examination

From this full mouth radiograph (Figure 8), generalized bone loss is evident with severe bone loss surrounding #4, #6, #7, and #30. Bone loss in the furcation area is evident for #17 and #30.

Diagnosis

According to the American Academy of Periodontology (AAP), patient LD would be diagnosed with generalized severe chronic periodontitis, which corresponds to an ADA diagnosis of Case Type IV.

Self-Study Questions

A. What dental history questions are important to consider for a periodontal patient?

B. What medical history questions are important to consider for a periodontal patient?

1. From a medical perspective for medical management of the patient
2. From a perspective of conditions that might affect the gingiva/periodontium

C. What constitutes a thorough periodontal examination?

D. How often and what type of radiographs should be exposed for a periodontal examination?

E. How does one come to a diagnosis for gingival and periodontal diseases?

Answers located at the end of the chapter.

Diagnosis (ADA)

Case Type I. Gingivitis

- No attachment loss
- Bleeding may or may not be present
- Pseudopockets may be present
- Only the gingival tissues have been affected by the inflammatory process
- No radiographic evidence of bone loss
- The crestal lamina dura is present
- The alveolar bone level is within 1–2 mm of the CEJ area

Case Type II. Early Periodontitis

- Bleeding on probing may be present in the active phase
- Pocket depths or attachment loss of 3–4 mm
- Localized areas of recession
- Possible class I furcation invasion areas
- Horizontal type of bone loss is most common
- Slight loss of the interdental septum
- Alveolar bone level is 3–4 mm from the CEJ area

Case Type III. Moderate Periodontitis

- Pocket depths or attachment loss of 4–6 mm
- Bleeding on probing
- Grade I and/or grade II furcation invasion areas
- Tooth mobility of class I
- Horizontal or vertical bone loss may be present
- Alveolar bone level is 4–6 mm from the CEJ area
- Radiographic furcations of grade I and/or grade II

- Crown to root ratio is 1 : 1 (loss of a third of supporting alveolar bone)

Case Type IV. Advanced Periodontitis

- Bleeding on probing
- Pocket depths or attachment loss >6 mm
- Grade II, grade III furcation invasion areas
- Mobility of class II or class III
- Horizontal and vertical bone loss
- Alveolar bone level is ≥6 mm from the CEJ area
- Radiographic furcations
- Crown to root ratio is ≥2 : 1 (loss of more than a third of the supporting alveolar bone)

Source: American Academy of Periodontology: Current Procedural Terminology for Periodontics and Insurance Reporting Manual, 7th ed.

References

1. Academy Reports position paper: Tobacco use and the periodontal patient. J Periodontol 1999;70:1419–1427.
2. Haber J, Wattles J, et al. Evidence of cigarette smoking as a major risk factor for Periodontitis. J Periodontol 1993;64:16–23.
3. Emrich LJ, Shlossman M, et al. Periodontal disease in non-insulin dependent diabetes mellitus. J Periodontol 1991;62:123–131.
4. Nelson RG, Shlossman M, et al. Periodontal disease and NIDDM in Pima Indians. Diabetes Care 1990;13:836–840.
5. Academy Reports informational paper: Drug associated gingival enlargement. J Periodontol 2004;75:1424–1431.

6. Rose L, Mealey B. Periodontics: Medicine, Surgery, and Implants. St. Louis, MO: Elsevier Mosby, 2004.
7. Association Report: The use of dental radiographs. Update and Recommendations. JADA 2006;137:1304–1312.
8. American Academy of Periodontology. Current procedural terminology for periodontics and insurance reporting manual. 7th ed. Chicago, IL: AAP, 1995.
9. Armitage G. Development of a classification system for periodontal diseases and conditions. Ann Periodontol 1999;4:1–6.
10. Armitage G. Periodontal diagnoses and classification of periodontal disease. Periodontology 2000 2004;34:9–21.

TAKE-HOME POINTS

A. The patient should be asked if he or she has a history of bleeding gums, loose teeth, or if there is a history of periodontal disease in the family. Bleeding of the gums spontaneously or on brushing or flossing can either indicate a systemic problem or a gingival/periodontal problem. Most patients with "bleeding gums" most likely have plaque-associated gingivitis or a form of aggressive/chronic periodontitis. If the bleeding does not resolve after initial phase therapy and home care instructions, the dentist/periodontist should refer the patient for a medical workup. Examples of diseases that may involve bleeding gums include leukemia or hemophilia. Loose teeth can either indicate an advanced stage of periodontitis or trauma from occlusion. A family history of periodontal disease should be considered in cases of localized aggressive periodontitis. Patients should also be asked if they have had prior periodontal therapy and when the last visit to a dentist took place. This history can indicate a past history of treatment for periodontal problems, or it might indicate the patient has had irregular care in the past. One must also ask patients how regularly they brush/floss and if they use any other aids. This can indicate dental neglect or good oral hygiene practices.

For this portion of the examination, it is also important to ask patients if they have a history of smoking or are currently smoking, if they have diabetes or a family history of diabetes, and if they are taking any medications. Smoking and uncontrolled diabetes are both factors that put patients at higher risk for getting periodontitis [1–4]. Because smoking and diabetes are known to affect periodontal health, it is vital that we question patients about these issues. If the patients smoke, they should be given information about how smoking affects oral health and advised to consider smoking cessation. If a patient has diabetes, he or she should be under the care of a physician who regularly monitors the condition.

B. **(1)** As discussed, a history of smoking and uncontrolled diabetes can reveal risk factors for periodontal disease. Any major systemic conditions or illnesses that a patient has need to be incorporated in the treatment plan. For example, complex medical issues or conditions may need to be treated in a hospital setting. If a patient is hypertensive, the AHA guidelines should be followed before any treatment. If a patient has bleeding disorders or is taking blood thinners (Coumadin, Plavix), a consultation with a physician before any surgeries should be completed. **(2)** Certain drugs such as nifedipine, cyclosporine, and phenytoin are known to cause gingival hyperplasia [5]. Oral contraceptives can affect the gingiva as well. If patients are taking any medications such as these, they should be informed that their prescription medication may cause changes in their gingiva.

C. A complete periodontal examination involves filling out a periodontal chart. This chart can include information on (1) probing depths (PDs), (2) bleeding on probing (BOP), (3) distance from the gingival margin to the cementoenamel junction (GM-CEJ), (4) clinical attachment loss (CAL), (5) recession, (6) furcation, (7) mobility, (8) ridge defects, and (9) plaque and calculus [6].

1. P obing Depths

To obtain probing depths, the periodontal probe is placed in the sulcus in six different locations around each tooth. These locations are the mesiobuccal, straight buccal, distobuccal, distolingual, straight lingual, and mesiolingual. The probe is gently placed to the depth of the gingival sulcus, and the distance from the base of the pocket to the gingival margin is measured in millimeters using the markings on the instrument.

2. Bleeding on Probing

Following periodontal probing, bleeding on probing should be noted. Some sites will experience bleeding immediately or a few moments afterward. Bleeding on probing or the lack of bleeding should be recorded on the periodontal chart.

3. Distance from Gingival Margin to Cementoenamel Junction

With the use of the periodontal probe, the distance from the CEJ to the gingival margin must be measured in the same locations as the periodontal probing depths. If there is recession, this distance should be measured and recorded as a positive number. If the gingival margin is above the CEJ, which occurs in gingival health or when there is gingival hyperplasia, the probe should be used to feel the CEJ subgingivally, and the measurement should be recorded as a negative number.

4. Clinical Attachment Loss

The CAL calculated using the numbers obtained after periodontal probing and after determining the distance from the gingival margin to the CEJ. The probing depth number is added to the GM-CEJ measurement. For example, if the probing depth is 2 mm and there is 2 mm of recession (GM-CEJ = +2), the CAL will be 4 mm. If the probing depth is 3 mm, and the gingival margin is 1 mm above the CEJ (GM-CEJ = −1), the CAL will be 2 mm. The values calculated for CAL are necessary for diagnosing periodontal disease.

5. Recession

Recession occurs when the gingival margin is below the CEJ. The Miller classification for recession defects may be used to categorize the recession, as follows:

Miller Class 1: Recession that does not extend to the mucogingival junction with no periodontal bone loss in the interdental areas.

Miller Class 2: Recession that extends to or beyond the mucogingival junction, with no interdental bone loss.

Miller Class 3: Recession that extends to or beyond the mucogingival junction, with some periodontal attachment loss in the interdental area or malpositioning of teeth.

Miller Class 4: Recession that extends to or beyond the mucogingival junction, with severe bone and/or soft tissue loss in the interdental area and/or severe malpositioning of teeth.

6. Furcation

Furcation classifications for maxillary molars, maxillary first premolars, and mandibular molars should be recorded. According to the Glickman classification for furcations, it should be recorded as grade 1, 2, 3, or 4.

Grade 1: There is incipient furcation involvement involving mostly soft tissue. Early bone loss may have occurred but is not visible radiographically.

Grade 2: There is a horizontal component to the bone loss in the furcation area resulting in an area that can be probed. Some bone does remain attached to the tooth.

Grade 3: There is no attached bone in the furcation area, resulting in a through-and-through tunnel. Soft tissue may still occlude the furcation.

Grade 4: There is a visible through-and-through tunnel that is easily probed.

7. Mobility

The mobility of each tooth should be tested using the blunt ends of two instruments. Depending on the mobility, the tooth should be classified using the Miller classification system as having class 1, 2, or 3 mobility.

Miller Class 1: Tooth can be moved <1 mm in the buccolingual or mesiodistal direction.

Miller Class 2: Tooth can be moved ≤1 mm in the buccolingual or mesiodistal direction but not in the apico-coronal direction.

Miller Class 2: Tooth can be moved ≤1 mm in the buccolingual or mesiodistal direction, and movement in the apico-coronal direction is present as well.

8. Ridge Defects

In edentulous areas, the remaining ridge may be classified as a Siebert class 1, 2, or 3 ridge defect if there is bone loss in the area.

Seibert Class 1: Loss of bone in the buccolingual direction with normal adequate bone in the apico-coronal direction.

Seibert Class 2: Loss of bone in the apico-coronal direction with adequate bone in the buccolingual direction.

Seibert Class 3: Loss of bone in both the buccolingual and apico-coronal direction.

9 Plaque and Calculus

The presence of plaque and calculus should also be recorded on the periodontal chart as absent, mild, moderate, or abundant.

D. To obtain an accurate picture of a patient's periodontal health, radiographs should be taken and analyzed as a part of the periodontal examination. Typically a full mouth series of radiographs should be taken every 5 years and a set of bite-wing radiographs should be taken every 2 years [7]. Bite-wing radiographs provide a way to assess the crestal bone and observe bone loss in the posterior. If there is severe bone loss that cannot be seen in a horizontal bite wing, vertical bite-wing radiographs should be taken. Periapical radiographs are useful for viewing the bone level as well, but especially for determining the crown-to-root ratio, which helps in assigning a tooth's prognosis. Furcation involvement can also be seen in radiographs.

E. Diagnosis (American Academy of Periodontology [8])

If ≤30% of the sites are affected, the disease is localized.

If >30% of sites are affected, the disease is generalized

According to the AAP, patients are diagnosed based on their clinical attachment level.

If CAL = 0 mm, the patient is diagnosed with gingivitis.

If CAL = 1–2 mm, the patient is diagnosed with slight/mild periodontitis.

If CAL = 3–4 mm, the patient is diagnosed with moderate periodontitis.

If CAL = ≥5, the patient is diagnosed with severe periodontitis.

If the clinical attachment loss has occurred gradually for years, the disease is chronic.

If the clinical attachment loss has occurred rapidly, the disease is aggressive.

Figure 9–14 further describe the classification of periodontal diseases and conditions [9,10].

Table 1: Classification of periodontal diseases and conditions

I.   Gingival Diseases
  A. Dental plaque-induced gingival diseases
     1. Gingivitis associated with dental plaque only
        a. without other local contributing factors
        b. with local contributing factors
     2. Gingival diseases modified by systemic factors
        a. associated with the endocrine system
           1) puberty-associated gingivitis
           2) menstrual cycle-associated gingivitis
           3) pregnancy associated
              a) gingivitis
              b) pyogenic granuloma
           4) diabetes mellitus-associated gingivitis
        b. associated with blood-dyscrasias
           1) leukemia-associated gingivitis
           2) other
     3. Gingival diseases modified by medications
        a. drug-influenced gingival diseases
           1) drug-influenced gingival enlargements
           2) drug-influenced gingivitis
              a) oral contraceptive-associated gingivitis
              b) other
     4. Gingival diseases modified by malnutrition
        a. ascorbic acid-deficiency gingivitis
        b. other
  B. Non-plaque-induced gingival lesions
     1. Gingival lesions of specific bacterial origin
        a. *Neisseria gonorrhea*-associated lesions
        b. *Treponema pallidum*-associated lesions
        c. streptococcal species-associated lesions
        d. other
     2. Gingival diseases of viral origin
        a. herpesvirus infections
           1) primary herpetic gingivostomatitis
           2) recurrent oral herpes
           3) varicella-zoster infections
        b. other
     3. Gingival diseases of fungal origin
        a. *Candida*-species infection
           1) generalized gingival candidosis
        b. linear gingival erythema
        c. histoplasmosis
        d. other
     4. Gingival lesions of genetic origin
        a. hereditary gingival fibromatosis
        b. other
     5. Gingival manifestations of systemic conditions
        a. mucocutaneous disorders
           1) lichen planus
           2) pemphigoid
           3) pemphigus vulgaris
           4) erythema multiforme
           5) lupus erythematosus
           6) drug-induced
           7) other

        b. allergic reactions
           1) dental restorative materials
              a) mercury
              b) nickel
              c) acrylic
              d) other
           2) reactions attributable to
              a) toothpastes/dentifrices
              b) mouthrinses/mouthwashes
              c) chewing gum additives
              d) foods and additives
           3) other
     6. Traumatic lesions (factitious, iatrogenic, accidental)
        a. chemical injury
        b. physical injury
        c. thermal injury
     7. Foreign body reactions
     8. Not otherwise specified (NOS)
II. Chronic Periodontitis
  A. Localized
  B. Generalized
III. Aggressive Periodontitis
  A. Localized
  B. Generalized
IV. Periodontitis as a Manifestation of Systemic Diseases
  A. Associated with hematological disorders
     1. Acquired neutropenia
     2. Leukemias
     3. Other
  B. Associated with genetic disorders
     1. Familial and cyclic neutropenia
     2. Down Syndrome
     3. Leukocyte adhesion deficiency syndromes
     4. Papillon-Lefèvre syndrome
     5. Chediak-Higashi syndrome
     6. Histiocytosis syndromes
     7. Glycogen storage disease
     8. Infantile genetic agranulocytosis
     9. Cohen syndrome
     10. Ehlers-Danlos syndrome (Types IV and VIII)
     11. Hypophosphatasia
     12. Other
  C. Not otherwise specified (NOS)
V.   Necrotizing Periodontal Diseases
  A. Necrotizing ulcerative gingivitis (NUG)
  B. Necrotizing ulcerative periodontitis (NUP)
VI. Abscesses of the Periodontium
  A. Gingival abscess
  B. Periodontal abscess
  C. Pericoronal abscess
VII. Periodontitis Associated With Endodontic Lesions
  A. Combined periodontic-endodontic lesions

(Continued)

Table 1: (*Continued*)

VIII. Developmental or Acquired Deformities and
Conditions
 A. Localized tooth-related factors that modify or
  predispose to plaque-induced gingival diseases/
  periodontitis
   1. Tooth anatomic factors
   2. Dental restorations/appliances
   3. Root fractures
   4. Cervical root resorption and cemental tears
 B. Mucogingival deformities and conditions around
  teeth
   1. Gingival/soft tissue recession
    a. facial or lingual surfaces
    b. interproximal (papillary)
   2. Lack of keratinized gingiva
   3. Decreased vestibular depth
   4. Aberrant frenum/muscle position

   5. Gingival excess
    a. pseudopocket
    b. inconsistent gingival margin
    c. excessive gingival display
    d. gingival enlargement
   6. Abnormal color
 C. Mucogingival deformities and conditions on
  edentulous ridges
   1. Vertical and/or horizontal ridge deficiency
   2. Lack of gingiva/keratinized tissue
   3. Gingival/soft tissue enlargement
   4. Aberrant frenum/muscle position
   5. Decreased vestibular depth
   6. Abnormal color
 D. Occlusal trauma
   1. Primary occlusal trauma
   2. Secondary occlusal trauma

Reprinted from Armitage, 1999, with permission from the American Academy of Periodontology.

Table 2: Main clinical features and characteristics of chronic periodontics (1999 Classification)

* Most prevalent in adults, but can occur in children and adolescents
* Amount of destruction is consistent with the presence of local factors
* Subgingival calculus is a frequent finding
* Associated with a variable microbial pattern
* Slow to moderate rate of progression, but may have periods of rapid progression
* Can be associated with local predisposing factors (e.g., tooth–related or iatrogenic factors)
* May be modified by and/or associated with systemic diseases (e.g., diabetes mellitus)
* Can be modified by factors other than systemic disease such as cigarette smoking and emotional stress

Reprinted from Armitage, 2004, with permission from the American Academy of Periodontology.

Table 3: Features of aggressive periodontitis that are common to both the localized and generalized forms of the disease (1999 Classification)

P imary features
– Except for the presence of periodontitis, patients are otherwise clinically healthy
– Rapid attachment loss and bone destruction
– Familial aggregation

Secondary features (often present)
– Amounts of microbial deposits are inconsistent with the severity of periodontal tissue destruction
– Elevated proportions of *Actinobacillus actinomycetemcomitans* and, in some populations, *Porphyromonas gingivalis* may be elevated
– Phagocyte abnormalities
– Hyperresponsive macrophage phenotype, including elevated levels of prostaglandin E2 (PGE2) and interleukin-1β (IL-1β)
– Progression of attachment loss and bone loss may be self-arresting

Reprinted from Armitage, 2004, with permission from the American Academy of Periodontology.

Table 4: Specific features of localized and generalized aggressive periodontitis (1999 Classification)

Localized aggressive periodontitis

- Circumpubertal onset
- Robust serum antibody to infecting agents
- Localized first molar/incisor presentation with interproximal attachment loss on at least two permanent teeth, one of which is a first molar, and involving no more than two teeth other than first molars and incisors

Generalized aggressive periodontitis

- Usually affecting persons under 30 years of age, but patients may be older
- Poor serum antibody response to infecting agents
- Pronounced episodic nature of the destruction of attachment and alveolar bone
- Generalized interproximal attachment loss affecting at least three permanent teeth other than first molars and incisors.

Reprinted from Armitage, 2004, with permission from the American Academy of Periodontology.

Table 5: Comparison of the main clinical characteristics of chronic periodontitis, localized aggressive periodontitis, and generalized aggressive periodontitis.

Chronic periodontitis

- Most prevalent in adults, but can occur in children
- Slow to moderate rates of progression
- Amount of microbial deposits consistent with severity of destruction
- Variable distribution of periodontal destruction; no discernible pattern
- No marked familial aggregation
- Frequent presence of subgingival calculus

Localized aggressive periodontitis

- Usually occurs in adolescents (circumpubertal onset)
- Rapid rate of progression
- Amount of microbial deposits not consistent with severity of destruction
- Periodontal destruction localized to permanent first molars and incisors
- Marked familial aggregation
- Subgingival calculus usually absent

Generalized aggressive periodontitis

- Usually affects people under 30 years of age, but patients may be older
- Rapid rate of progression (pronounced episodic periods of progression).
- Amount of microbial deposits sometimes consistent with severity of destruction
- Periodontal destruction affects many teeth in addition to permanent molars and incisors
- Marked familial aggregation
- Subgingival calculus may or may not be present

Reprinted from Armitage, 2004, with permission from the American Academy of Periodontology.

Case 2

Plaque-Induced Gingivitis

CASE STORY

A 27-year-old Caucasian male presented with the chief complaint of: "My gums bleed." The patient noticed blood in the gingiva whenever he brushed (A). He also noted that his gums bled when he flossed (A). There had never been any swelling or pain associated with his gums, and the patient had never had an episode like this before. The patient claimed to brush his teeth once daily, and he flossed two to three times a week (B).

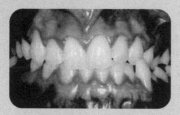

Figure 1: Preoperative presentation.

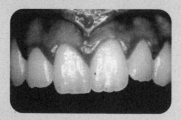

Figure 2: Preoperative maxillary anteriors.

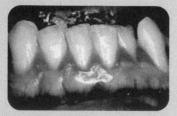

Figure 3: Preoperative mandibular anteriors.

LEARNING GOALS AND OBJECTIVES

- To be able to diagnose gingivitis
- To identify the possible etiology for the same condition and to address them
- To understand the importance of oral hygiene in preventing gingivitis

Medical History

There were no significant medical problems. The patient had no known allergies or medical illnesses. On questioning the patient stated he was taking no medications and he had no allergies.

Review of Systems

- Vital signs
  - Blood pressure: 120/65 mm Hg
  - Pulse rate: 72 beats/minute (regular)
  - Respiration: 15 breaths/minute

Social History

The patient did not drink alcohol. He did smoke (started at age 23 and currently smoked half a pack of cigarettes daily).

Extraoral Examination

No significant findings. The patient had no masses or swelling, and the temporomandibular joint was within normal limits.

Intraoral Examination

- The soft tissues of the mouth (except gingiva) including the tongue appeared normal.
- A gingival examination revealed a mild marginal erythema, with rolled margins and swollen papillae (Figures 1–3).

- A hard tissue and soft tissue examination were completed (Figure 4) (F).

Occlusion

There were no occlusal discrepancies or interferences.

Radiographic Examination

A full mouth set of radiographs was ordered (G). (See Figure 5 for the patient's bite-wing radiographs.)

Diagnosis

After reviewing the history and both the clinical and radiographic examinations, a differential diagnosis was generated (H).

Treatment Plan

The treatment plan of the periodontal problems for this patient includes an initial phase of scaling with polishing and a 6-week reevaluation.

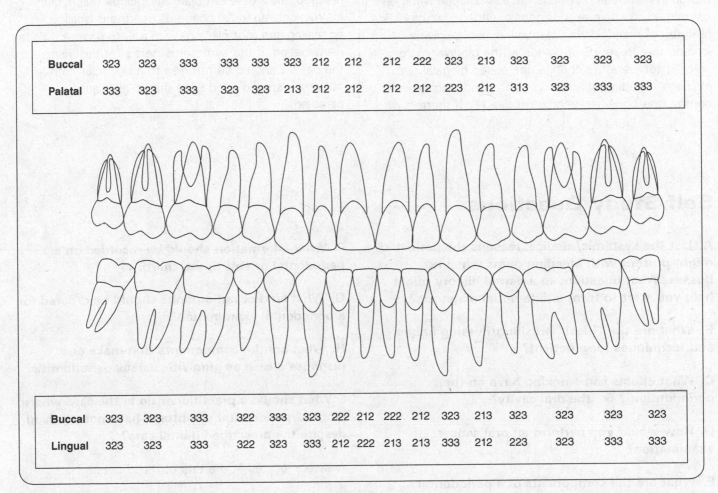

Buccal	323	323	333	333	333	323	212	212	212	222	323	213	323	323	323	323
Palatal	333	323	333	323	323	213	212	212	212	212	223	212	313	323	333	333

Buccal	323	323	333	322	333	323	222	212	222	212	323	213	323	323	323	323
Lingual	323	323	333	322	323	333	212	222	213	213	333	212	223	323	333	333

Figure 4: Probing pocket depth measurements.

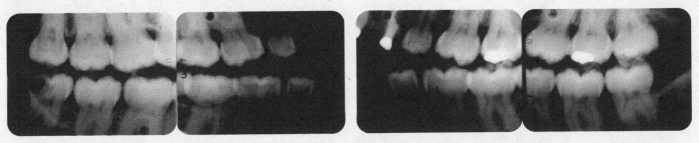

Figure 5: Bite-wing radiographs depicting the interproximal bone levels.

Treatment

The patient received a scaling and polishing. At the 6-week reevaluation, the clinical signs and symptoms had not improved, even though the patient claimed to be practicing excellent oral hygiene as per your instructions (I).

Discussion

Most patients who present with these symptoms (bleeding gums) have a plaque-induced gingivitis. A thorough history and periodontal examination must be completed to arrive at a diagnosis. Other characteristic features associated with plaque-induced gingivitis include the presence of plaque at the gingival margin, sulcular temperature change, increased gingival exudate, bleeding on probing. With good plaque control, the condition should resolve [1]. If there is a medical concern, it is typically identified by obtaining a thorough medical history. Conditions such as diabetes and leukemia have a profound effect on gingival health, and therefore the patient must be evaluated accordingly. In women, hormonal changes such as those that occur during the onset of puberty, pregnancy, or menstruation have a transient effect on the inflammatory status of these patients [2], which when combined with poor plaque control will lead to severe gingivitis [3,4]. After a diagnosis is reached, the treatment plan will include oral hygiene instructions, an initial phase of treatment (scaling or scaling and root planing) with a 4- to 6-week reevaluation. If the symptoms persist at this visit, the patient should be referred to a physician to rule out any systemic conditions that might cause bleeding.

Self-Study Questions

A. List the systemic/medical reasons the patient might present with bleeding gums when he flosses. What questions in a dental history might help you start to form a differential diagnosis?

B. What are the "ideal" brushing/flossing habits and techniques for a patient?

C. What effects can smoking have on the periodontium? On the oral cavity?

D. How would you perform an oral cancer examination?

E. What are the components of a periodontal examination?

F. What information should be recorded on a periodontal or soft tissue charting?

G. What kind of radiographs should be ordered for a periodontal examination?

H. What are the components that make one diagnose a case as gingivitis versus periodontitis?

I. What should a practitioner do in the case where gingival/periodontal symptoms have not resolved despite the prescribed dental care?

Answers located at the end of the chapter.

References

1. Mariotti A. Dental plaque-induced gingival diseases. Ann Periodontol 1999;4:7–17.
2. Mariotti A. Sex steroid hormones and cell dynamics in the periodontium. Crt Rev Oral Biol Med 1994;5:27–53.
3. Hugoson A. Gingivitis in pregnant women. A longitudinal clinical study. Odontologisk Revy 1971;22:25–42.
4. Loe H. Periodontal changes in pregnancy. J Periodontol 1965;36:209–216.
5. Moran JM, Addy M, et al. A comparative study of stain removal with electric tooth brushes and a manual tooth brush. J Clin Dent 1995;6:188–193.
6. Tritten CB, Armitage GC. Comparison of a sonic and a manual toothbrush for efficacy in supra gingival plaque removal and reduction of gingivitis. J Clin Periodontol 1996;23:641–648.
7. Grossi SG, Zambon JJ, et al. Assessment of risk for periodontal disease. I. Risk indicators for attachment loss. J Periodontol 1994;65:260–267.
8. Mullally B, Breen B, et al. Smoking and patterns of bone loss in early-onset periodontitis. J Periodontol 1999;70:394–401.
9. Rose LF, Mealy BL, et al. Periodontics: Medicine, Surgery, and Implants. St. Louis, MO: Mosby, 2004. Chapter 34 p871.
10. Blot WJ, McLaughlin JK, et al. Smoking and drinking in relation to oral and pharyngeal cancers. Cancer Res 1988;48:3282–3287.
11. Neville BW, Damm DD, et al. Oral and Maxillofacial Pathology. Philadelphia, PA: Lippincott, 2005. Chapter 10 p356–362.

TAKE-HOME POINTS

A
a. Bleeding disorders
   Idiopathic thrombocytopenic purpura
b. Medications
   Use of blood thinners
   Use of oral contraceptives
c. Systemic conditions
   Hormonal changes during pregnancy and puberty
   Gingivitis associated with diabetes mellitus
   Leukemia
   Vitamins C and/or K deficiency
d. Others
   Ill-fitting dental appliances or from its components (e.g., clasps)
   Questions to help develop a differential diagnosis include the following:
• How often do you brush or floss?
• Do you bruise easily?
• When you wake up do you notice any blood in your mouth?
• When you cut yourself, do you tend to clot within a normal amount of time?
• What medicines are you taking currently?
• Are you pregnant (for female patients)?
• Are you a mouth breather?/Do you have difficulty breathing through your nose?

B. A patient should ideally brush twice daily and floss once daily. Evidence indicates that the use of rotary brushes is better than manual brushes for interproximal plaque removal and stain removal [5,6]. A toothbrush with soft bristles is strongly recommended. The bristles should be positioned at a 45-degree angle to the junction of the tooth and marginal gingiva, and then the brushing should be initiated using short circular gentle motions (Bass method of brushing). The same technique should be repeated for the rest of the mouth. If a patient has gingival recession, coronal sweeping motion of bristles from the gingiva to the teeth is recommended to prevent the progression of recession (modified Stillman's technique).

C. Smoking has been identified as a risk factor for periodontitis [7]. The number of cigarettes an individual smokes per day and the number of years an individual has been smoking are two important parameters strongly associated with the degree of attachment loss [8]. It is well established that smoking affects the host immune response, causes local tissue ischemia, and also alters the bacterial profile, shifting the plaque ecology and increasing the periodontal pathogens in the host [9]. This risk factor is "behavioral" and can be modified.

Smoking causes an increased risk for oral and throat cancers [10]. Oral cancer is the sixth most common cancer in males and the twelfth most common cancer in women in the United States [11].

D. A thorough extraoral examination should be conducted. Visualization and palpation of the soft tissues of the head and neck should be completed including palpation of the muscles and lymph nodes.

The intraoral examination should consist of visualization and palpation of the tongue. The tongue represents the most common site (50%) for oral cancer and ventral and lateral surfaces (20%), in particular, have a higher predilection for cancer than the dorsal surface of the tongue (4%) [11]. The floor of the mouth is the second most common site for oral cancer, and therefore careful examination of this area of the mouth should be a part of cancer screening. Other areas that should be examined specifically for oral cancer include the soft palate, gingiva, and buccal and labial mucosa [11].

E. A periodontal examination includes looking at and describing the gingival color, contour, consistency, texture, presence or absence of exudates from sulcus, and bleeding on probing. Six probing depths (mesiobuccal, midbuccal, distobuccal, mesiolingual, midlingual, and distolingual) per tooth should be recorded. Areas of recession, mobility, and furcation involvement are also recorded and graded according to the established classifications for each of these conditions. Radiographs and study models are also important because they offer valuable information that is not obtained from the clinical oral examination.

F. The following are essential components of a periodontal chart:
- Name of the patient and the date of recording
- Missing teeth should be recorded
- Probing pocket depth: measured on six surfaces of each tooth in the mouth using a periodontal probe
- Degree of recession: measured using periodontal probe
- Mobility: measured using two flat ends of dental instruments such as dental mirror and/or periodontal probe and pushing the teeth with one instrument against the second instrument.

- Fremitus: measured by placing the inner pad of the fingers on the gingiva of the teeth in question and asking the patient to tap teeth three or four times. In traumatic occlusion, fremitus is usually felt by the examiner's fingers, which is then recorded.
- Degree of furcation involvement: examined using Naber's probe
- Mucogingival complex: the width of the mucogingival complex should be measured from the gingival margin to the apical-most part of the attached gingiva in every tooth, using a periodontal probe, and recorded.

G. Radiographs form an essential component of a periodontal examination. Apart from giving information about the periodontium of the tooth in question, other valuable information such as root length, root form, periapical lesions, and root proximity can be ascertained. The American Dental Association recommends a full mouth set of radiographs should be taken for a full diagnosis (typically every 5 years). A set of four bite wings should be exposed every 2 years. The diagnosis of periodontal disease can be made using periapical radiographs and bite-wing radiographs. Bite-wing radiographs are the most diagnostic for reading bone height because the head of the x-ray tube is perpendicular to the film. Vertical bite wings are recommended for areas with extensive bone loss. In general, paralleling technique is recommended over bisecting angle technique because it reduces the errors associated with film angulations.

H. Clinical attachment loss (CAL) (distance from the cementoenamel junction to the base of a periodontal pocket) and bone loss as seen on a radiograph are the gold standards used to help distinguish a patient with periodontitis versus gingivitis. Patients with gingivitis do not exhibit CAL and bone loss (radiographically), whereas if the diseases progresses to periodontitis, CAL and bone loss are characteristically observed.

I. A referral to physician should be made to rule out any systemic conditions.

Case 3

Non–Plaque-Induced Gingivitis

CASE STORY
A 41-year-old Latin American female presented with a chief complaint of: "My gums and teeth are sensitive." She had been referred by her general dentist for periodontal treatment. She reported a 5-year history of gingival sensitivity and progressive gingival recession. She experienced lingering pain after drinking hot and cold liquids and also noted sensitivity when brushing.

LEARNING GOALS AND OBJECTIVES
- To be able to distinguish desquamative gingivitis from plaque-induced gingivitis
- To formulate a differential diagnosis for common causes of desquamative gingivitis
- To be able to arrive at a definitive diagnosis and properly manage a patient with desquamative gingivitis

Medical History
There were no significant findings found in the patient's medical history. The patient saw her physician for an annual physical. She did not currently take any medications and she had no known drug allergies.

Review of Systems
- Vital signs
  - Blood pressure: 120/70 mm Hg
  - Heart rate: 78 beats/minute
  - Respiration: 15 breaths/minute

Dental History
The patient had received sporadic general dental care and orthodontics in Brazil and was unsure if the city water she consumed in her childhood was fluoridated. She had received dental care more regularly since moving to the United States 13 years ago. She had her teeth cleaned twice yearly. She reported that her teeth and gums were very sensitive and that local anesthesia was often needed during her cleanings.

Social History
The patient had been born and raised in Brazil and had moved to the United States when she was 28 years old. She was married and had two daughters. She worked as a housecleaner. The patient consumed one to three alcohol drinks per week and denied the use of tobacco products.

Family History
Both of the patient's parents currently resided in Brazil and were in good health. She had one brother who lived in the United States and was also in good health. The patient was unaware of any dental problems in the members of her immediate family.

Extraoral Examination
The patient had no detectable lesions, masses or swelling. The temporomandibular joint was within normal limits.

Intraoral Examination
- The buccal mucosa adjacent to the mandibular third molars demonstrated diffuse white reticulations.
- Generalized gingival erythema was present with desquamation of the gingiva in the maxillary and mandibular anterior regions (Figure 1).

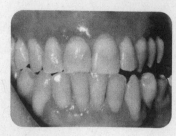

Figure 1: Frontal view.

Hard Tissue Examination

- The patient had had several restorations in her posterior dentition. All of the restorations appeared clinically and radiographically sound.
- No carious lesions were detected.

Periodontal Examination

- The periodontal examination revealed probing depths of 1–4 mm with generalized bleeding on probing.
- There was diffuse gingival erythema with varying degrees of mucosal sloughing and erosion.
- There was generalized mild to moderate gingival recession on the buccal and lingual/palatal surfaces of her teeth.
- The patient had mild plaque accumulations on her posterior teeth.

Occlusion

- The patient had class III occlusion with an open bite on the posterior left side.

Radiographic Examination

- A full mouth set of radiographs was taken.
- There were no carious lesions present.

- There was generalized mild horizontal bone loss.
- There were no other pathologic findings noted.

Diagnosis

Following review of the history and clinical evaluation, a clinical diagnosis of desquamative gingivitis was rendered.

Treatment Plan

Desquamative gingivitis is not a definitive diagnosis but a nonspecific clinical term associated with one of a variety of underlying conditions. To arrive at a definitive diagnosis, a tissue biopsy is required. The patient will receive a dental scaling with oral hygiene instructions. The treatment of her desquamative gingivitis will be determined after a definitive diagnosis is established.

Discussion

Once a clinical diagnosis of desquamative gingivitis has been rendered, a definitive diagnosis must be made. In this case, punch biopsies of the gingiva and buccal mucosa were performed and submitted for pathologic evaluation. One sample was placed in 10% formalin for hematoxylin and eosin staining and the second in Michel's medium for direct immunofluorescence. The pathology report was signed out as oral lichen planus (LP). After the diagnosis was established, the patient was prescribed a topical corticosteroid (fluocinonide gel 0.05%) and instructed to apply it two to three times daily. The patient returned after 2 weeks of treatment with a reduction in gingival erythema. The patient was informed that because there is no cure for her condition, the medication would need to be reapplied whenever she became symptomatic.

Self-Study Questions

A. How are non–plaque-induced gingival lesions classified?

B. What is desquamative gingivitis, and how does it differ from plaque-induced gingivitis?

C. What is the differential diagnosis for desquamative gingivitis?

D. How is desquamative diagnosis managed?

E. What is the presentation and prevalence of oral LP

F. How is a diagnosis of oral LP rendered?

G. What is the etiology of oral LP

H. What are the histopathologic features of oral LP

I. How is oral lichen planus managed?

J. What is the long-term prognosis for oral LP

Answers located at the end of the chapter.

References

1. Holmstrup P. Non-plaque induced gingival lesions Ann Periodontol 1999;4:20–29
2. American Academy of Periodontology Position Paper: Oral features of mucocutaneous disorders. J Periodontol 2003;74:1545–1556
3. Neville BW, Damm DD, et al. Oral and Maxillofacial Pathology. Philadelphia, PA: Saunders; 2009. Chapter 4, p162–163.
4. Scully C, Porter SR. The clinical spectrum of desquamative gingivitis. Semin Cutan Med Surg 1997;16:308.
5. Guiglia R, Di Liberto C, et al. A combined treatment regimen for desquamative gingivitis in patients with oral lichen planus. J Oral Pathol Med 2007;36(2):110–116.
6. Chams-Davatchi D, et al. Pemphigus: analysis of 1209 cases. Int J Dermatol 2005;44:470–476.
7. Axell T, Rundquist L. Oral lichen planus – a demographic study. Community Dent Oral Epidemiol 1987;15:52–56.
8. Scully C, Almeida OPD, et al. Oral lichen planus in childhood. Br J Dermatol 1994;130:131–133.
9. Scully C, Beyli M, et al. Update on oral lichen planus: etiopathogenesis and management. Crit Rev Oral Biol Med 1998;9:86–122.
10. Thorn JJ, Holmstrup P, et al. Course of various clinical forms of oral lichen planus. A prospective follow-up study of 611 patients. J Oral Pathol 1988;17:213–218.
11. Ingafou M, Leao JC, Porter SR, Scully C, et al. Oral lichen planus: a retrospective study of 690 British patients. Oral Dis 2006;12:463–468.
12. Neville BW, Damm DD, et al. Oral and Maxillofacial Pathology. Philadelphia, PA: Saunders; 2009. Chapter 9 p347–350.
13. Eversole LR. Immunopathology of oral mucosal ulcerative, desquamative and bullous diseases. Oral Surg Oral Med Oral Pathol 1994;77:555–571.
14. Holmstrup P, Schiotz AW, et al. Effect of dental plaque control on gingival lichen planus. Oral Surg Oral Med Oral Pathol 1990;69:585–590.
15. Neville BW, Damm DD, et al. Oral and Maxillofacial Pathology. Philadelphia, PA: Saunders; 2009. Chapter 16, p782–792.

TAKE-HOME POINTS

A. According to the American Academy of Periodontology 1999 World Workshop on the classification of periodontal disease, the etiology of the non–plaque-induced gingival lesions can be divided into several categories [1]. It should be emphasized that even though the direct cause of the lesions in these cases is not plaque, the severity of the inflammation often depends on the interaction with the bacterial plaque present.

- Gingival lesions of infectious origin (e.g., herpes simplex, candidiasis)
- Gingival lesions of genetic origin (e.g., hereditary gingival fibromatosis)
- Gingival manifestations of systemic conditions (LP, mucous membrane pemphigoid, pemphigus vulgaris)
- Traumatic lesions (e.g., factitious, iatrogenic, accidental)

Arriving at a specific diagnosis may be a complex process and requires taking a detailed history along with the specific clinical presentation of a particular patient.

B. Desquamative gingivitis (DG) is a clinical term used to describe a condition characterized by intense erythema, desquamation, and ulceration of the gingiva [2]. A variety of different conditions can manifest as desquamative gingivitis, but it is most often associated with one of the vesiculoerosive diseases (see answer to question C).

Plaque-induced gingivitis is a response to inadequate oral hygiene practices and generally presents with inflammation at the gingival margin. This inflammation often causes the tissue to become erythematous and edematous. There is commonly bleeding on probing and an increase in gingival crevicular fluid or exudate. The clinical signs and symptoms of plaque-induced gingivitis are usually reversed after removing the primary etiology of bacteria-laden plaque. Refer to Chapter 1, Case 2, for a detailed description on plaque-induced gingivitis.

C. Desquamative gingivitis can be a manifestation of any of a number of dermatologic conditions,

most commonly oral LP, benign mucous membrane pemphigoid, or pemphigus vulgaris [3]. Other conditions that can present as desquamative gingivitis include chronic ulcerative stomatitis, bullous pemphigoid, linear immunoglobulin A disease, dermatitis herpetiformis, or lupus erythematosus [4]. Once a clinical diagnosis of desquamative gingivitis is rendered, a definitive diagnosis must be established.

D. Regardless of the underlying cause of DG, it has been shown that improved oral hygiene can decrease the severity of the lesions [5]. However, this will not bring about complete resolution and, more importantly, does not address the underlying cause. A biopsy of the lesion must be taken to establish a definitive diagnosis. The biopsy should include perilesional tissue because the center of an ulceration histologically reveals only nonspecific granulation tissue. A second specimen submitted for immunofluorescence studies may aid in the diagnosis.

The symptoms of desquamative gingivitis are managed based on the underlying cause of the condition. In most cases, the oral lesions themselves may be managed with topical corticosteroids. A common first line of treatment is 0.05% fluocinonide gel, which may be applied to the lesions three times daily. This may be delivered directly to the gingiva or, in the case of widespread lesions, placed in a custom-fabricated tray analogous to a bleaching tray typically used for tooth whitening. Alternatively, a dexamethasone elixir may be prescribed for patients to swish and expectorate three times daily. It is important to monitor the patients for signs of oral candidiasis that may develop in the setting of steroid use.

In the case of a diagnosis of mucous membrane pemphigoid, the patient should be referred to an ophthalmologist who is familiar with the ocular lesions of this condition to guard against vision loss. Although corticosteroid therapy has helped to reduce the mortality rate associated with pemphigus vulgaris to less than 10% [6], patients with this diagnosis should be evaluated by their primary care physicians or dermatologists for the evaluation of cutaneous lesions.

E. Oral LP is one of the most common mucocutaneous diseases manifesting on the gingiva. Oral involvement alone is common; concomitant skin lesions in patients with oral lesions have been found in 5–44% of cases [7]. Most patients who present with oral LP are middle aged. Children are rarely affected [8]. A predilection for women is shown in most series of cases by a ratio of 3:2 over men. The prevalence of oral LP in various populations has been found to be 0.1–4% [9].

Oral LP has traditionally been divided into reticular and erosive forms. Simultaneous presence of more than one type of lesion is common [10]. The reticular form is much more common than the erosive and often goes unnoticed by the patient. It generally involves the posterior buccal mucosa bilaterally, but any area of the oral mucosa may be affected. Reticular LP is named because of its characteristic pattern of interlacing white lines (Wickham striae). Erosive/erythematous LP is less common but more significant for the patient because the lesions are usually symptomatic. Clinically there are erythematous areas with or without ulcerations. The periphery is usually bordered by the fine white radiating striae of reticular LP. Erythema and/or ulceration involving the gingiva produce desquamative gingivitis.

F. The most characteristic clinical manifestations of oral LP are white interlacing white striae appearing bilaterally on the posterior buccal mucosa [11]. A diagnosis of reticular LP can often be made based on the clinical presentation alone of the lesions. Erosive LP can be more challenging to diagnose based on clinical features alone. Unilateral lesions or presentations lacking typical radiating white striae may be difficult to distinguish from other ulcerative or erosive diseases. If the diagnosis is in question after clinical examination, a biopsy is necessary to confirm a diagnosis.

G. The etiology of most oral LP cases is idiopathic. Oral lichenoid lesions can also be associated with various types of medications including nonsteroidal anti-inflammatory drugs, antihypertensive agents, antimalarials, gold salts, and penicillamine [12]. Unilateral oral lichenoid lesions are rare and may be secondary to contact with amalgam dental restorations.

H. Oral LP presents histologically with varying degrees of orthokeratosis and/or parakeratosis. There is disruption of the basal cells and transmigration of T lymphocytes into the basal and parabasal cell layers of the epithelium. Degenerating keratinocytes termed *Civatte bodies* (colloid bodies) are often found at the junction of the epithelium and connective tissue. There is characteristically a subepithelial bandlike accumulation of T lymphocytes and macrophages characteristic of a type IV hypersensitivity reaction [13] (Figure 2). These features are characteristic but not specific to oral LP. Other interface processes including lupus erythematous and chronic ulcerative stomatitis have similar histopathologic presentations.

I. Reticular LP often causes no symptoms and need not be treated. The first line of treatment for symptomatic erosive LP is topical corticosteroids. Fluocinonide gel applied to the most symptomatic

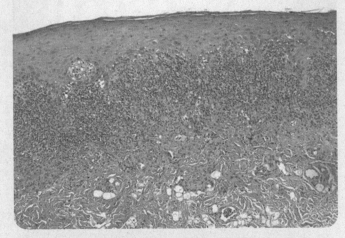

Figure 2: Characteristic histopathology of lichen planus demonstrates parakeratinized and/or orthokeratinized stratified squamous epithelium with sawtooth-shaped rete ridges, squamatization of basal cells, and a bandlike infiltrate of lymphocytes in the superficial connective tissue.

areas or dexamethasone elixir used as a mouthrinse three to four times per day is often sufficient to induce healing within 1–2 weeks. Patients should be informed that the lesions will likely return and the corticosteroids should be reapplied. Patients should be monitored for their response and for the possibility of candidiasis induced by the use of the steroids. Another important part of the therapeutic regimen in patients with desquamative gingivitis is meticulous plaque control, which results in significant improvement in many patients [14].

J. LP is a chronic condition with lesions that wax and wane over time. The erosive form should be monitored and treated as necessary to improve patient comfort. Some investigators suggest that patients with erosive LP be evaluated every 3 months, particularly if the lesions are not typical. Cases of malignant transformation of LP have been reported, but a clear association is lacking in evidence. If the potential for malignant transformation does exist, it appears to be small and generally confined to patients with the erosive form of LP [15].

Case 4

Gingival Enlargement

CASE STORY

A 35-year-old Caucasian female presented with a chief complaint of: "My gums are swollen and bleed." The patient noticed swelling of the gingiva 2 months after she started taking phenytoin (Dilantin) for epilepsy, which was first diagnosed 13 years ago. The patient did not brush or floss her teeth consistently.

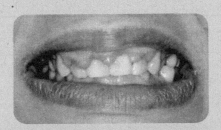

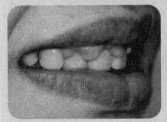 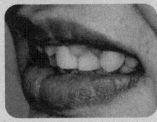

Figure 1: Initial presentation of a patient with phenytoin-induced gingival enlargement: smile frontal, right, and left views.

LEARNING GOALS AND OBJECTIVES

■ To be able to diagnose gingival overgrowth
■ To identify the etiology and to address it in the treatment plan
■ To understand the difference between true pockets and pseudo-pockets

Medical History

The patient had been diagnosed with epilepsy about 13 years ago. Since that time she had been taking Dilantin 500 mg daily. Additionally, the patient currently took 2000 mg Depakote daily (1000 mg bid) and 10 mg Zyprexa at bedtime. There were no other significant medical problems and the patient had no known allergies.

Social History

The patient did not smoke or drink alcohol.

Extraoral and Intraoral Examinations

- There were no significant findings on extraoral examination. The patient had no masses or swelling and the temporomandibular joint was within normal limits.
- With the exception of the gingiva, the soft tissues of the mouth including the tongue appeared normal.
- Examination of the gingiva revealed generalized marginal erythema, edema, rolled margins, enlarged papillae, and bleeding on probing (Figures 1 and 2). Probing depths ranged from 2 to 5 mm (pseudo-pockets due to gingival overgrowth; Figure 3).
- The hard tissue examination found multiple restorations.

Occlusion

Angle class II, division 2 occlusion with tooth #12 in cross-bite due to arch incongruence.

Radiographic Examination

A full mouth set of radiographs revealed normal levels of alveolar bone throughout the mouth including the maxillary and mandibular anterior where clinical gingival enlargement was present (Figure 4).

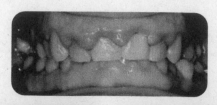
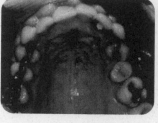
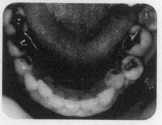

Figure 2: Initial presentation of a patient with phenytoin-induced gingival enlargement: buccal view in occlusion, maxilla and mandible occlusal views. Note that gingival enlargement is localized to anterior and facial segments on both maxilla and mandible.

Diagnosis

After reviewing the history and the clinical and radiographic examinations, the patient was diagnosed with phenytoin-associated gingival overgrowth and a differential diagnosis was generated (A).

Treatment Plan

The treatment plan for the phenytoin-associated gingival overgrowth includes interdisciplinary consultation (to include the primary care physician regarding alternative medication for treatment of epilepsy), oral hygiene instructions, initial phase therapy consisting of supra- and subgingival scaling with polishing, reevaluation at 6 weeks, and surgical phase (gingivectomy) if gingival overgrowth persists. Routine maintenance therapy should be performed every 3 months following resolution of the gingival overgrowth (G).

Treatment

The patient received full-mouth scaling and polishing. The patient was referred to a restorative dentist for

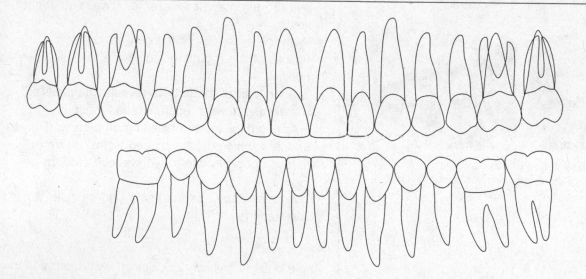

| Buccal | - | 423 | 323 | 433 | 423 | 434 | 435 | 534 | 434 | 524 | 314 | 424 | 324 | 423 | 323 | - |
| Palatal | - | 433 | 322 | 323 | 333 | 322 | 222 | 322 | 322 | 223 | 323 | 323 | 334 | 323 | 333 | - |

| Buccal | - | - | 323 | 333 | 323 | 424 | 434 | 334 | 434 | 424 | 323 | 333 | 323 | 333 | 333 | - |
| Lingual | - | - | 333 | 333 | 323 | 333 | 333 | 323 | 323 | 223 | 223 | 222 | 323 | 323 | 333 | - |

Figure 3: Probing pocket depth measurements.

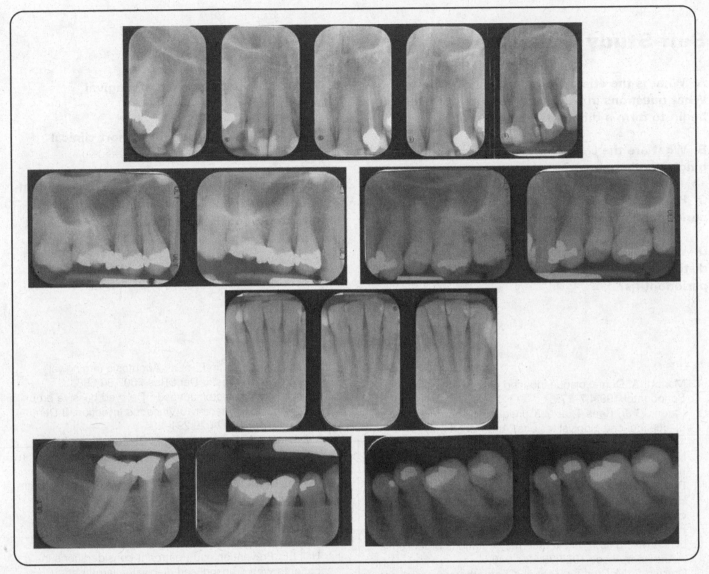

Figure 4: Peri-apical radiographs depicting the interproximal bone levels.

detailed hard tissue examination and treatment of active decay. At 6-week reevaluation, the patient demonstrated excellent oral hygiene, but the clinical signs and symptoms had improved only slightly. Therefore, gingivectomy and gingivoplasty were performed to restore gingival contours (G; Chapter 3, Case 1). The patient is currently on 3-month recall.

Discussion

Most patients who have gingival enlargement present with the chief complaint of an unaesthetic smile. Comprehensive medical and dental histories (A) as well as a complete periodontal examination are needed to come to the appropriate diagnosis. Most commonly, gingival overgrowth is a dental plaque–induced gingival

disease modified by medications, such as phenytoin, cyclosporine A, or calcium channel blockers. In some rare cases, a non–plaque-induced gingival enlargement called hereditary gingival fibromatosis (A) may be seen.

Once the diagnosis is determined, the treatment plan includes oral hygiene instructions, an initial phase of treatment (scaling and polishing), and communication with the primary care physician for potential alternative medication to address the systemic condition (G). Phase 1 therapy is followed by periodontal reevaluation at 4–6 weeks. If the gingival enlargement persists at this visit, surgical excision of excessive gingiva is recommended with subsequent reinforcement of home care oral hygiene and a periodontal maintenance every 3 months is instituted (G).

Self-Study Questions

A. What is the etiology for gingival overgrowth? What questions in a dental history might help you begin to form a differential diagnosis?

B. What are the characteristics of drug-induced gingival enlargement?

C. How would you differentiate between a "true" periodontal pocket and a "pseudo-pocket"?

D. What are the clinical characteristics that distinguish gingival enlargement versus periodontitis?

E. What is the pathogenesis of gingival enlargement?

F. What is another reason for a short clinical crown?

G. What is the current treatment for patients with drug-induced gingival enlargement? What is the long-term prognosis with treatment for these patients?

Answers located at the end of the chapter.

References

1. Mariotti A. Dental plaque-induced gingival diseases. Ann Periodontol 199;4:7–17.
2. Caton JG Jr, Rees T, et al. Consensus report: Non-plaque-induced gingival lesions. Ann Periodontol 1999;4:30–31.
3. Hart TC, Pallos D, et al. Evidence of genetic heterogeneity for hereditary gingival fibromatosis. J Dent Res 2000;79:1758–1764.
4. Hart TC, Zhang Y, et al. A mutation in the SOS1 gene causes hereditary gingival fibromatosis type 1. Am J Hum Genet 2002;70:943–954.
5. Lynch MA, Ship II. Initial oral manifestations of leukemia. J Am Dent Assoc 1967;75:932–940.
6. Dreizen S, McCredie KB, et al. Chemotherapy-associated oral hemorrhages in adults with acute leukemia. Oral Surg Oral Med Oral Pathol 1984;57:494–498.
7. Listgarten MA. Periodontal probing: what does it mean? [review]. J Clin Periodontol 1980;7:165–176.
8. Trackman PC, Kantarci A. Connective tissue metabolism and gingival overgrowth. Crit Rev Oral Biol Med 2004;15;165–175.
9. Black SA Jr, Palamakumbura AH, et al. Tissue-specific mechanisms for CCN2/CTGF persistence in fibrotic gingiva: interactions between cAMP and MAPK signaling pathways, and prostaglandin E2-EP3 receptor mediated activation of the c-JUN N-terminal kinase J Biol Chem 2007;282:15416–15429.
10. Kantarci A, Black SA, et al. Epithelial and connective tissue cell CTGF/CCN2 expression in gingival fibrosis. J Pathol 2006;210:59–66.
11. Uzel MI, Kantarci A, et al. Connective tissue growth factor in drug-induced gingival overgrowth. J Periodontol 2001;72:921–931.
12. Kantarci A, Augustin P, et al. Apoptosis in gingival overgrowth tissues. J Dent Res 2007;86:888.
13. Volchansky A, Cleaton-Jones P. Delayed passive eruption – A predisposing factor to Vincent's Infection. J Dent Assoc S Africa 1974;29:291–294.
14. Volchansky A, Cleaton-Jones P. The position of the gingival margin as expressed by clinical crown height in children ages 6–16 years J Dent 1975; 4:116–122.
15. Goldman HM, Cohen DW. Periodontal Therapy. 4th ed. St. Louis, MO: Mosby, 1968.
16. Marshall RI, Bartold PM. A clinical review of drug-induced gingival overgrowths. Aust Dent J 1999;44:219–232.
17. Hall EE. Prevention and treatment considerations in patients with drug-induced gingival enlargement. Curr Opin Periodontol 1997;4:59–63.
18. Ilgenli T, Atilla G, et al. Effectiveness of periodontal therapy in patients with drug-induced gingival overgrowth. Long-term results. J Periodontol 1999;70:967–972.
19. Ciancio SG, Bartz NW Jr, et al. Cyclosporine-induced gingival hyperplasia and chlorhexidine: a case report. Int J Periodontics Restorative Dent 1991;11:241–245.
20. Prasad VN, Chawla HS, et al. Folic acid and phenytoin induced gingival overgrowth – is there a preventive effect? J Indian Soc Pedod Prev Dent 2004;22:82–91.
21. Chand DH, Quattrocchi J, et al. Trial of metronidazole vs. azithromycin for treatment of cyclosporine-induced gingival overgrowth. Pediatr Transplant 2004;8:60–64.

TAKE-HOME POINTS

A. Gingival overgrowth or enlargement is a common side effect and unwanted outcome of certain systemic medication. Drug-influenced gingival enlargement refers to an abnormal growth of the gingiva secondary to use of systemic medication and is classified by the America Academy of Periodontology as a form of dental plaque–induced gingival disease modified by medications [1]. Currently three pharmaceutical categories of medication (anticonvulsants, immunosuppressants, and calcium channel blockers) are associated with gingival enlargement. However, a strong association has been noted only with phenytoin (when used in a chronic regimen to control epileptic seizures), cyclosporine A (powerful immunoregulator drug primarily used in the prevention of organ transplant rejection), and nifedipine (commonly prescribed as antihypertensive, antiarrhythmic, and antianginal agent). The prevalence of the gingival overgrowth varies widely: the prevalence related to use of phenytoin is approximately 50%, whereas cyclosporine and nifedipine produce significant gingival changes in about 25% of the patients treated.

Among the non–plaque-induced gingival lesions, gingival fibromatosis of genetic origin has been also described as associated with gingival overgrowth [2]. Hereditary gingival fibromatosis (HGF) is an uncommon disorder that can occur as an isolated finding or as part of a genetic syndrome. HGF is most frequently reported to be transmitted as an autosomal dominant trait, but autosomal recessive inheritance has also been reported [3]. The clinical presentation of HGF is variable, both in the distribution (number of teeth involved) and in the degree (severity) of expression [3]. Affected individuals have a benign slowly progressive, nonhemorrhagic, fibrous enlargement of the oral masticatory mucosa [4]. A mutation in the Son of Sevenless-1 (SOS1) gene was reported to cause hereditary gingival fibromatosis type 1 [4]. HGF usually develops before the person reaches 10 years of age, often at or about the time of eruption of the permanent incisors. However, cases have been reported to occur during the eruption of the deciduous dentition and even to appear at birth [3].

Gingival enlargement has been found to be one of the oral manifestations associated with acute leukemias [5], in addition to cervical adenopathy, petechiae, mucosal ulcers and gingival inflammation. Gingival bleeding is a common and usually the initial oral sign and/or symptom in 17.7% and 4.4% of patients with acute and chronic leukemias, respectively [5]. Gingival inflammation in leukemic patients presents as swollen, glazed, and spongy tissues that are red to deep purple in appearance [6]. Gingival enlargement has been associated with leukemia beginning at the interdental papilla and extending to the marginal and attached gingiva [6].

Questions important in the development of a differential diagnosis include:
- When did your gingiva start to swell?
- Did anybody in your family describe a similar pattern of gingival enlargement?
- Are you taking any medication?
- How long have you been taking the specific medication?
- Do your gums bleed easily?

B. As detailed in the Annals of Periodontology 1999 [1], the common clinical characteristics of drug-related gingival enlargement include a variation in interpatient and intrapatient pattern (such as genetic predisposition), predilection for anterior and facial segments, higher prevalence in children (due to phenytoin most often used in young patients and having the highest prevalence of all medication-induced gingival enlargement), onset within 1–3 months of drug use, change in gingival contour leading to modification of gingival size, enlargement starting at the interdental papilla, change in gingival color, pronounced inflammatory response of gingiva in association with bacterial plaque and reduction in severity with decrease in dental plaque, bleeding upon provocation, increased gingival exudate, and found in gingiva with or without bone loss but is not associated with attachment loss. Patients with this diagnosis are usually taking one of the following: phenytoin, cyclosporine A, or certain channel blocker drugs.

C. The probing depth is the distance from the gingival margin to the bottom of the gingival sulcus. The normal sulcus, measuring between 1 and 3 mm is normally measured to the nearest millimeter by means of a graduated periodontal probe with a standardized tip diameter of approximately 0.4–0.5 mm. The measurements recorded clinically with the periodontal probe have generally been considered a reasonably accurate estimate of sulcus or pocket depth. A probing of the sulcus depth (PPD) of ≥4 mm suggests a diseased state and represents a true periodontal pocket. A "true" periodontal pocket is the measurement from the gingival margin to the bottom of the pocket, recording an increased value (PPD ≥4 mm) beyond that found in the normal gingival sulcus. This depth increase is the result of apical migration of the junctional epithelium subsequent to alveolar bone resorption in patients with periodontitis.

Pocket depths >3–4 mm may also be caused by the swelling of the gingiva without a concomitant apical migration of dentogingival epithelium from the cementumenamel junction (CEJ), as the case of gingival enlargement. This increase in pocket depth is called a "pseudo-pocket" because it is not associated with bone loss or apical migration of the junctional epithelium.

Probing depth, in fact, is a histologic term expressing the distance from the gingival margin to the most coronal level of the junctional epithelium. Clinical probing depth measured from the gingival margin seldom corresponds to sulcus or pocket depth. The discrepancy is least in the absence of inflammation and increases with increasing degrees of inflammation [7]. In the presence of periodontitis the probe tip passes through the inflamed tissues to stop at the level of the most coronal intact dentogingival fibers, approximately 0.3–0.5 mm apical to the apical termination of the junctional epithelium. Decreased probing depth measurements following periodontal therapy

may be in part due to decreased penetrability of the gingival tissues by the probe. Therefore, a distinction should be made between the histologic and the clinical PPD to differentiate between the actual depth of anatomic defect and the measurement recorded by the periodontal probe [7].

D. Gingival enlargement is usually associated with certain medications (i.e., Dilantin, nifedipine, cyclosporine A), and the clinical presentation is typically characteristic: papillary and free marginal gingiva is enlarged, mostly localized in anterior facial segments, increased probing depth with normal bone levels generally; possibly there are signs of inflammation.

Periodontitis is characterized by plaque-induced inflammation localized at the marginal gingiva, with bleeding on probing, increased probing depth with loss of periodontal tissues – cementum, periodontal ligament along with crestal bone resorption – therefore "true" periodontal pockets. Depending on the degree of clinical attachment loss, periodontitis can be mild, moderate, or severe.

Diagnosis of each disease type is critical due to distinct treatment that is needed to restore form and function and/or stabilize the periodontal disease progression, as mainly in the case of periodontitis.

E. The biologic origins for gingival overgrowth are complex. Recent studies indicate that molecular markers and clinical features of gingival overgrowth differ in their response to medication and that multiple genetic loci are linked to the inherited forms of gingival overgrowth [8].

Multiple hypotheses have been suggested and tested to better understand the molecular mechanisms underlying the clinical features of drug-induced gingival overgrowth. One leading theory is that substances that cause gingival overgrowth may do so by altering the normal balance of cytokines in gingival tissues because abnormally high levels of specific cytokines were found in enlarged gingival tissues. Among the cytokines and growth factors found to be at elevated levels in human drug-induced gingival overgrowth are interleukin (IL)-6, IL-1β, platelet-derived growth factor-B, fibroblast growth factor-2, transforming growth factor-β, and connective tissue growth factor [8].

Connective tissue growth factor (CTGF, or CCN2), is a 38-kDa secreted protein belonging to the CCN family of growth factors. It has been shown to promote the synthesis of various components of the extracellular matrix, and its overexpression is associated with the onset and progression of fibrosis in many organs including human gingiva [9]. Moreover, fibrotic human gingival tissues express CTGF/CCN2 in both epithelium [10] and connective tissues [11], suggesting that interactions between epithelial and connective tissues could contribute to gingival fibrosis.

It has also been suggested that variations in the balance between cell proliferation and apoptosis contribute to the etiology of gingival overgrowth. Increased fibroblast proliferation and a simultaneous decrease in apoptosis were found to contribute to gingival overgrowth [12].

F. Short clinical crowns associated with healthy-appearing gingiva can be due to gingival tissue located more incisally or occlusally on the anatomic crown. Volchansky and Cleaton-Jones described this condition as delayed passive eruption [13,14]. They reported an incidence of 12% of patients examined demonstrating delayed passive eruption. Goldman and Cohen also described this condition where the gingival margin fails to recede to the CEJ during tooth eruption as altered (retarded) passive eruption [15].

G. The treatment of patients with drug-induced gingival enlargement consists of oral hygiene instructions, supra- and subgingival scaling and polishing, and referral to the primary care physician for possible substitution of one medication for another (i.e., phenytoin can be replaced with carbamazepine or valproic acid, cyclosporine with tacrolimus, and nifedipine with one of many dihydropteridines) not as strongly associated with gingival overgrowth. If the previously described treatment does not result in significant resolution of gingival enlargement, surgical excision of the excessive gingiva is performed using a classic external bevel gingivectomy or an internal bevel gingivectomy approach [16] (Chapter 3, Case 1). The internal bevel approach provides primary closure and reduction of postoperative bleeding, discomfort, and infection. More recently, a carbon dioxide laser has been used for surgical excision and provides rapid hemostasis and compatibility with a host with underlying medical conditions. It also has been reported to reduce surgical time [16].

Having the patient in a rigorous home plaque control regimen as well as regular 3-month periodontal maintenance are strongly recommended [17] and may considerably reduce the risk of recurrence. In a study of 38 individuals, 18 months after surgical therapy, the recurrence rate of gingival overgrowth in patients taking cyclosporin A or nifedipine was 34%. Age, gingival inflammation, and attendance at periodontal maintenance visits were all significantly related to recurrence, and they suggest that regular re-motivation and professional care at frequent recall appointments are of great importance in patients with a history of drug-induced gingival overgrowth [18]. To prevent postsurgical recurrence, a chlorhexidine rinse twice daily is recommended [19].

Several medications have been shown to ameliorate gingival enlargement such as systemic or topical folic acid [20] or a short course of metronidazole or azithromycin. The latter drugs work particularly well for significant resolution of cyclosporine-induced gingival overgrowth [21]. The mechanism of action for these antibiotics is not clear, but it is suggested they may contribute to inhibition of collagen fiber proliferation in addition to their antimicrobial action.

Case 5

Aggressive Periodontitis

CASE STORY

A 23-year-old African American female presented with a chief compliant of: "Bleeding gums on brushing and swollen gingiva in specific areas of the mouth." The patient's dentist had observed 7- to 10-mm probing depths in several teeth in all four quadrants of the mouth and referred her to a periodontist for a periodontal consultation.

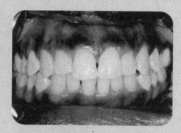

Figure 1: Preoperative frontal view.

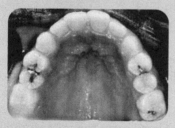

Figure 2: Preoperative maxillary dentition.

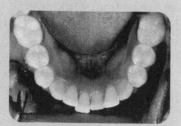

Figure 3: Preoperative mandibular dentition.

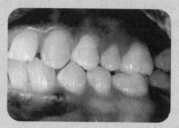

Figure 4: Preoperative left occlusal view.

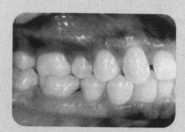

Figure 5: Preoperative right occlusal view.

LEARNING GOALS AND OBJECTIVES

- To be able to understand the definition and diagnostic criteria of aggressive periodontitis
- To understand the various treatment options available for this condition
- To understand the prognosis of periodontal and implant treatment in these patients

Medical History

No relevant medical history was noted, and the patient did not report any allergies to food or to drugs. The patient was not taking any medications.

Review of Systems

- Vital signs
  - Blood pressure: 120/80 mm Hg
  - Pulse rate: 73 beats/minute (regular)
  - Respiration: 15 breaths/minute

Social History

The patient was a nonsmoker and reported that she did not consume alcohol.

Extraoral Examination

There were no significant findings. The patient had no masses or swelling, and the temporomandibular joint was within normal limits.

Intraoral Examination

- No abnormal findings with respect to tongue, floor of the mouth, palate, and buccal mucosa were observed.
- A gingival examination revealed mild marginal erythema with areas of rolled margins and swollen papillae in relation to all first molars and mandibular incisors (Figures 1 and 3).
- A periodontal charting was completed (Figures 4 and 5). Tooth #3, 14, 19, and 30 exhibited probing depths >7 mm, especially in the interproximal areas. Mandibular incisors also exhibited probing depths in the range of 6–7 mm (Figures 6 and 7).
- Grade 3 mobility was observed in teeth #23 to 26.
- The teeth other than incisors and molars exhibited probing depths in the range of 2–4 mm.
- Grade II furcation involvements were recorded for all the affected molars.
- The patient's oral hygiene was good.

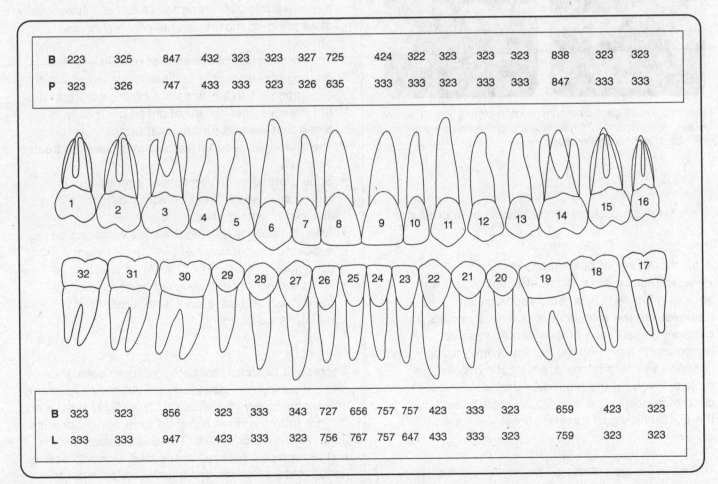

Figure 6: Probing pocket depth measurements during phase I revaluation. B, buccal; P, palatal; L, lingual.

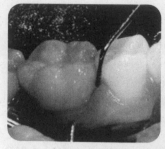 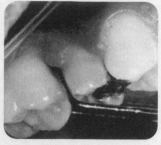

Figure 7: Intraoral clinical photographs depicting deeper probing depth associated with maxillary and mandibular molars.

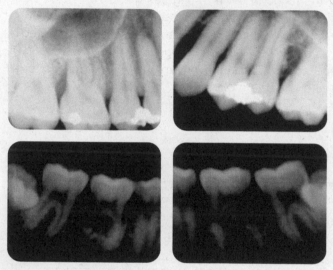

Figure 8: Periapical radiographs demonstrating the intrabony defects surrounding all four molars and the relatively normal premolars and second molars.

Occlusion

There were no occlusal discrepancies or interferences.

Radiographic Examination

A full-mouth set of radiographs was ordered. Periapical radiographs of the affected molars are shown in Figure 8. The radiographs clearly demonstrate the involvement of all first molars, the classical presentation of localized aggressive periodontitis (LAP). All the defects were intrabony and confined to interproximal areas of the maxillary molars, involving the proximal furcations, and are circumferential in the mandibular molars involving the buccal or lingual furcation areas.

Diagnosis and Prognosis

The patient's age, ethnicity, history, and clinical and radiographic examinations led to the diagnosis of LAP.

Molars are not mobile, and the defects surrounding them are intrabony, which are highly amenable to regeneration by bone grafting or by guided tissue regeneration. Moreover, the patient had very good oral hygiene and was highly compliant. Therefore, these molars will have a good prognosis after treatment. With respect to mandibular incisors, the long-term prognosis will be questionable because the sites exhibit severe destruction of the periodontium with bone loss almost up to the apex of the teeth.

Treatment Plan

The treatment plan for a typical case of LAP consists of the following phases:

- The diagnostic phase consists of a comprehensive periodontal examination, radiographs, and study models. In some cases, microbial testing and genetic testing are performed.
- The disease control phase includes oral hygiene instruction, splinting of the mandibular incisors, and scaling/root planing of all the affected areas with adjunctive antibiotics (amoxicillin 500 mg and metronidazole 250 mg tid for 14 days). Extractions of all the third molars can be included in this phase.
- The reevaluation phase consist of revisiting her probing pocket depths and her overall periodontal condition plus treatment planning for sites that did not improve after the initial phase of therapy or those that warrant further treatment.
- The sites that need further treatment will be treated surgically.
- Bone grafting or guided tissue regeneration is commonly used to treat intrabony defects associated with molars.
- After the surgical phase, the sites will again be evaluated for improvement in the periodontal condition.
- Once the periodontal condition is stabilized, the patient will be placed on a 3- to 4-month maintenance protocol.

Discussion

Aggressive periodontitis, categorized as a separate class of periodontal disease in the American Academy of Periodontology classification [1] is highly unique and distinct from the most common form of periodontitis (i.e., chronic periodontitis). The characteristic clinical and radiographic features associated with aggressive periodontitis allow the oral health care provider to diagnose the condition without much difficulty. The case presented here exhibits the classical clinical and radiographic features of LAP. Therefore a clear-cut diagnosis of LAP was made. In some cases, microbiologic and immunologic tests can be used as an adjunct to diagnose this disease. Increased levels of *Actinobacillus actinomycetemcomitans* (especially serotype b) microbes and a robust antibiotic response to the same microorganism are expected in such testings. After completing phase I therapy consisting of scaling and root planing, a drastic improvement in probing depth reduction and clinical attachment gain are expected in deeper pockets. Residual pockets (>6 mm) remaining after phase I therapy are usually treated with surgical periodontal therapy. Adequate oral hygiene is critical in the successful outcome of any periodontal therapy. Usually patients with LAP

tend to exhibit insignificant amount of local factors such as plaque and calculus and tend to have good oral hygiene. Even in the case described in this chapter, the patient had insignificant amounts of local factors (Figures 1–5). With respect to outcomes of surgeries performed in patients with aggressive periodontitis, long-term stability after regenerative therapy has been shown but mostly in the form of case reports [2,3]. The success rates of dental implants in patients with aggressive periodontitis in not conclusive. Considering the defect in host response in these patients, it is reasonable to expect lower implant survival rates in these patients. Some studies have indicated that the success rates in these patients are slightly lower (10%) than in patients with chronic periodontitis [4–6].

Self-Study Questions

A. How do you define aggressive periodontitis and how do you classify it?

B. What are the other terms used to describe aggressive periodontitis?

C. What are the characteristic clinical presentations common to LAP and generalized aggressive periodontitis (GAP?

D. What are the features that distinguish localized from generalized periodontitis?

E. How common is aggressive periodontitis, and which sector of the population is more susceptible to this disease?

F. What are the etiologic agents responsible for aggressive periodontitis?

G. How do you treat patients with aggressive periodontitis?

H. In aggressive periodontitis patients, what will be the prognosis after treatment?

Answers located at the end of the chapter.

References

1. Armitage GC. Development of a classification system for periodontal diseases and conditions. Ann Periodontol 1999;4:1–6.
2. Sant'Ana AC, Passanezi E, et al. A combined regenerative approach for the treatment of aggressive periodontitis: long-term follow-up of a familial case. Int J Periodontics Restorative Dent 2009;29:69–79.
3. Mengel R, Soffner M, et al. Bioabsorbable membrane and bioactive glass in the treatment of intrabony defects in patients with generalized aggressive periodontitis:
   results of a 12-month clinical and radiological study. J Periodontol 2003;74:899–908.
4. De Boever AL, Quirynen M, et al. Clinical and radiographic study of implant treatment outcome in periodontally susceptible and non-susceptible patients: a prospective long-term study. Clin Oral Implants Res 2009;20:1341–1350.
5. Mengel R, Schroder T, et al. Osseointegrated implants in patients treated for generalized chronic periodontitis and generalized aggressive periodontitis: 3- and 5-year results of a prospective long-term study. J Periodontol 2001;72:977–989.

6. Al-Zahrani MS. Implant therapy in aggressive periodontitis patients: a systematic review and clinical implications. Quintessence Int 2008;39:211–215.

7. Meng H, Xu L, et al. Determinants of host susceptibility in aggressive periodontitis. Periodontol 2000 2007;43:133–159.

8. Brown LJ, Albandar JM, et al. Early-onset periodontitis: progression of attachment loss during 6 years. J Periodontol 1996;67:968–975.

9. Orban B. A diffuse atrophy of the alveolar bone (periodontosis). J Periodontol 1942;13:31.

10. Baer PN. The case for periodontosis as a clinical entity. J Periodontol 1971;42:516–520.

11. Lang N, Bartold PM, et al. Consensus report: aggressive periodontitis. Ann Periodontol 1999;4:53.

12. Benjamin SD, Baer PN. Familial patterns of advanced alveolar bone loss in adolescence (periodontosis). Periodontics 1967;5:82–88.

13. Carvalho RP, Mesquita JS, et al. Relationship of neutrophil phagocytosis and oxidative burst with the subgingival microbiota of generalized aggressive periodontitis. Oral Microbiol Immunol 2009;24:124–132.

14. Cainciola LJ, Genco RJ, et al. Defective polymorphonuclear leukocyte function in a human periodontal disease. Nature 1977;265:445–447.

15. Asman B. Peripheral PMN cells in juvenile periodontitis. Increased release of elastase and of oxygen radicals after stimulation with opsonized bacteria. J Clin Periodontol 1988;15:360–364.

16. Kantarci A, Oyaizu K, et al. Neutrophil-mediated tissue injury in periodontal disease pathogenesis: findings from localized aggressive periodontitis. J Periodontol 2003;74:66–75.

17. Shaddox L, Wiedey J, et al. Hyper-responsive phenotype in localized aggressive periodontitis. J Dent Res 2010;89:143–148.

18. Eres G, Saribay A, et al. Periodontal treatment needs and prevalence of localized aggressive periodontitis in a young Turkish population. J Periodontol 2009;80:940–944.

19. Loe H, Brown LJ. Early onset periodontitis in the United States of America. J Periodontol 1991;62:608–616.

20. Marazita ML, Burmeister JA, et al. Evidence for autosomal dominant inheritance and race-specific heterogeneity in early-onset periodontitis. J Periodontol 1994;65:623–630.

21. Hart TC, Marazita ML, et al. Re-interpretation of the evidence for X-linked dominant inheritance of juvenile periodontitis. J Periodontol 1992;63:169–173.

22. Fine DH, Markowitz K, Furgang D, et al. *Aggregatibacter actinomycetemcomitans* and its relationship to initiation of localized aggressive periodontitis: longitudinal cohort study of initially healthy adolescents. J Clin Microbiol 2007;45:3859–3869.

23. Haraszthy VI, Hariharan G, et al. Evidence for the role of highly leukotoxic *Actinobacillus actinomycetemcomitans* in the pathogenesis of localized juvenile and other forms of early-onset periodontitis. J Periodontol 2000;71:912–922.

24. Faveri M, Figueiredo LC, et al. Microbiological profile of untreated subjects with localized aggressive periodontitis. J Clin Periodontol 2009;36:739–749.

25. Zambon JJ, Christersson LA, et al. *Actinobacillus actinomycetemcomitans* in human periodontal disease. Prevalence in patient groups and distribution of biotypes and serotypes within families. J Periodontol 1983;54:707–711.

26. Schacher B, Baron F, et al. *Aggregatibacter actinomycetemcomitans* as indicator for aggressive periodontitis by two analysing strategies. J Clin Periodontol 2007;34:566–573.

27. Xajigeorgiou C, Sakellari D, et al. Clinical and microbiological effects of different antimicrobials on generalized aggressive periodontitis. J Clin Periodontol 2006;33:254–264.

28. Guerrero A, Griffiths GS, et al. Adjunctive benefits of systemic amoxicillin and metronidazole in non-surgical treatment of generalized aggressive periodontitis: a randomized placebo-controlled clinical trial. J Clin Periodontol 2005;32:1096–1107.

29. Pavicic MJ, van Winkelhoff AJ, et al. Microbiological and clinical effects of metronidazole and amoxicillin in *Actinobacillus actinomycetemcomitans*-associated periodontitis. A 2-year evaluation. J Clin Periodontol 1994;21:107–112.

30. Winkel EG, van Winkelhoff AJ, et al. Additional clinical and microbiological effects of amoxicillin and metronidazole after initial periodontal therapy. J Clin Periodontol 1998;25:857–864.

31. Buchmann R, Nunn ME, Van Dyke TE, Lange DE. Aggressive periodontitis: 5-year follow-up of treatment. J Periodontol 2002;73:675–683.

32. Kamma JJ, Baehni PC. Five-year maintenance follow-up of early-onset periodontitis patients. J Clin Periodontol 2003;30:562–572.

33. Mros ST, Berglundh T. Aggressive periodontitis in children: a 14–19-year follow-up. J Clin Periodontol 2010;37:283–287.

34. Mengel R, Schreiber D, et al. Bioabsorbable membrane and bioactive glass in the treatment of intrabony defects in patients with generalized aggressive periodontitis: results of a 5-year clinical and radiological study. J Periodontol 2006;77:1781–1787.

35. Kaner D, Bernimoulin JP, et al. Minimally invasive flap surgery and enamel matrix derivative in the treatment of localized aggressive periodontitis: case report. Int J Periodontics Restorative Dent 2009;29:89–97.

TAKE-HOME POINTS

A. Aggressive periodontitis is a rapidly progressing form of periodontitis, characterized by early onset and familial aggregation; affected individuals are otherwise clinically healthy [1,7].

Aggressive periodontitis is subclassified into localized (LAP) and generalized (GAP) forms. LAP is defined as the interproximal loss of attachment localized to at least two permanent first molars/incisors, one of which is a first molar, and involving no more than two teeth other than first molars and incisors. When the interproximal loss of attachment extends to at least three permanent teeth other than first incisors and molars, the condition is called generalized aggressive periodontitis. If left untreated, 35% of originally classified LAP may progress to GAP [8].

B. Aggressive periodontitis was formerly called "Periodontosis" [9,10] and later called "early-onset periodontitis" (EOP). EOP includes prepubertal, juvenile, and rapidly progressive periodontitis. Because aggressive periodontitis generally affects young patients, there was a tendency to consider it a childhood disease. The current diagnosis is recommended to be based on clinical, radiographic, historical, and/or laboratory findings, rather than the age of the patient [1].

LAP and GAP replace the former terms *localized prepubertal/juvenile periodontitis* and *generalized prepubertal/juvenile periodontitis*, respectively. The patients who were classified with rapidly progressive periodontitis (RPP) are now be assigned to either GAP or "chronic severe periodontitis" based on the clinical presentation.

Most of the patients diagnosed with "generalized prepubertal periodontitis" in the 1989 American Academy of Periodontics (AAP) classification actually had been found to be associated with systemic conditions and should now be placed under the category of "periodontitis as a manifestation of systemic diseases."

C. The Following are primary features common to both LAP and GAP [11]:
- Rapid attachment loss accompanied with severe bone destruction. The progression rate of aggressive periodontitis is about three to four times faster than that of chronic periodontitis. The rapidly progressive vertical bone loss is often half-moon shaped and symmetric to the contralateral tooth [12].
- Patients are usually medically healthy.
- Familial aggregation is a common to both LAP and GAP.

Secondary features that are frequently but not always present in LAP and GAP include the following:
- Inconsistency in the relationship between the amount of microbial deposits and the severity of periodontal destruction.
- Elevated levels of *A. actinomycetemcomitans* and/or *Porphyromonas gingivalis*.
- Patients usually exhibit phagocyte abnormalities (e.g., abnormal polymorphonuclear neutrophil in adherence, chemotaxis, phagocytosis, superoxide (O_2^-) production and bactericidal activity [13–16].
- Elevated levels of inflammatory cytokines (e.g., prostaglandin E2, interleukin [IL]-1α, and IL-1β) from primed macrophages.
- Progression of attachment loss and bone loss may be self-arresting and remain stationary for years.

D.

Table 1: Features distinguishing localized aggressive periodontitis from generalized aggressive periodontitis

Features	LAP	GAP
Age of onset	Circumpubertal	<30 years of age but may be older
Clinical manifestation	Involves no more than two teeth other than incisors and first molars	Involves at least three teeth other than incisors and first molars
Serum antibody response to infecting agents [17]	Robust response	Poor response

LAP, localized aggressive periodontitis; GAP, generalized localized aggressive periodontitis.

E. The prevalence of aggressive periodontitis varies among racial and geographic groups and ranges from 0.1% to 35% [18]. The prevalence is about 0.2% in white populations and about 2.6% for people of African descent [19]. Early studies showed that aggressive periodontitis was more common in females than in males. However, the high incidence in females is believed due to the high number of females in the study populations. The proportion of affected males and females is now believed to be similar [20,21].

F. Nonmotile gram-negative anaerobic rods such as *A. actinomycetemcomitans, P. gingivalis* [22,23], and red and some orange complex species [24] are the most numerous and prevalent periodontal pathogens in aggressive periodontitis and present in most of the diseased sites compared with healthy sites. *A. actinomycetemcomitans* (especially serotype b) was found in higher numbers and frequency when compared with other pathogens in aggressive periodontitis [25,26].

G. The general treatment methods should be similar to those used for chronic periodontitis, including oral hygiene instruction/reinforcement, plaque control, scaling and root planing, and occlusal adjustment (if necessary).

Additional treatments that may be required in certain patients include:

- General medical evaluation to determine the presence of any systemic diseases. Consultation with the physician may be indicated.
- Counseling of family members.
- Adjunctive antimicrobial therapy combined with scaling and root planing. Tetracycline is contraindicated in young patients due to the problem of tooth staining. Systemic administration of amoxicillin 500 mg plus metronidazole 250 mg/500 mg tid or metronidazole 500 mg alone tid for 7 days resulted in significant clinical improvement and reduction of the levels of key periodontal pathogens for up to 6 months in deep pockets of GAP patients [27,28].
- Periodontal maintenance with short intervals may be needed.

Teeth with poor prognosis are usually extracted mostly in phase 1 or sometimes in phase 2 of

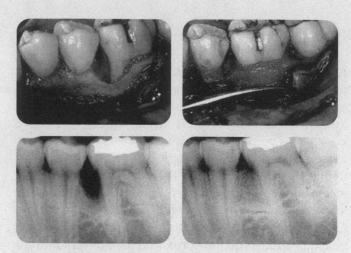

Figure 9: Classical intrabony defect affecting a mandibular first molar in another patient with LAP (top left). Guided tissue regeneration (GTR) was performed to regenerate the periodontal defect using bone grating and membrane (top right). Periapical radiographs depicting the vertical bony defect before (lower left) and after (lower right) GTR therapy. Significant radiographic bone fill was obtained after GTR therapy.

periodontal therapy. Most of the intrabony defects that result from aggressive periodontitis and that are amenable to regeneration are surgically treated using either guided tissue regeneration (GTR) or using bone grafts (Figure 9). See the appropriate chapters in this textbook for more details on these surgical techniques.

H. Scaling and root planing in combination with amoxicillin 375 mg and metronidazole 250 mg (tid for 7 days) in patients with *Actinobacillus actinomycetemcomitans*–associated periodontitis or aggressive periodontitis improved clinical parameters and suppressed *A. actinomycetemcomitans* below cultivable levels in most of the patients for up to 2 years with supportive periodontal therapy once every 3–6 months [29,30]. Long-term stabilization of periodontal health also has been reported after administering amoxicillin 500 mg and metronidazole 250 mg along with periodontal surgeries with a small percentage (5–10%) of recurrence in 5 years [31,32].

Treated LAP patients, when followed for 15 years, have been shown to have limited recurrence rate even in the absence of maintenance [33].

Successful treatment outcomes also have been shown following GTR [2,3,34] or enamel matrix derivative [35] in LAP.

The success rates in patients with aggressive periodontitis is not conclusive. Considering the defect in host response in these patients, it is reasonable to expect lower survival rates of the teeth in these patients, compared with chronic periodontitis patients. Some studies have indicated that the success rates in these patients are slightly lower (10%) than in patients with chronic periodontitis [4–6].

Case 6

Chronic Periodontitis

CASE STORY

The patient had been referred by his general dentist for periodontal treatment. Although he had a long history of dental treatment, he had never been diagnosed with periodontal disease. At the time of his first visit he had no chief complaint. He did report occasional gingival bleeding during toothbrushing.

LEARNING GOALS AND OBJECTIVES

■ To be able to identify the clinical features and overall characteristics of chronic periodontitis
■ To be able to list difficulties in the proper diagnosis of early chronic periodontitis
■ To understand possible overlaps with the diagnosis of aggressive periodontitis
■ To know what clinical changes can be anticipated in the response of chronic periodontitis to anti-infective therapy

Medical History

There were no significant medical problems, and the patient had no known allergies. He had been previously hospitalized for a day surgery to remove polyps from his vocal cords. At the time of his first appointment he was not taking any medication.

Review of Systems

- Vital signs
  - Blood pressure: 120/75 mm Hg
  - Pulse rate: 70 beats/minute (regular)

Social History

The patient was a 43-year-old white man, originally from Texas, but had been living in Massachusetts for the past 10 years. He drank alcohol socially, quit smoking 10 years ago, and reported not consuming recreational drugs. He was a musician, divorced, and has no children. His mother had heart disease, and his father died of lung cancer.

Extraoral Examination

His extra-oral examination was unremarkable: skin, head, neck, temporomandibular joint, and muscles were all within normal limits.

Intraoral Examination

The oral cancer screen was negative. His gingiva was pink, firm, with pointed papillae on the buccal aspect (Figure 1). The lingual and palatal aspects, though, presented with signs of inflammation, with erythematous and edematous gingival margins. Adequate amounts of attached tissue were present around most teeth. Gingival recession was present at several sites (see periodontal chart for details). Supra- and subgingival calculus could be detected on several tooth surfaces, particularly on the buccal surface of upper molars and lingual surfaces of lower incisors. There was generalized plaque accumulation. Saliva was of normal flow and consistency.

The periodontal chart presented in Figure 2 includes the following periodontal parameters: (1) probing pocket depth (PD) in millimeters; (2) measurement from the cementoenamel junction (CEJ) to the gingival margin (GM) in millimeters (gingival recession was recorded as a negative value); (3) clinical attachment level (CAL), which was calculated by subtracting the CEJ-GM distance from the PD; and (4) presence (1) or absence (0) of bleeding on probing (BOP). Each clinical

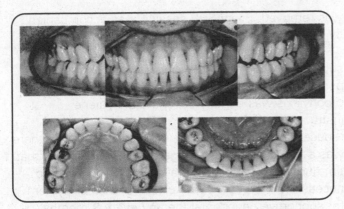

Figure 1: Clinical presentation of the case at initial visit. Courtesy of Dr. Eduardo Sampaio and Dr. Marcelo Faveri.

parameter was measured at six sites per tooth excluding third molars. Probing values were colored in blue, green, or red to highlight shallow (<4mm), intermediate (4–6mm), and deep pockets (>6mm), respectively. Bleeding on probing was detected in 68% of sites, and the mean values for PD and CAL were 3.2mm and 2.7mm, respectively.

Occlusion

There were no signs of trauma from occlusion, no major occlusal discrepancies and interferences, and no significant mobility.

Radiographic Examination

A full mouth set of radiographs (Figure 3) was exposed. There was generalized moderate to severe

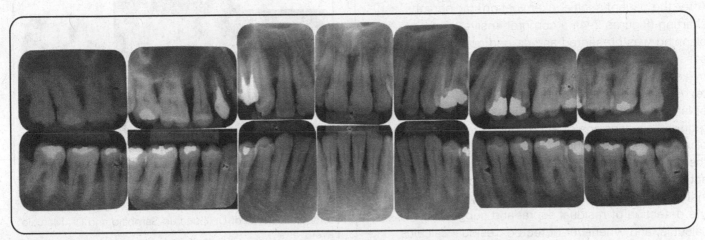

Figure 2: Periodontal chart, initial visit. Courtesy of Dr. Eduardo Sampaio and Dr. Marcelo Faveri.

Visit: Initial Exam

Surface — Buccal

Tooth	2	3	4	5	6	7	8	9	10	11	12	13	14	15
PD	8 3 4	5 3 4	7 2 5	4 2 4	4 2 3	5 1 3	3 1 4	4 1 2	3 1 3	4 1 4	4 1 6	5 2 6	6 2 6	6 2 7
CEJ-GM	2 -2 -1	-1 -2 -1	1 -1 1	1 1 -1	1 2 0	0 1 0	0 0 0	1 2 -1	-1 0 0	0 1 0	2 2 -1	2 1 -1	2 2 2	-2 -1 1
CAL	6 5 5	6 5 5	6 3 4	3 3 3	2 2 3	4 1 3	3 1 3	3 2 3	3 1 2	2 2 4	2 4 4	3 4 4	4 5 5	5 3 5
BOP	1 1 1	1 1 1	1 1 1	0 0 1	0 1 0	1 1 0	0 0 0	1 1 0	0 0 0	0 0 1	1 1 0	1 1 1	1 1 1	1 1 1

Surface — Palatal

Tooth	2	3	4	5	6	7	8	9	10	11	12	13	14	15
PD	8 2 7	7 2 6	7 2 5	5 2 5	4 3 4	5 4 4	3 2 3	3 3 3	4 3 4	3 3 3	3 2 4	5 2 7	6 3 7	7 3 8
CEJ-GM	2 0 2	2 -1 2	2 0 2	2 0 2	2 1 1	1 1 1	1 0 1	1 0 0	0 0 1	1 0 1	1 1 1	1 0 2	2 0 2	2 1 2
CAL	6 2 5	5 3 4	5 2 3	3 2 3	2 2 3	4 3 3	2 2 2	2 3 3	4 3 3	2 3 2	2 1 3	4 2 5	4 3 5	5 2 6
BOP	1 1 1	1 1 1	1 1 1	1 1 1	1 1 0	0 1 1	1 1 1	1 1 1	1 1 0	1 1 1	1 1 1	1 1 1	1 1 1	1 1 1

Surface — Buccal

Tooth	31	30	29	28	27	26	25	24	23	22	21	20	19	18
PD	3 2 3	5 1 1	3 1 3	1 1 2	2 1 1	1 1 1	1 1 2	2 1 2	1 1 1	1 1 1	1 2 1	2 1 2	1 3 3	1 3
CEJ-GM	3 0 2	2 -1 0	1 0 1	0 -2 1	0 0 -1	-1 0 -2	-2 0 -2	-2 0 -1	1 1 0	0 0 -1	1 1 -1	1 1 0	1 1 -1	2
CAL	0 2 1	3 2 1	2 1 2	1 3 1	2 1 2	2 1 3	3 1 4	4 1 4	2 1 1	0 1 1	1 2 0	1 2 1	1 1 1	2 2 1
BOP	1 0 1	1 0 1	1 1 0	0 0 0	0 0 0	0 0 0	0 0 0	0 0 0	0 0 0	0 0 0	0 0 1	0 1 1	0 1 1	0 1

Surface — Lingual

Tooth	31	30	29	28	27	26	25	24	23	22	21	20	19	18
PD	4 2 6	6 4 5	5 4 4	4 1 2	3 1 3	3 2 2	1 2 2	2 3 4	4 3 3	4 1 3	4 2 5	6 3 5	4 2 6	6 3 2
CEJ-GM	4 2 2	2 1 2	2 2 2	2 0 2	2 0 1	1 -1 -2	-2 -3 -3	-3 -3 -2	-2 -1 0	2 1 2	1 0 2	2 2 2	2 2 2	2 2 2
CAL	0 0 4	4 3 3	3 2 2	2 1 0	1 1 2	2 3 4	4 4 5	5 6 6	6 4 3	2 0 1	3 2 3	4 1 3	2 0 4	4 1 0
BOP	1 1 1	1 1 1	1 1 1	1 1 1	1 1 1	1 1 0	1 1 1	1 1 1	1 1 1	1 0 1	1 1 1	0 1 1	1 1 1	1 1 1

Figure 3: Full-mouth periapical radiographs of the case at initial visit. Courtesy of Dr. Eduardo Sampaio and Dr. Marcelo Faveri.

horizontal bone loss. There was furcation involvement seen in teeth #1, 2, 3, 14, 15, 16, 18, 19, and 30. There was a periapical radiolucency noted on tooth #5. There were root canal treatments seen on teeth #5/12. There were several amalgam restorations and recurrent decay noted on tooth #13.

Treatment Plan

The treatment plan for this case consisted primarily of four to six sessions of scaling and root planning accompanied by oral hygiene instructions. A reassessment of the case was planned for 3 months after the completion of this initial phase when the need for additional therapy would be decided.

Treatment

After the patient's initial examination, radiographs, and charting (Figures 2–4), a comprehensive treatment planning was presented and agreed upon. The first session involved full-mouth gross scaling and oral hygiene instructions on the proper toothbrushing technique and use of dental floss. Due to the presence of large amounts of subgingival calculus, the patient required six sessions of subgingival scaling and root planing (SRP) under local anesthesia (one sextant of the mouth was instrumented per session). During this active phase of anti-infective therapy, previously instrumented sextants were constantly reexamined for the detection of residual supra- and subgingival calculus, and whenever detected, residual calculus

was removed. Every SRP session was accompanied by reinforcement of the oral hygiene instructions.

Three months after the last SRP session, the subject was reexamined (Figures 4 and 5), residual pockets ≥4 mm received additional SRP, a full-mouth prophylaxis was performed, and oral hygiene instructions reinforced. Mean PD and CAL were reduced to 2.3 mm and 2.4 mm, respectively, and there was a reduction in percentage of BOP to 13%. At that time no additional periodontal therapy was deemed necessary. The patient was placed in a recall system for supportive periodontal therapy every 3 months.

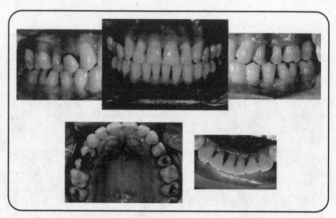

Figure 4: Clinical presentation of the case 3 months after therapy. Courtesy of Dr. Eduardo Sampaio and Dr. Marcelo Faveri.

Visit: 3 months post-therapy

Surface	Buccal																																									
Tooth	2			3			4			5			6			7			8			9			10			11			12			13			14			15		
PD	6	2	3	4	3	3	4	1	3	2	2	2	2	2	3	3	1	2	2	1	2	2	1	2	2	1	2	2	1	2	2	1	3	3	2	4	4	2	4	4	2	4
CEJ-GM	0	-3	-3	-2	-2	-1	-1	-2	-1	-1	-1	-1	1	0	0	-1	-1	-2	-1	-1	0	-1	-1	-1	-1	-1	-1	0	0	0	0	-1	-2	-1	-1	-1	0	-2	-1	-2	-2	0
CAL	6	5	6	6	5	4	5	3	4	3	3	3	1	2	3	4	2	4	3	2	2	3	2	3	3	2	3	2	1	2	2	2	5	4	3	5	4	4	5	6	4	4
BOP	1	0	0	0	0	0	0	1	0	0	0	0	0	0	0	0	0	0	0	0	0	0	0	0	0	0	0	0	0	0	0	0	0	0	0	1	0	1	1	0	1	
Surface	Palatal																																									
Tooth	2			3			4			5			6			7			8			9			10			11			12			13			14			15		
PD	5	2	4	3	2	4	4	2	4	3	2	3	2	3	2	3	2	3	2	3	2	2	3	3	2	3	3	2	3	4	2	4	4	2	4	4	2	5				
CEJ-GM	1	0	1	2	-1	1	1	0	1	2	0	2	1	1	1	1	1	1	1	0	1	1	0	0	0	0	1	1	0	1	1	1	1	1	0	1	1	0	1	2	1	1
CAL	4	2	3	1	3	3	3	2	3	1	2	1	1	2	1	2	1	1	1	2	2	2	1	2	3	3	2	2	2	2	2	1	2	3	2	3	3	2	3	2	1	4
BOP	0	0	1	0	0	0	1	0	0	0	0	0	0	0	0	0	0	0	0	0	0	0	0	0	0	0	0	0	0	0	0	0	0	0	0	0	1	1	0	1		
Surface	Buccal																																									
Tooth	31			30			29			28			27			26			25			24			23			22			21			20			19			18		
PD	3	2	3	4	1	1	2	1	2	1	1	2	2	1	1	1	1	1	1	1	2	2	1	2	1	1	1	1	1	1	1	1	1	1	2	1	2	2	1	2		
CEJ-GM	2	0	1	0	-1	0	-1	-1	0	0	-2	1	0	0	-1	-1	0	-2	-2	0	-2	-2	0	-2	-1	0	0	0	0	0	-1	0	-1	-2	-1	0	0	0	0	-1	0	
CAL	1	2	2	4	2	1	3	2	2	1	3	1	2	1	2	2	1	3	3	1	4	4	1	4	2	1	1	1	1	1	2	1	2	3	2	2	1	2	2	2	2	
BOP	1	0	1	1	0	0	0	0	0	0	0	0	0	0	0	0	0	0	0	0	0	0	0	0	0	0	0	0	0	0	0	0	0	0	0	0	1	1	0	1		
Surface	Lingual																																									
Tooth	31			30			29			28			27			26			25			24			23			22			21			20			19			18		
PD	3	2	4	4	3	4	3	2	3	3	1	2	3	1	3	2	2	2	2	1	2	2	1	2	2	1	2	2	2	3	4	2	3	3	2	4	4	2	2			
CEJ-GM	3	2	1	1	0	1	2	3	2	2	0	2	2	0	0	-1	-2	-2	-2	-3	-3	-3	-3	-2	-2	-2	0	0	1	1	0	1	1	1	1	2	2	2	1	2	2	
CAL	0	0	3	3	3	3	1	-1	1	1	1	0	1	1	3	3	4	4	4	4	5	5	4	4	4	3	2	2	1	1	1	2	2	3	1	2	1	0	2	3	0	0
BOP	1	0	0	0	0	0	0	0	0	1	0	0	0	0	0	0	0	0	0	0	0	0	0	0	0	0	0	0	0	0	0	0	0	0	0	0	1	0	0	1	0	1

Figure 5: Periodontal chart, 3 months after therapy. Courtesy of Dr. Eduardo Sampaio and Dr. Marcelo Faveri.

Figures 6 and 7 illustrate the clinical presentation and the periodontal parameters 1 year after completion of periodontal therapy.

Discussion

Chronic periodontitis is diagnosed based on the clinical signs of inflammation and clinical evidence of periodontal tissue destruction. Radiographs also help to determine the extent of bone loss. Chronic periodontitis is distinguished from gingivitis primarily on the basis of the presence of loss of attachment and resorption of alveolar bone. Therefore, in addition to

signs such as redness, swelling, bleeding tendency, and suppuration, the diagnosis of periodontitis requires the presence of periodontal pockets associated with clinical loss of attachment. Alveolar bone loss is also a hallmark of the pathology and can be detected radiographically. It is not uncommon to detect extensive accumulation of dental plaque and calculus, although this can also be found in gingivitis cases [1]. According to the American Academy of Periodontology, the severity of the condition can be categorized into slight, moderate, and severe. Strict criteria for these distinctions are not provided, but guidelines suggest a loss of clinical attachment of 1–2 mm, 3–4 mm, and ≥5 mm for each clinical category of severity, respectively [2]. The disease can also be described in terms of its extent as localized (≤30% of sites present involved) or generalized (>30% of sites present affected) [2]. Based on these criteria, the present case would be diagnosed as chronic, severe, generalized periodontitis.

Although the diagnosis of chronic periodontitis for cases such as the one presented here is straightforward, the determination of cases at the beginning of the disease process and the distinction between advanced generalized cases and aggressive forms of periodontitis is not always easy. The distinction between early periodontitis and advanced gingivitis is complicated by difficulties in determining early clinical attachment loss in the absence of radiographic evidence of alveolar bone loss, mainly in

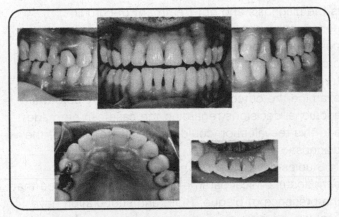

Figure 6: Clinical presentation of the case 1 year after therapy. Courtesy of Dr. Eduardo Sampaio and Dr. Marcelo Faveri.

Visit: 1 year post-therapy

Surface	Buccal													
Tooth	2	3	4	5	6	7	8	9	10	11	12	13	14	15
PD	6 2 3	4 3 3	5 1 3	2 2 2	2 2 3	3 1 2	2 1 2	2 1 2	2 1 2	2 1 2	2 1 2	2 1 3	3 2 4	4 2 5 5 3 4
CEJ-GM	0 -3 -3	-2 -2 -1	0 -2 -1	-1 -1 -1	1 0 0	-1 -1 -2	-1 -1 0	-1 -1 -1	-1 -1 -1	0 0 0	0 -1 -2	-1 -1 -1	0 -2 0	-1 -1 0
CAL	6 5 6	6 5 4	5 3 4	3 3 3	1 2 3	4 2 4	3 2 2	3 2 3	3 2 3	2 1 2	2 2 5	4 3 5	4 4 5	6 4 4
BOP	0 0 0	1 0 0	1 0 0	0 0 0	0 0 0	0 0 0	0 0 0	0 0 0	0 0 0	0 0 0	0 0 0	0 0 1	1 0 1	1 0 1

Surface	Palatal													
Tooth	2	3	4	5	6	7	8	9	10	11	12	13	14	15
PD	5 2 5	4 2 4	4 2 4	3 2 3	2 3 2	3 2 3	2 2 3	2 3	2 3 3	2 3 3	2 3 4	2 4 4	2 5 5	2 5
CEJ-GM	1 0 2	2 -1 1	1 0 1	2 0 2	1 1 1	1 1 1	1 1 0	1 1	0 0 0	1 1 0	1 1 1	1 1 0	1 1 0	1 2 1 1 1
CAL	4 2 3	2 3 3	3 2 3	1 2 1	1 2 1	2 1 1	2 2 2	1 2 3	3 2 2	2 2 2	2 1 2	3 2 3	2 3 3	2 4 3 1 4
BOP	1 0 1	0 0 0	1 0 1	0 0 0	0 0 0	0 0 0	0 0 0	0 0 0	0 0 0	0 0 0	0 0 0	0 0 0	1 0 1	1 0 0

Surface	Buccal													
Tooth	31	30	29	28	27	26	25	24	23	22	21	20	19	18
PD	3 2 3	4 1 1	2 1 2	1 1 2	2 1 1	1 1 1	1 1 2	2 1 2	1 1 1	1 1 1	1 1 1	1 1 1	2 1 2	2 1 2
CEJ-GM	2 0 1	0 -1 0	-1 -1 0	0 -2 1	0 0 -1	-1 0 -2	-2 0 -2	-2 0 -2	-1 0 0	0 0 0	-1 0 -1	-2 -1 0	0 0 0	-1 0
CAL	1 2 2	4 2 1	3 2 2	1 3 1	2 1 2	2 1 3	3 1 4	4 1 4	2 1 1	1 1 1	1 2 1	2 3 2	2 1 2	2 2 2
BOP	1 0 0	1 0 0	0 0 0	0 0 0	0 0 0	0 0 0	0 0 0	0 0 0	0 0 0	0 0 0	0 0 0	0 0 0	0 0 1	0 0 1

Surface	Lingual													
Tooth	31	30	29	28	27	26	25	24	23	22	21	20	19	18
PD	3 2 5	5 3 4	3 2 3	1 2 3	1 3 2	2 2 2	1 2 2	1 2 2	1 2 1	2 1 2	2 2 3	4 2 3	3 2 4	4 2 2
CEJ-GM	3 2 2	1 0 1	2 3 2	2 0 2	2 0 0	-1 -2 -2	-2 -3 -3	-3 -3 -2	-2 -2 0	0 0 1	1 0 1	1 1 1	2 2 2	1 2 2
CAL	0 0 3	4 3 3	1 -1 1	1 1 0	1 1 3	3 4 4	4 4 5	5 4 4	4 3 2	2 1 1	1 2 3	1 2 1	0 2 3	0 0
BOP	1 0 1	1 0 1	0 0 1	1 0 0	0 0 0	0 0 0	0 0 0	0 0 0	0 0 0	1 0 1	1 0 1	1 0 1		

Figure 7: Periodontal chart, 1 year after periodontal therapy. Courtesy of Dr. Eduardo Sampaio and Dr. Marcelo Faveri.

areas where severe gingival inflammation causes hyperplasia of the gingival margin.

The issue is further complicated by the existence of areas of incidental attachment loss [3] not caused by the bacterial-induced inflammation characteristic of periodontitis. For instance, isolated sites of gingival recession caused by toothbrush trauma should not be confused as a sign of chronic periodontitis. These lesions are easily distinguishable from recession of the gingival margin as a consequence of chronic periodontitis on the basis of their clinical features. They involve primarily the buccal surface of teeth, with no loss of adjacent interproximal tissue; they are primarily associated with teeth with thin buccal soft tissues such as maxillary canines and premolars. The presence of these isolated lesions is not sufficient for the diagnosis of chronic periodontitis, even though they are associated with attachment and alveolar bone loss.

Other common examples of incidental attachment loss lesions are the bone loss associated with restorations invading the biologic width and the defects on the distal aspect of second molars caused by the malposition of unerupted or partially erupted third molars. The mesial tipping of teeth can also lead to a clinically deepened sulcus and a radiographic image suggestive of a vertical bone loss. This appearance is the consequence of the apical displacement of the mesial CEJ and should not lead to the erroneous diagnosis of chronic periodontitis. As one can see, there are several circumstances where the diagnosis of early chronic periodontitis can be complicated.

The distinction between chronic and aggressive periodontitis can also be difficult. The two conditions are differentiated based on rates of progression and the age of onset [4]. Chronic forms of periodontitis are characterized by a relatively slow progression of attachment and bone loss starting around 30 years of age, whereas, as the term implies, aggressive periodontitis shows a faster rate of tissue loss. However, clinicians rarely have the opportunity to measure rates of disease progression. Therefore, although both conditions can affect individuals of any age, chronological age remains an essential component of the differential diagnosis. If a younger individual presents with advanced attachment and bone loss, it is concluded that these subjects are presenting a faster rate of progression.

The classic form of localized aggressive periodontitis presents several clinical features that make it easily distinguishable from chronic periodontitis, such as age of onset, only firsts molars and incisors are affected by the disease, and an overall lack of clinical signs of inflammation and minimal amounts of gross plaque and calculus accumulation despite severe bone loss around the affected teeth [3]. The lesions associated with the first molars also tend to manifest as infrabony angular defects.

The treatment of chronic periodontitis as discussed in later chapters depends on the ability of the clinician to remove plaque and calculus from the root surfaces allowing for proper healing of the gingival tissues and on the capacity of the patient to perform proper plaque control. These are the cornerstones of periodontal therapy. Although the focus of this chapter is the diagnosis and not treatment of chronic periodontitis, the results obtained with anti-infective periodontal therapy will determine the long-term prognosis of the case and the need for additional treatment. Therefore, it is essential that clinicians examine the outcome of the initial therapy before any additional decisions regarding the case can be made, and this reevaluation could be considered part of the diagnostic process.

Studies examining the prognostic ability of periodontal clinical parameters have demonstrated that the presence of plaque, BOP, and suppuration have very low positive predictive values but very high negative predictive values [5,6]. This indicates that sites without clinical signs of inflammation are at very low risk for disease progression and might not require additional therapy. In addition, the accumulation of information regarding the clinical parameters for a given site over time increases the prognostic value of these parameters. Sites with constant BOP have a much higher chance of progression than sites that bleed sporadically [6]. It is also well established that the prognosis of chronic periodontitis directly depends on the patient's ability to control plaque accumulation. A longer time of follow-up will afford the clinician a better assessment of the patient's oral hygiene skills.

The presence of residual pockets after initial therapy, rather than the presence of deep pockets at the initial examination, is associated with an increased risk of future attachment loss. This information is readily available to periodontists and can add great insights into the long-term prognosis of the case. When clinicians are trying to assess the outcome of their initial periodontal therapy, another key piece of information is how much improvement one can anticipate. In other words, what should be the realistic expectation of a therapist regarding the treatment outcome? This clearly will depend on the severity and extent of the periodontal condition at the beginning of the treatment. Several longitudinal studies have been conducted, and guidelines regarding the amount of pocket depth reduction and clinical attachment gains for each initial pocket depth are available and should be used to keep the outcome of treatment in perspective [7,8]. It is unrealistic, for instance, to expect a 9-mm pocket to convert to a 3-mm sulcus after SRP.

Self-Study Questions

A. What are the clinical features that differentiate incidental loss of attachment resulting from mechanical trauma from periodontitis-induced loss of attachment?

B. If a clinician cannot decide on the final diagnosis for the case (i.e., generalized (severe) chronic or generalized aggressive periodontitis), how should he or she proceed?

C. What are the possible therapeutic consequences of a differential diagnosis between generalized

severe chronic periodontitis and generalized aggressive periodontitis?

D. If the initial outcome of a periodontal anti-infective therapy is below standards indicated by the literature, what should the therapist suspect and how should he or she proceed?

E. How should the periodontist proceed if, by the reexamination, the case has several residual pockets?

Answers located at the end of the chapter.

References

1. Page RC, Eke PI. Case definitions for use in population-based surveillance of periodontitis. J Periodontol 2007;78:1387–1399.
2. Flemmig TF. Periodontitis. Ann Periodontol 1999;4:32–38.
3. Tonetti MS, Mombelli A. Early-onset periodontitis. Ann Periodontol 1999;4:39–53.
4. Armitage GC. Development of a classification system for periodontal diseases and conditions. Ann Periodontol 1999;4:1–6.
5. Claffey N, Nylund K, et al. Diagnostic predictability of scores of plaque, bleeding, suppuration and probing depth for probing attachment loss. 3 1/2 years of observation following initial periodontal therapy. J Clin Periodontol 1990;17:108–114.
6. Lang NP, Adler R, et al. Absence of bleeding on probing. An indicator of periodontal stability. J Clin Periodontol 1990;17:714–721.
7. Hung HC, Douglass CW. Meta-analysis of the effect of scaling and root planing, surgical treatment and antibiotic therapies on periodontal probing depth and attachment loss. J Clin Periodontol 2002;29:975–986.
8. Heitz-Mayfield LJ, Trombelli L, et al. A systematic review of the effect of surgical debridement vs non-surgical debridement for the treatment of chronic periodontitis. J Clin Periodontol 2002;29(Suppl 3):92–102; discussion 160–162.
9. Dye BA, Tan S, et al. Trends in oral health status: United States, 1988–1994 and 1999–2004. Vital Health Stat 2007;11:1–92.
10. Mongardini C, van Steenberghe D, et al. One stage full-versus partial-mouth disinfection in the treatment of chronic adult or generalized early-onset periodontitis. I. Long-term clinical observations. J Periodontol 1999;70:632–645.
11. Claffey N, Egelberg J. Clinical indicators of probing attachment loss following initial periodontal treatment in advanced periodontitis patients. J Clin Periodontol 1995;22:690–696.
12. Nyman S, Rosling B, et al. Effect of professional tooth cleaning on healing after periodontal surgery. J Clin Periodontol 1975;2:80–86.

TAKE-HOME POINTS

A. Incidental loss of attachment associated with mechanical trauma has distinct clinical features that make it clearly distinguishable from infection/inflammation-induced attachment loss. It tends to be circumscribed to buccal surfaces, particularly in areas of a very thin soft tissue, and the neighboring papilla present normal height. The tissue surrounding the recession has a very healthy appearance, and it is not uncommon to have toothbrush abrasion associated with the gingival recession. The collapse of gingival tissues on buccal surfaces can also be associated with marginal gingival inflammation, but in this case, the presence of plaque and calculus is not an uncommon finding and the tissues surrounding the gingival recession tend to shown clinical signs of inflammation.

B. As discussed earlier, the distinction between the two diagnoses can be difficult at times. The differences are typically determined by the age of onset, rate of progression, and the patterns of bone loss. In general, chronic periodontitis starts at age 30–35 and progresses in random bursts in different sites throughout one's life. If the disease presents in younger patients or can be documented to have occurred in a short period, it tends to be classified as aggressive. Both diseases can occur in a localized or generalized pattern. Familial aggregation is also one of the features of aggressive forms of periodontitis; therefore, if this diagnosis is suspected, the clinician should inquire about the periodontal status of close relatives or suggest they receive an oral examination. Finally, if the clinician cannot decide on a diagnosis, the safe assumption is to define the case as chronic periodontitis, due to the much higher prevalence of this condition compared with aggressive forms of the disease [9].

C. Although it is not the intent of this chapter to address therapy, which is discussed extensively in other chapters of the book, the relevance of the distinction between chronic and aggressive forms of periodontitis depends on the assumption that these two clinical forms of the disease would require specific types of treatment. However, recent literature has indicated that subjects with generalized aggressive periodontitis and generalized chronic periodontitis with comparable extent and severity of the conditions tend to respond similarly to periodontal therapy [10]. This would imply that the prognosis of the case would depend more on the extent and severity of the periodontal disease than on its precise diagnosis as chronic or aggressive.

D. In these circumstances, the clinician should rule out any systemic causes for the disease (risk factors such as smoking or uncontrolled diabetes, immunocompromise, endocrine disorders, or syndromes). The next thing to check is the efficiency of the patient's plaque control. This can be easily ascertained by the gingival and plaque indices. In the presence of large amounts of plaque, reinfection of pockets occurs fast and healing is compromised. Once the level of oral hygiene of the patient has been assessed, provided it was not the problem, the next steps will depend greatly on the level of periodontal training of the therapist. If the clinician is an experienced periodontist, the chances are that therapy was properly executed and there is very little room for improvement. The clinician might be dealing with a rare case of refractory periodontitis, where the subject does not respond to conventional therapy. The next step would be to consider adjunctive or complementary approaches such as systemic antibiotics and/or periodontal surgery. If we are dealing with a less experienced clinician, the fair assumption is there was failure in calculus removal to a level compatible with resolution of the periodontal condition. Particularly for severe generalized forms of the disease this should not be a surprise because subgingival debridement of deep pockets is not an easy task and requires highly skilled and well-trained individuals. Residual pockets should be carefully reinstrumented, and this step should involve as many sessions as needed. A new period of 3 months of healing should be given before an assessment of the outcome of this new cycle of SRPs is conducted. Clinicians should keep in mind that there is very little risk to the patient in delaying a possible surgical phase of treatment and make every effort to guarantee an optimal outcome of the anti-infective therapy.

E. Although the presence of residual pockets has been demonstrated as a good predictor of future attachment loss [11], clinicians should interpret this information with caution. Several other clinical aspects will impact the prognosis of the case such as the level of plaque control by the subject, the presence of BOP, and the presence of furcation defects. Further, one must keep in mind that periodontal surgical procedures involve nonaffected periodontally diseased sites adjacent to residual pockets. If residual pockets are isolated nonbleeding lesions, they present a very low risk of progression and can be easily addressed with SRP during supportive periodontal therapy. Conversely, if residual pockets cluster around a few adjacent teeth and BOP is a recurrent finding over several sessions of maintenance, a surgical approach seems adequate. Periodontal surgery in the absence of proper plaque control exposes the periodontal patient to the risk of accelerated attachment loss [12] and should be avoided at all costs.

Case 7

Local Anatomic Factors Contributing to Periodontal Disease

CASE STORY

A 47-year-old female presented with a chief complaint of: "My gums around one of the lower right teeth hurts." The patient reported soreness and discomfort around tooth #30 from time to time, especially on the buccal side. On occasion, the patient experienced bleeding when brushing her teeth (Figures 1 and 2).

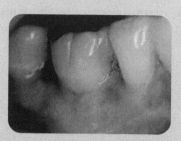

Figure 1: Clinical presentation of tooth #30.

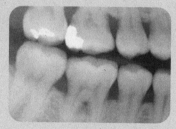 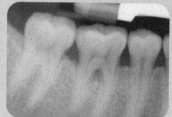

Figure 2: Radiographic presentation of tooth #30.

LEARNING GOALS AND OBJECTIVES

- To be able to identify local anatomic factors that may contribute to periodontal disease
- To understand the anatomy of the furcation and root
- To be able to diagnose a furcation invasion using a furcation classification system

Medical History

The patient's medical history was not significant, except for hypercholesterolemia that was controlled with simvastatin. The patient reported no allergies to any medication, metal, or food.

Review of Systems

- Vital signs
  - Blood pressure: 132/82 mm Hg
  - Pulse rate: 72 beats/minute
  - Respiration: 15 breaths/minute

Social History

The patient denied ever smoking, occasionally drank alcohol during social events, and denied the use of recreational drugs. The patient was happily married with a son and a daughter.

Oral Hygiene Status

The patient brushed twice a day and sometimes flossed.

Extraoral Examination

No significant findings were present.

Intraoral Examination

- Soft tissues including buccal mucosa, hard and soft palate, floor of the mouth, and tongue were all within normal limits.
- There was an adequate amount of attached keratinized gingiva present in general but with mild marginal erythema.
- Refer to Figure 3 for the periodontal charting.
- Tooth #30 exhibited a probing depth of 5mm on the midbuccal aspect and clinically had grade II furcation invasion. No significant mobility was detected.
- A cervical enamel projection (CEP) was detected at the buccal furcation area below the gingival margin on #30.

Occlusion

No occlusal interferences were detected.

Radiographic Examination

A full-mouth radiographic series was taken. Periapical and bite-wing radiographs of tooth #30 showed evidence of furcation invasion (Figure 2).

Diagnosis

A diagnosis of localized severe chronic periodontitis was made based on the clinical and radiographic examinations. The attachment loss and grade II furcation invasion on tooth #30 required definitive periodontal treatment. The prognosis of #30 was questionable because the grade II furcation made the patient's daily oral hygiene maintenance in this area very difficult [1].

Treatment Plan

The treatment plan and sequence were as follows.
- Diagnostic phase: comprehensive dental and periodontal examination, radiographic examination

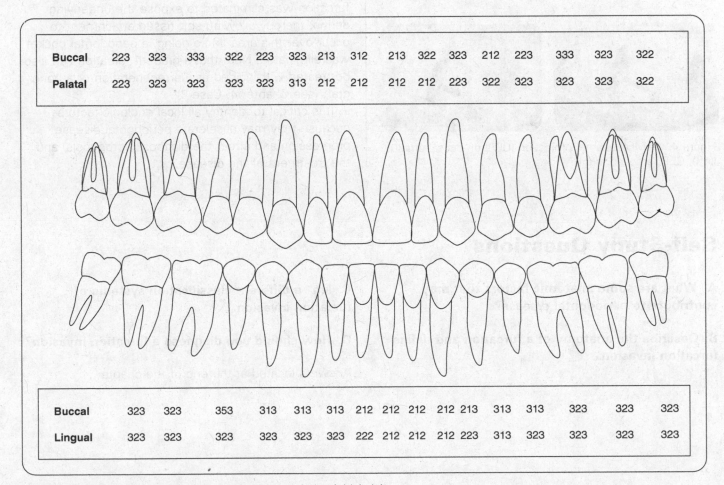

Buccal	223	323	333	322	223	323	213	312	213	322	323	212	223	333	323	322
Palatal	223	323	323	323	323	313	212	212	212	212	223	322	323	323	323	322

Buccal	323	323	353	313	313	313	212	212	212	212	213	313	313	323	323	323
Lingual	323	323	323	323	323	323	222	212	212	212	223	313	323	323	323	323

Figure 3: Periodontal probing depth measurements during initial visit.

- Disease control phase: oral hygiene instruction, adult prophylaxis, localized scaling, and root planing of the buccal furcation of tooth #30
- Reevaluation phase: periodontal reevaluation of tooth #30, oral hygiene evaluation and reinforcement
- Surgical phase: open flap debridement and removal of the CEP on the buccal aspect of tooth #30
- Maintenance phase: regular 3-month recall visits

Treatment

Localized scaling and root planing of tooth #30 was performed using a Cavitron and hand instruments. After a healing period of 6 weeks, periodontal reevaluation was done revealing a probing depth of 5mm with bleeding on probing on the midbuccal of #30. The treatment plan at this point included surgical treatment to remove the CEP. An intrasulcular incision was made from the mesial line angle of #29 to distal line angle of #31 using a #15 blade. Full-thickness buccal and lingual flaps were raised to expose the furcation area of #30 to allow adequate visualization and to give access to remove the CEP. As shown in

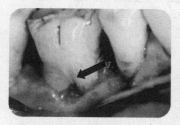 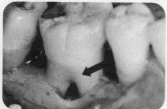

Figure 4: Cervical enamel projection (CEP) on buccal of #30 (left); CEP removed (right).

Figure 4, the CEP extended apically almost to the level of bone crest. A diamond burr was then used to remove the CEP completely (Figure 4), and the furca was debrided using a Cavitron and hand instruments. The flap was eventually sutured back to its original position. Postoperative instructions were given and the patient was seen 2 weeks afterward for a follow-up. Six months later, localized probing at tooth #30 showed a probing depth of 3mm without bleeding on probing.

Discussion

The patient presented with a probing depth of 5mm on the buccal furcation area of tooth #30 possibly due to the presence of a CEP that extended deep into the furcation. The presence of the CEP prevented proper soft tissue attachment at the furcal area, leading to the formation of a deep periodontal pocket. Bone loss at the furcal area is most likely due to the prolonged plaque accumulation in this periodontal pocket that subsequently led to chronic inflammation and hence attachment loss. By removing the CEP, enamel at furcation was eliminated to expose the underlying dentin, thereby allowing soft tissue attachment to occur over this area. In so doing, a periodontal pocket was eliminated. Note that a grade II furcation can also be treated with guided tissue regeneration or a bone graft (see Chapter 4, Case 3).

It is critical to identify all local etiologic factors because they may accelerate periodontal disease progression and affect the diagnosis, prognosis, and the treatment of the disease.

Self-Study Questions

A. What are some anatomic factors that may contribute to periodontal disease?

B. Describe the anatomy of a furcation and define furcation invasion.

C. Name different classification systems of furcation invasion.

D. How should you diagnose a furcation invasion?

Answers located at the end of the chapter.

ACKNOWLEDGMENT

We would like to thank Dr. David M for providing Figure 8.

References

1. McGuire MK, Nunn ME. Prognosis versus actual outcome. II. The effectiveness of clinical parameters in developing an accurate prognosis. J Periodontol 1996;67:658–665.
2. Masters DH, Hoskins SW. Projection of cervical enamel into molar furcations. J Periodontol 1964;35:49–53.
3. Bissada NF, Abdelmalek RG. Incidence of cervical enamel projections and its relationship to furcation involvement in Egyptian skulls. J Periodontol 1973;44:583–585.
4. Swan RH, Hurt WC. Cervical enamel projections as an etiologic factor in furcation involvement. J Am Dent Assoc 1976;93:342–345.
5. Moskow BS, Canut PM. Studies on root enamel (2). Enamel pearls. A review of their morphology, localization, nomenclature, occurrence, classification, histogenesis and incidence. J Clin Periodontol 1990;17:275–281.
6. Bower RC. Furcation morphology relative to periodontal treatment. Furcation root surface anatomy. J Periodontol 1979;50:366–374.
7. Haskova JE, Gill DS, et al. Taurodontism – a review. Dent Update 2009;36:235–236.
8. Everett FG, Jump EB, et al. The intermediate bifurcational ridge: a study of the morphology of the bifurcation of the lower first molar. J Dent Res 1958;37:162–169.
9. Burch JG, Hulen S. A study of the presence of accessory foramina and the topography of molar furcations. Oral Surg Oral Med Oral Pathol 1974;38:451–455.
10. Ben-Bassat Y, Brin I. The labiogingival notch: an anatomical variation of clinical importance. J Am Dent Assoc 2001;132:919–921.
11. Schwartz SA, Koch MA, et al. Combined endodontic-periodontic treatment of a palatal groove: a case report. J Endod 2006;32:573–578.
12. Vertucci FJ, Williams RG. Furcation canals in the human mandibular first molar. Oral Surg Oral Med Oral Pathol 1974;38:308–314.
13. Dunlap RM, Gher ME. Root surface measurements of the mandibular first molar. J Periodontol 1985;56:234–238.
14. Tal H. Relationship between the depths of furcal defects and alveolar bone loss. J Periodontol 1982;53:631–634.
15. Bower RC. Furcation morphology relative to periodontal treatment. Furcation entrance architecture. J Periodontol 1979;50:23–27.
16. Hermann DW, Gher ME Jr, et al. The potential attachment area of the maxillary first molar. J Periodontol 1983;54:431–434.
17. Gher MW Jr, Dunlap RW. Linear variation of the root surface area of the maxillary first molar. J Periodontol 1985;56:39–43.
18. Booker BW 3rd, Loughlin DM. A morphologic study of the mesial root surface of the adolescent maxillary first bicuspid. J Periodontol 1985;56:666–670.
19. Gher ME, Vernino AR. Root morphology – clinical significance in pathogenesis and treatment of periodontal disease. J Am Dent Assoc 1980;101:627–633.
20. Glickman I. Clinical Periodontology. 2nd ed. Philadelphia, PA: Saunders, 1958. pp 694–696.
21. Hamp SE, Nyman S, et al. Periodontal treatment of multirooted teeth. Results after 5 years. J Clin Periodontol 1975;2:126–135.
22. Tarnow D, Fletcher P. Classification of the vertical component of furcation involvement. J Periodontol 1984;55:283–284.
23. Hardekopf JD, Dunlap RM, et al. The "furcation arrow." A reliable radiographic image? J Periodontol 1987;58:258–261.
24. Ross IF, Thompson RH Jr. Furcation involvement in maxillary and mandibular molars. J Periodontol 1980;51:450–454.

TAKE-HOME POINTS

A.

P oximal Contact Relation

Open interproximal contacts or uneven marginal ridge relations may encourage food impaction between the teeth. If proper oral hygiene is absent, food impaction can lead to inflammation, thereby potentially resulting in attachment loss in the interproximal area (Figure 5).

Root P oximity

Close root proximity between the two adjacent teeth will render oral hygiene difficult to maintain for both the patient and the dental professionals. Hence without good oral hygiene there can be loss of attachment between the two teeth (Figure 6).

Cervical Enamel P ojct ions and Enamel Par ls

Cervical enamel projections (CEPs) refer to the extension of enamel to the furcal area of the root surface. CEPs may potentially predispose a furcation to attachment loss because they prevent connective tissue attachment at furcation. As such, a periodontal pocket may form, leading to plaque accumulation and possibly furcation invasion.

Most clinicians agree there is a correlation between CEPs and the incidence of furcation invasion. Masters and Hoskins reported that 90% of mandibular furcation invasions have CEPs [2]. Bissada and Abdelmalek reported a 50% correlation between CEPs and furcation invasion [3]. Swan and Hurt observed a statistically significant association between CEPs and furcation invasion [4].

In descending order of occurrence, CEPs are most commonly seen in mandibular second molars, maxillary second molars, mandibular first molars, and maxillary first molars. When CEPs are observed, they are usually seen on buccal aspects of molars [2] (Figure 7).

Enamel pearls are ectopic globules of enamel and sometimes pulpal tissue that often adhere to the cementoenamel junction (CEJ). They are present in roughly 2.7% of the molars and are mostly found on maxillary third and second molars [5]. Moskow and Canut suggested that enamel pearls may also predispose a furcation to attachment loss [5] (Figure 8).

Root Concavity

The furcal aspects of the roots frequently have concavities with a certain amount of depth (see Question B for details) that will encourage plaque

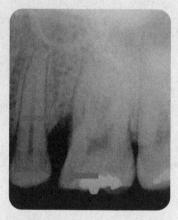

Figure 5: Interproximal open contact between #13 and #14 (indicated by the red arrows) and vertical bone loss on #14 mesial.

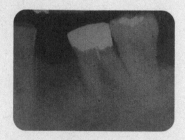

Figure 6: Close root proximity between #18 and #19.

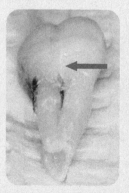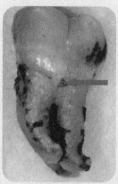

Figure 7: Cervical enamel projection (indicated by the red arrow).

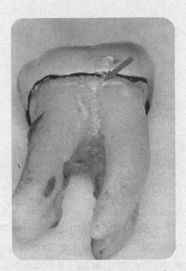

Figure 8: Enamel pearl (indicated by the red arrow).

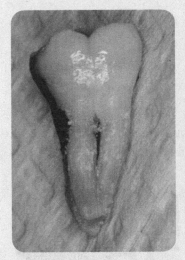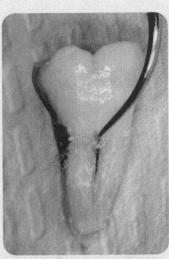

Figure 10: The size of the Cavitron tip is too big to enter the furcated area, rendering scaling and root planing in this area very difficult.

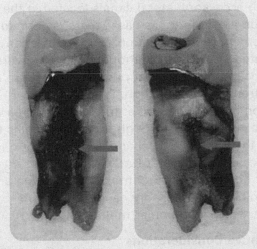

Figure 9: Mesial and distal root concavities of maxillary first premolar.

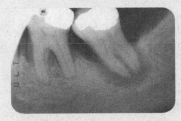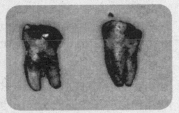

Figure 11: The root divergence of #19 is more prominent than #17.

accumulation and prevent proper instrumentation of furcation. Hence a root concavity may predispose the furcation to attachment loss (Figure 9).

Size of Furcation Entrance
Approximately 80% of all furcation entrances are <1.0 mm in diameter with about 60% of them <0.75 mm [6]. Because frequently used curettes and scalers have a face width of 0.75–1.10 mm, it is unlikely that effective removal of accretions at furcation can be achieved by using these

instruments alone. Hence a small furcation entrance may predispose a furcation to attachment loss (Figure 10).

Root Divergence and Root Fusion
The degree of root divergence in a multirooted tooth will influence the ability of the patient and dental professionals to control plaque level. Diverging roots allow easier instrumentation to the furcation area, whereas converging roots (e.g., root fusion) render the access to the furcation area very difficult, resulting in poor plaque control and possible attachment loss (Figure 11).

Root Trunk Length
The length of root trunk affects attachment loss. The longer a given root trunk, the less likely a furcation will be predisposed to attachment loss.

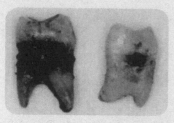 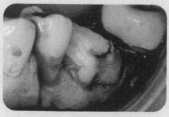

Figure 12: Long root trunk length (left) and short root trunk at #19 (right).

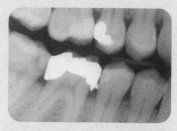

Figure 14: Overhangs on the mesial and distal of #30 that may eventually lead to bone loss on the mesial and distal of #30.

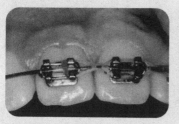 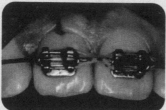

Figure 13: Buccal radicular groove present on #8 as indicated by the probe tip.

Teeth with Taurodontism usually have apically displaced furcation and longer root trunk length [7] (Figure 12).

Intermediate Bifurcation Ridge

Intermediate bifurcation ridges are ridges spanning across the bifurcation of mandibular molars in the mesiodistal direction. These ridges are present in 70–77% of the mandibular molars [8,9]. Just like other anatomic structures, the presence of an intermediate bifurcation ridge may hinder effective plaque control and root preparation by both the patient and dentist.

Buccal Radicular Groove and Palat o-Gingival Groove

Buccal radicular grooves and palato-gingival grooves are developmental phenomena that affect mainly the maxillary anterior teeth [10,11]. These grooves run on the roots in the coronal-apical direction. Due to their anatomy, the grooves frequently provide a plaque-retentive area that is very difficult to instrument, making teeth with these developmental grooves more prone to attachment loss (Figure 13).

Accessory Pulpal Canals

Accessory pulpal canals are small endodontic canals branching off from the main root canal that

may furnish a communication between the pulpal chamber and the periodontal ligament. These accessory canals are usually located near the root apex; however, they can also be found anywhere along the root, including the furcation area. There is a theory that some periodontal infections can originate from endodontic sources, traveling through accessory/lateral canals located in the furcation areas. In these cases there is periodontal involvement in the furcation, but the infection originated in the pulp. Although still controversial, it has been proposed that periodontal disease can result from pulpal infection. An endodontic infection may be present at the furcation area when the infection travels through accessory canals that end at the furca. Vertucci and Williams reported that accessory canals at furcations are present in 46% of human lower first molars [12]. Burch and Hulen observed accessory canals in 76% of maxillary and mandibular molars [9].

Restorative Considerations

Dental restorations with overhangs or open margins are plaque-retentive areas that may result in gingival inflammation and attachment loss. Restorative margins are most compatible with the periodontium when located either supragingivally or at the level of gingival margin. Should the restorative margin violate the biologic width, the resulting inflammatory process may lead to gingival recession, bone loss, and the exposure of the restorative margin. The restorative contour (e.g., crown contour) should follow the root surface contour rather than accentuating the cervical bulge to support periodontal health. In the case of bridges, the design of the pontic can affect its ability to be cleaned and hence the periodontal health of the teeth (Figure 14).

B. A furcation is an anatomic area where the roots of a multirooted tooth start to diverge. Mandibular molars and maxillary first premolars are bifurcated because they each have two roots. Maxillary molars are trifurcated because they each have three roots.

A furcation consists of two parts: (1) root separation area: the area where alveolar bone begins to separate the roots and (2) fluting area: the part of the root that is directly coronal to the root separation area.

There are often concavities in the furcal side of the roots. In mandibular molars, all the mesial roots have concavities on the furcal side with each concavity averaging 0.7 mm in depth [13]. Likewise, 99% of the distal roots of mandibular molars have concavities on the furcal side with an average depth of 0.5 mm [13]. The root trunk, which is the distance from the CEJ to the level of root separation, is about 4.0 ± 0.7 mm in mandibular first molars [13,14].

In maxillary molars, 94% of the mesio-buccal roots have concavities on the furcal side, with each concavity averaging 0.3 mm in depth [15]. Roughly a third (31%) of the mesio-distal roots and a quarter (17%) of the palatal roots have concavities, and each concavity is about 0.1 mm in depth [15]. The length of root trunks of maxillary molars is 3.6 mm, 4.2 mm, and 4.8 mm on the mesial, buccal, and distal surfaces, respectively [16,17].

All bifurcated maxillary first premolars have a mesial and distal root trunk of about 8 mm. In addition, almost all the buccal roots have "developmental depressions" also known as "buccal furcation groove" present at the 9.4-mm level on the furcal side [18,19].

Furcation invasion is defined as a loss of attachment within a furcation. When there is a loss of clinical attachment, the presence of concavities on these roots at furcation will hinder effective plaque control at these areas.

C. There are a number of different classification systems of furcation invasion. The three most commonly used systems are as follows.
1. The Glickman classification [20] describes both the vertical and horizontal components of the furcation invasion:

Grade I: pocket formation into the fluting area but with intact interradicular bone

Grade II: pocket formation into the root separation area with interradicular bone loss that is not completely through to the opposite side of the furcation

Grade III: same as grade II but with a through-and-through interradicular bone loss (the soft tissue still covers part of the entrance of the furcation)

Grade IV: same as grade III but with gingival recession making furcation clinically visible

2. The Hamp et al classification [21] describes the horizontal component of the furcation invasion.

Degree I: horizontal bone loss going into the furcation <3 mm

Degree II: horizontal bone loss going into the furcation >3 mm but not to the opposite side

Degree III: a through-and-through horizontal bone loss in the furcation

3. The Tarnow and Fletcher classification [22] describes the vertical component of the furcation invasion.

Subclass A: vertical attachment loss 0–3 mm in furcation

Subclass B: vertical attachment loss of 4–6 mm in furcation

Subclass A: vertical attachment loss of >7 mm

D. The most effective way to diagnose a furcation invasion is to use a combination of clinical examination and radiographic evaluation. The clinical examination involves using periodontal and furcation probes to detect the furcation invasion.

Radiographs must be taken with a paralleling technique to minimize the distortion of the images. Note that radiographically the palatal root of maxillary molars may leave a grade III furcation invasion undetected due to the overlapping of the palatal root with mesio-buccal and distobuccal roots. In addition, the presence of a furcation arrow (a triangular show seen either at the mesial or distal roots in the interproximal area on maxillary molars) may possibly suggest the presence of grade II–III furcation invasion on maxillary molars [23] (Figure 15). The more extensive a given furcation invasion, the higher the likelihood of observing the furcation arrow. However, it must be noted that the absence of furcation arrow does not necessarily suggest the absence of a furcation invasion.

Generally interproximal surfaces of the maxillary molars are more prone to furcation invasion than buccal surfaces [24].

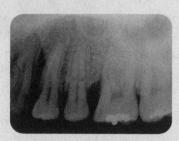

Figure 15: Furcation arrow as indicated by the red arrow is showing furcal involvement on the mesial of #14 radiographically.

2

Nonsurgical Periodontal Therapy

Clinical Cases in Periodontics, First Edition. Nadeem Karimbux.
© 2012 John Wiley & Sons, Inc. Published 2012 by John Wiley & Sons, Inc.

Case 1

Hand and Automated Instrumentation

CASE STORY

A 25-year-old Caucasian male presented with a chief compliant of: "I need a cleaning." The patient had noticed significant staining as well as plaque and calculus buildup, particularly in the mandibular anterior region (Figures 1, 2, and 3).

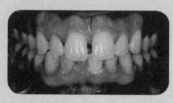

Figure 1: Frontal view.

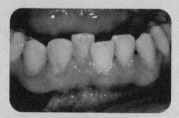

Figure 2: Buccal view, mandibular anterior.

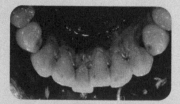

Figure 3: Lingual view, mandibular anterior.

LEARNING GOALS AND OBJECTIVES

- To identify appropriate instruments that may be used for scaling and/or scaling and root planing
- To learn the importance of Initial phase, reevaluation, and maintenance therapy
- To learn the advantages and disadvantages of hand versus power instrumentation
- To understand the limitations of these instruments in the nonsurgical management of periodontal disease

Medical History

The patient reported a history of asthma and used an albuterol inhaler once per day. Otherwise, there were no significant medical problems, and the patient had no known allergies.

Review of Systems

- Vital signs
  - Blood pressure: 120/65 mm Hg
  - Pulse rate: 72 beats/minute (regular)
  - Respiration: 15 breaths/minute

Social History

The patient did not drink alcohol. He reported smoking one time per week.

Extraoral Examination

No significant findings. The patient had no masses or swelling and the temporomandibular joint was within normal limits.

Intraoral Examination

- The soft tissues of the mouth, including the tongue, appeared normal.

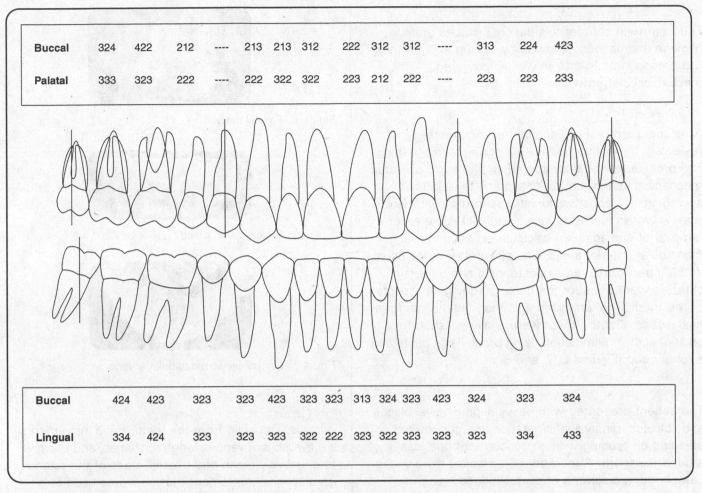

Buccal	324	422	212	----	213	213	312	222	312	312	----	313	224	423
Palatal	333	323	222	----	222	322	322	223	212	222	----	223	223	233

Buccal	424	423	323	323	423	323	323	313	324	323	423	324	323	324
Lingual	334	424	323	323	323	322	222	323	322	323	323	323	334	433

Figure 4: Probing pocket depth measurements

- A gingival examination revealed a localized marginal erythema, with rolled margins and some inflamed papillae (Figures 1, 2, and 3).
- Periodontal examination and charting were completed (Figure 4).

Occlusion
There were no occlusal discrepancies or interferences.

Radiographic Examination
Bite-wing radiographs were ordered given that the patient was young, and there was no history of caries (Figure 5).

Diagnosis
After reviewing the patient's history as well as the clinical and radiographic examination, a differential diagnosis of generalized moderate gingivitis was made.

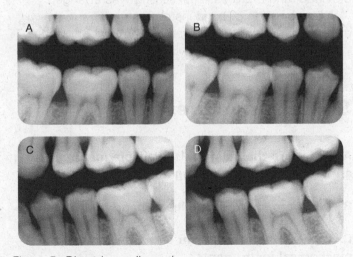

Figure 5: Bite-wing radiographs

Treatment Plan

The treatment plan for this patient includes oral hygiene instructions, followed by scaling and polishing using hand instruments as well as powered mechanical instruments.

Treatment

After thorough oral hygiene instructions were reviewed, the patient received a scaling and polishing. The procedure was started with an ultrasonic-powered mechanical instrument to loosen any tenacious supragingival deposits and initial stain removal. Hand scalers were then used, including a sickle scaler for removal of supragingival calculus and stain in the mandibular anterior areas, Gracey curettes were used in the interproximal areas posteriorly, and universal curettes were used for the buccal and lingual aspects of the teeth. The ultrasonic was then used again for a final lavage, and the teeth were finally polished for any additional stain elimination using prophylaxis paste and a rubber cup (Figures 6, 7, and 8).

Discussion

The patient presented with heavy supragingival plaque and calculus, gingival inflammation and generalized bleeding on probing with no concurrent bone loss around the teeth. After a detailed medical history was completed, a diagnosis of plaque-induced gingivitis was given. To restore the patient to periodontal health, comprehensive oral hygiene instructions were provided, and a professional scaling was arranged.

A combination of hand instruments and power-driven instruments were used for removal of plaque,

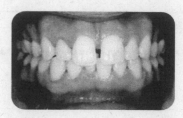

Figure 6: Frontal view.

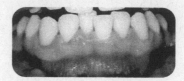

Figure 7: Buccal view, mandibular anterior.

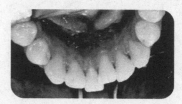

Figure 8: Lingual view, mandibular anterior.

calculus, and stain from the teeth. Hand instruments are available in various lengths, shapes, and designs to effectively reach and treat all areas of the teeth. An ultrasonic instrument (Cavitron) was used as an adjunct for stain removal, mechanical debridement, lavage, and cavitation. Regularly scheduled reevaluations and prophylaxis in addition to routine home care are recommended for maintaining optimal oral hygiene and periodontal health in this patient.

Self-Study Questions

A. What are the chief tools available in our armamentarium for scaling and root planing?

B. What are some examples of hand instruments?

C. What is the mechanism of action of powered mechanical instruments?

D. What are the limitations to prophylaxis and scaling and root planing?

E. Are there any contraindications to using power mechanical instruments?

F. Are there differences in efficacy of treatment between hand scalers and automated scalers?

G. What are some advantages and disadvantages of hand instruments versus power mechanical instruments?

Answers located at the end of the chapter.

References

1. Ewen SJ, Glickstein BA. Ultrasonic Therapy in Periodontics. Springfield, IL: Charles C. Thomas, 1968. pp.12–34.
2. Clarke PR, Hill CR. Physical and chemical aspects of ultrasonic disruption of cells. J Acoust Soc Am 1970;47:649–653.
3. Waerhaug J. Healing of the dento-epithelial junction following subgingival plaque control II: as observed on extracted teeth. J Periodontol 1978;49:119–134.
4. Caffesse RG, Sweeney PL, et al. Scaling and root planing with and without periodontal flap surgery. J Clin Periodontol 1986;13:205–210.
5. Lindhe J, Socransky S, et al. Critical probing depths in periodontal therapy. J Clin Periodontol 1982;9:323–336.
6. Philstrom BL, McHugh RB, et al. Comparison of surgical and nonsurgical treatment of periodontal disease. A review of current studies and additional results after 6½ years. J Clin Periodontol 1983;10:524–541.
7. Isidor F, Karring T. Long-term effect of surgical and non-surgical periodontal treatment. A 5-year clinical study. J Periodontal Res 1986;21:462–472.
8. Gantes BG, Nilveus R. The effects of different hygiene instruments on titanium surfaces: SEM observations. Int J Periodontics Restorative Dent 1991;11:225–239.
9. Miller CS, Leonelli FM, et al. Selective interference with pacemaker activity by electrical dental devices. Oral Surg Oral Med Oral Pathol Oral Radiol Endod 1998;85:33–36.
10. Breininger D, O'Leary T, et al. Comparative effectiveness of ultrasonic and hand scaling on removal of subgingival plaque and calculus. J Periodontol 1987;58:9–18.
11. Thornton S, Garnick J. Comparison of ultrasonic to hand instruments in the removal of subgingival plaque. J Periodontol 1982;53:35–37.
12. Baeni P, Thilo B, et al. Effects of ultrasonic and sonic scalers on dental plaque microflora in vitro and in vivo. J Clin Periodontol 1992;19:455–459.
13. Nishimine D, O'Leary TJ. Hand instrumentation versus ultrasonics in the removal of endotoxins from root surface. J Periodontol 1979;50:345–349.
14. Hunter R, P'Leary T, et al. The effectiveness of hand versus instrumentation in open-flap root planing. J Periodontol 1984;55:697–703.
15. Matia J, Bissada N, et al. Efficiency of scaling the molar furcation area with and without surgical access. Int J Periodontics Restorative Dent 1986;6:24–35.
16. Gellin R. The effectiveness of the Titan-S sonic scaler versus curettes in the removal of subgingival calculus. A human evaluation. J Periodontol 1986;57:672–680.
17. Bower RC. Furcation morphology relative to periodontal treatment – furcation entrance architecture. J Periodontol 1979;50:23–27.
18. Dragoo M. A clinical evaluation of hand and ultrasonic instruments on subgingival debridement. Part I. With unmodified and modified ultrasonic inserts. Int J Periodontics Restorative Dent 1992;12:311–313.
19. Leon L, Vogel R. A comparison of the effectiveness of hand scaling and ultrasonic debridement in furcations as evaluated with dark-field microscopy. J Periodontol 1987;58:86–94.
20. Ritz L, Hefti A, et al. An in vitro investigation on the loss of root substance in scaling with various instruments. J Clin Periodontol 1991;18:643–647.
21. Larato DC, Ruskin PF, et al. Effect of an ultrasonic scaler on bacterial counts in air. J Periodontol 1967;38:550–554.

TAKE-HOME POINTS

The most fundamental objective of primary phase nonsurgical therapy is to reestablish periodontal health in a patient by reduction of putative periodontal pathogens from the periodontium. Literature has shown that instrumentation can effectively decrease these periodontal pathogens and restore a healthier bacterial flora in the mouth.

A. In our armamentarium the chief tools available for scaling and root planing include:
a. Manual mechanical instrumentation: scalers and curettes
b. Powered mechanical instrumentation: ultrasonics (magnetostrictive, piezoelectric)
c. Air abrasives/rubber cups (for stain removal)

B. Manual instrumentation is an essential skill that dental practitioners need to obtain good results from initial nonsurgical therapy. This involves a thorough understanding of the available tools:
• Scalers are designed for removal of supragingival calculus. They include two straight cutting edges and a pointed toe (e.g., sickle scalers; Figures 9A and B).

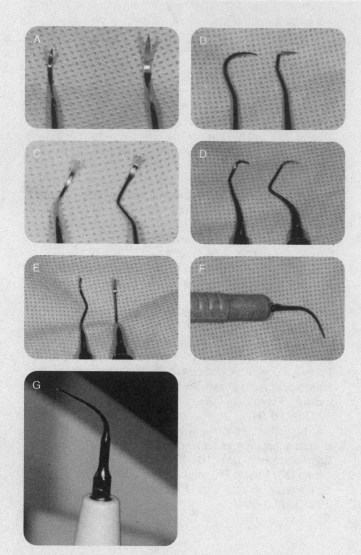

Figure 9: (A,B) Sickle scalers; (C) universal curettes; (D,E) Gracey curettes; (F) magnetorestrictive ultrasonic scalers; (G) piezoelectric ultrasonic scalers.

• Curettes are designed for subgingival instrumentation but can be used for supragingival scaling as well.
  i. Universal curettes have two cutting edges (Figure 9C)
  ii. Area-specific curettes have only one cutting edge (i.e., Gracey curettes; Figures 9D and E)

C. Powered mechanical instruments such as sonic and ultrasonic scalers have been used by practitioners to remove plaque, calculus, and stain from tooth and root surfaces. These automated scalers work by way of vibration; as the tip oscillates, it helps break apart adherent deposits that may be present on the teeth. The tip also sprays a jet of water that flushes away any debris and helps dissipate heat produced by the instrument. Additionally, when the water passes over the vibrations of the oscillating tip of an ultrasonic instrument, cavitation is observed. Cavitation is a process by which formation and destruction of small air cavities releases energy that may disrupt bacterial cell membranes [1,2].

Powered mechanical instruments are classified based on their frequencies, and are very effective for nonsurgical debridement of teeth:

• Sonic scalers operate at a frequency of 3000–8000 cycles per second and are driven by compressed air from the dental unit. A rotor system is then activated and the sonic tip oscillates in an elliptical to circular pattern.

• Ultrasonic scalers can be further classified into:
  i. Magnetorestrictive ultrasonic scalers: Operate inaudibly, and the tip oscillates at 18,000–42,000 kHz (cycles per second). The motion of the tip is elliptical to circular in motion, and all surfaces of the tip are useful in debridement (Figure 9F).
  ii. Piezoelectric ultrasonic scalers: Operate inaudibly, and the tip oscillates at 24,000–45,000 kHz (cycles per second). The motion of the tip is linear, so unlike the magnetorestrictive ultrasonics, only its lateral surfaces are useful in debridement (Figure 9G)

D. Although hand and power instruments are effective in treating periodontal and gingival disease as a part of the initial phase of therapy, there are some limitations. The literature has shown that even with all currently available instrumentation, there is a certain pocket depth up to which we can effectively eliminate subgingival plaque and calculus [3]. Caffesse and associates found that the extent of residual calculus is directly related to pocket depth; as pocket depth increased, the percentage of the tooth surfaces completely free of calculus gradually decreased [4]. This probing depth, referred to as the "critical probing depth," is 2.9 mm for scaling and root planing. Any probing depth beyond 4.2 mm benefits from surgical periodontal therapy rather than nonsurgical treatment due to the limits of the effectiveness of hand or powered instruments [5]. Nonsurgical treatments are usually attempted first; if appropriate results are not achieved at reevaluation, surgical treatment should be pursued. Whether nonsurgical or surgical periodontal treatment modalities are used, longitudinal studies show that if treated appropriately and followed closely, patients with periodontal disease can be maintained in the long term [6,7].

E. Concerns that the practitioner should be aware of if using powered mechanical instruments are both dental and medical in nature.

Dental

Sonic and ultrasonic instruments should *not* be used on dental implants because the metal tips can scratch the softer titanium. Ideally, hand periodontal scalers made of plastic, teflon, wood, titanium, or gold-plated scalers should be used for cleaning dental implants [8]. If used too vigorously, these instruments may damage certain restorative margins. As with manual instrumentation, these mechanical instruments may remove excessive tooth structure causing subsequent hypersensitivity.

Medical

Cardiac pacemakers, particularly those placed before the mid-1980s, may get electromagnetic interference from *magnetorestrictive* ultrasonics (piezoelectric scalers are a safe alternative) [9]. Patients with significant respiratory problems may be intolerant to the aerosols produced during power instrumentation. Powered mechanical instruments should be avoided in patients with infectious diseases that may be transmitted through aerosol production.

F. Several studies have looked at the efficacy of plaque and calculus removal using manual versus automated instrumentation. Studies have demonstrated that both hand instrumentation and ultrasonic instrumentation are very effective in plaque removal [10]. There are no significant differences found between the use of manual instruments and ultrasonic instruments [11] or between sonic and ultrasonic instrumentation in terms of the ability to remove plaque [12]. Some studies have shown that manual instrumentation is more effective than ultrasonic instrumentation in calculus removal [13,14]. However, power instruments have been shown to access concavities and furcations of roots better than manual instruments [15]. According to Gellin, using these methods concurrently is more effective than using either method alone [16].

G. See Table 1.

Table 1: Advantages and Disadvantages of Using Hand Instruments versus Power Mechanical Instruments

	Advantages	Disadvantages
Hand instruments	* Not as damaging to porcelain and composite restorations * More effective at removing endotoxin from periodontally involved root surfaces [13]	* Larger tip than furcation width [17] * Fatigue [18] * Longer scaling times [18]
Bw er mechanical instruments	* Lavage effect of irrigation * Cavitation [1,2] * Slightly shorter scaling times [18] * Less skill required to be competent [18] * More effective in class II and III furcations [19] * Less removal of tooth structure [20] * Require no sharpening	* May be contraindicated for patients with older cardiac pacemakers [9] * Production of aerosols (30-fold increase of airborne microorganisms in the treatment room) [21]

Case 2

Local Drug Delivery

CASE STORY

A 35-year-old Caucasian male presented with a chief compliant of: "My dentist told me I have gum disease." The patient had not experienced pain, discomfort, or swelling associated with his gums; however, he had noticed slight bleeding whenever he brushes and flosses. The patient claimed to brush his teeth at least once daily and he flossed once a week (Figures 1, 2, and 3).

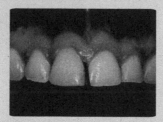

Figure 1: Preoperative view of maxillary anterior teeth and a15-mm periodontal probe demonstrating a 5-mm probing on mesial of tooth #8 with bleeding on probing.

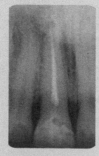

Figure 2: Preoperative periapical radiograph of tooth #8 demonstrating localized mild vertical bone loss.

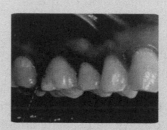

Figure 3: Preoperative view of maxillary posterior teeth and a15-mm periodontal probe demonstrating a 4-mm probing on the distal of tooth #3. with bleeding on probing.

LEARNING GOALS AND OBJECTIVES

- To be able to diagnose periodontitis
- To identify the possible etiological and contributing factors and to address them
- To be able to elaborate an initial treatment plan with a comprehensive phase 1 therapy to achieve initial periodontal stability
- To be able to identify the different local chemotherapeutic agents and how, when, and why to use them

Medical History

There were no significant medical problems and the patient had no known allergies. He had no known medical illnesses. On questioning the patient stated he was not taking any medications and he had no allergies.

Review of Systems

- Vital signs
  - Blood pressure: 128/83 mm Hg
  - Pulse rate: 69 beats/minute (regular)
  - Respiration: 16 breaths/minute

Social History

The patient did not smoke and drank alcohol twice a month in social gatherings.

Extraoral Examination

There were no significant findings. The patient had no masses or swelling, and the temporomandibular joint was within normal limits.

Intraoral Examination

- The soft tissues of the mouth (except gingiva) including the tongue appeared normal.

- A gingival examination revealed a mild marginal erythema and swollen papillae (Figures 1 and 3).
- The patient exhibited localized areas with bleeding on probing as well as localized areas with probing depths of 4 and 5 mm (Figures 1 and 3).
- A periodontal chart was completed. Note that the clinical attachment levels (CALs) are not displayed because all gingival margins are at the level of the cementoenamel junction, thus the CAL equals probing depth (Figure 4).

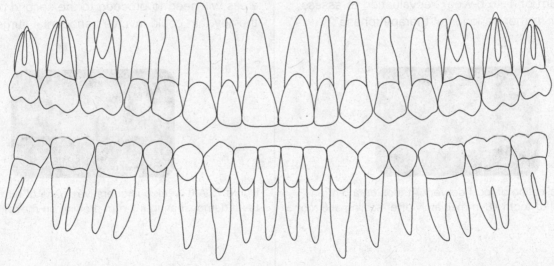

BUCCAL																
PD Pre-op	423	324	423	323	313	323	212	425	323	322	323	413	324	424	323	323
PD Re-eval	323	313	322	213	323	213	312	212	212	312	323	223	323	323	223	323
BOP Pre-op	1--1	1--1	1--1	1--1	1--1	111	---1	111	1--1	1--1	---1	---1	---1	1--1	1--1	1---
LINGUAL																
PD Pre-op	323	324	433	313	323	323	212	424	212	212	323	213	323	324	423	323
PD Re-eval	322	223	312	312	313	223	212	212	213	312	223	212	223	322	323	323
BOP Pre-op	---1	1--1	1--1	1--	---1	1--1	---1	1--1	1--1	1---	---1	1--1	----	---1	1--1	1---
Tooth #	1	2	3	4	5	6	7	8	9	10	11	12	13	14	15	16

Tooth #	32	31	30	29	28	27	26	25	24	23	22	21	20	19	18	17
LINGUAL																
PD Pre-op	324	324	423	313	323	323	312	212	212	222	313	213	324	424	424	423
PD Re-eval	323	322	222	213	222	322	212	211	112	212	213	212	322	323	323	323
BOP	---1	1--1	1---	---1	1--1	----	----	----	1---	---1	----	---1	---1	1--1	1--	1---
BUCCAL																
PD Pre-op	323	314	423	423	313	322	222	222	212	212	222	214	224	324	324	323
PD Re-eval	323	323	223	313	312	222	212	212	212	222	212	213	222	223	322	323
BOP	---1	1--1	1--1	1--1	1--1	---1	----	----	1--1	---1	---1	---1	1--1	1--1	1--1	1---

Figure 4: Probing pocket depth measurements.

Occlusion

There were no occlusal discrepancies or interferences.

Radiographic Examination

A full-mouth set of radiographs was ordered; there were localized areas of mild vertical bone loss on the mesial and distal surfaces of tooth #8 (Figure 2).

Diagnosis

After reviewing the history and the clinical and radiographic examinations, the periodontal diagnosis was localized chronic mild periodontitis. The American Dental Association diagnosis is type II.

Treatment Plan

The treatment plan consisted of addressing the primary etiology that causes the periodontal disease for this patient (phase 1) in the following order: oral hygiene instruction, subgingival scaling and root planing of all sites with initial probing depths >3 mm, and supragingival scaling and polishing of all other surfaces; concomitant administration of a local antibiotic immediately after scaling (Figures 5 and 6) and only for sites with probing depths >3 mm followed by a minimum of 4- to 6-week reevaluation to assess the need for further periodontal therapy (phase 2).

Reevaluation of Post-Initial Treatment

At the 6-week reevaluation, the clinical parameters had improved, and certain probing depths that were initially >3 mm were reduced (Figures 7 and 8). Thus no further periodontal treatment is needed; only periodontal maintenance therapy every 3 months is required.

Discussion

Elements that will lead to a successful outcome include an accurate diagnosis based on a thorough history and a periodontal examination, as well as the knowledge of the etiologic factors that lead to disease. Next, a variety of treatment choices must be selected with the understanding that the primary goal will be to provide initial stability of the disease or condition – in this particular case, periodontitis. Once the initial stability has been achieved, either one can proceed to further treatment such as restorative procedures or have the patient on a 3-month periodontal maintenance protocol. However, initial therapy or phase 1 with or without the concomitant use of local chemotherapeutics may not achieve the optimal periodontal stability desired, and thus, it is the responsibility of the treating clinician to identify what areas will need to proceed to the second phase of therapy that could involve periodontal surgery.

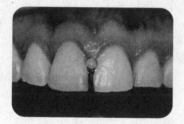

Figure 5: Application of local delivery Atridox on a 5-mm pocket mesial of tooth #8 immediately after scaling and root planing.

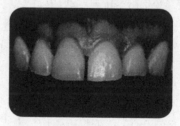

Figure 7: A 6-week postoperative image of maxillary anterior teeth demonstrating a 2-mm probing on mesial of tooth #8.

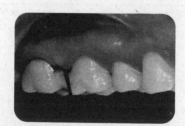

Figure 6: Application of local delivery Atridox on a 4-mm pocket distal of tooth #3 immediately after scaling and root planing.

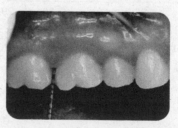

Figure 8: A 6-week postoperative image of maxillary posterior teeth demonstrating a 3-mm probing on distal of tooth #3.

Self-Study Questions

A. What is the rationale for using local antibiotics and other agents for the treatment of periodontal disease?

B. Which local drug delivery agents are available?

C. What type of patients will benefit from the use of a local antibiotic?

D. What is the existing research that justifies the use of local drug delivery?

E. What are the techniques and devices used to deliver local antibiotics?

F. What are the considerations for patients to observe after receiving the local antibiotic?

G. What are the determinants of success in local drug delivery therapy?

H. What does rescue therapy mean, and how can local antibiotics help patients with periodontal disease that recurs over time?

Answers located at the end of the chapter.

ACKNOWLEDGMENTS
Thanks to Dr. Campo Elias Perez for his contribution to this chapter.

References
1. Haffajee AD, Arguello EI, et al. Controlling the plaque biofilm. Int Dent J 2003;53(Suppl 3):191–199.
2. Haffajee AD, Socransky SS. Introduction to microbial aspects of periodontal biofilm communities, development and treatment Periodontol 2000 2006;42:7–12.
3. Hanes P, Purvis J. Local anti-infective therapy: pharmacological agents. A systematic review. Ann Periodontol 2003;8:79–98.
4. Golub LM, Goodson JM, et al. Tetracyclines inhibit tissue collagenases. J Periodontol 1985;56(Suppl):93–97.
5. Slot DE, Kranendonk AA, et al. The effect of a pulsed Nd:YAG laser in non-surgical periodontal therapy. J Periodontol 2009;80:1041–1056.
6. Sanz M, Teughels W; Group A of European Workshop on Periodontology. Innovations in non-surgical periodontal therapy: Consensus Report of the Sixth European
Workshop on Periodontology. J Clin Periodontol 2008;35(8 Suppl):3–7.
7. Armitage GC. Development of a classification system for periodontal diseases and conditions. Ann Periodontol 1999;4:1–6.
8. Caffesse RG, Sweeney PL, et al. Scaling and root planing with and without periodontal flap surgery. J Clin Periodontol 1986;13:205–210.
9. Cobb CM. Non-surgical pocket therapy: mechanical. Ann Periodontol 1996;1:443–490.
10. Goodson IM, Holborow D, et al. Monolithic tetracycline-containing fibres for controlled delivery to periodontal pockets. J Periodontol 1983;54:575–579.
11. Bonito A, Lux L, et al. Impact of local adjuncts to scaling and root planing in periodontal disease therapy: a systematic review. J Periodontol 2005;76:1227–1236.
12. Tanner ACR, Goodson JM. Sampling of microorganisms associated with periodontal disease. Oral Microbiol Immunol 1986;1:15–20.
13. Haffajee AD, Uzel NG, et al. Clinical and microbiological changes associated with use of combined antimicrobial therapies to treat "refractory" periodontitis. J Clin Periodontol 2004;31:869–877.
14. Magnusson I. The use of locally-delivered metronidazole in the treatment of periodontitis. Clinical results. J Clin Periodontol 1998;25:959–963.

TAKE-HOME POINTS

A. To understand the use of local antibiotics and other agents in the treatment of periodontal disease, one should understand the etiology of this disease, the bacterial colonization as well as the biofilm development. Bacterial colonization reaches a saturation gradient from the supragingival plaque, and it migrates vertically to colonize the subgingival sulcus or periodontal pocket. Bacteria in the supragingival plaque are composed mainly of gram-positive aerobes, and bacteria in the subgingival plaque are made up mainly of gram-negative anaerobes. These diverse bacterial communities that interact and exist with each other are called biofilms. Although bacterial biofilms exist in very diverse settings, it is well known that biofilm infections in the medical field are challenging to treat because of the complexity of the bacterial organization [1]. Periodontal disease is caused by a biofilm infection, and although some of the main causative bacteria have been isolated such as the so-called red complex (*Porphyromonas gingivalis, Treponema denticola,* and *Tannerella forsythia*) as described by Haffajee and Socransky, periodontal disease has multiple variables. These variables include the host–immune response and risk factors such as a genetic predisposition and environmental factors such as smoking [2].

The use of antibiotics as well as other agents for the treatment of periodontal diseases has been widely studied, and the aim of these therapies is to minimize the bacterial colonization within the biofilm, allowing a positive host response. The concomitant use of local antibiotics delivered into the sulcus, when combined with a mechanical debridement of the supra and subgingival plaque, reduce this bacterial burden, increase the attachment level, and reduce the pocket depth in patients with periodontal disease [3]. However, it should be noted that the use of local antibiotics and other agents should be considered as an adjunct therapeutic approach and that this approach is just one of many that can help in slowing down the progression of this complex disease.

B. The most common local drug delivery agents used today in dental practice are antibiotics such as tetracyclines and tetracycline derivatives such as doxycycline and minocycline. These are broad-spectrum antibiotics that are effective against both gram-positive and gram-negative bacteria; however, the concentration of the local drug is usually higher than those used systemically. In addition, tetracyclines inhibit matrix metalloproteinases (MMPs), enzymes that degrade the extracellular matrix like collagen [4] and are produced by the bacteria that are associated with periodontal disease. These commercially available antimicrobials are Arestin (minocycline microspheres), Atridox (10% doxycycline hyclate in a gel), and Actisite (12.7 mg tetracycline in an ethylene/vinyl acetate copolymer fiber).

In addition to the category just described, another antibiotic that has been widely studied is metronidazole, which targets anaerobic bacteria by affecting their DNA but not the aerobic microorganisms. The brand name of the local delivery form is Elyzol, which consists of a.gel containing metronidazole benzoate in a mixture of monoglycerides and triglycerides [14]. It should be noted that not all the local antibiotics mentioned here are still available in all markets.

There are some other agents, nonantibiotics, which have been proven effective in the management of the disease by affecting the host response, inflammation, and, to a certain extent, the bacterial burden. An example of this is PerioChip (chlorhexidine gluconate 2.5 mg in a biodegradable matrix of hydrolyzed gelatin cross-linked with glutaraldehyde). This product is also indicated as an adjunct to scaling and root planing procedures in patients with periodontitis or during a periodontal maintenance program. Chlorhexidine is active against broad-spectrum microorganisms that due to its positive charge reacts with the microbial cell surface and destroys the integrity of the cell membrane and precipitates the cytoplasm, causing cell death.

Other nondrug delivery devices that have been used as adjuncts to periodontal therapy are lasers and photodynamic light therapy. The word *laser* is an acronym for "light amplification by stimulated emission of radiation"; lasers are categorized according to the medium used to provide atoms to the emitting system. Although existing research has shown that lasers at a specific wave lengths can kill bacteria, the conclusions of current systematic reviews and consensus reports stated that there is insufficient evidence to support the clinical application of CO_2, Nd:YAG, Nd:YAP, or other diode lasers to treat periodontal disease. This is because the available clinical studies that used these laser applications as adjuncts to mechanical debridement did not demonstrate significant added clinical value [5,6]. The use of these devices is not discussed in this chapter.

C. The successful treatment of periodontal disease depends on the control and management of multiple variables as previously discussed. However, the appropriate diagnosis constitutes the primary step in selecting the treatment modality that is most appropriate for each case. The current reference to help the clinician formulate the proper diagnosis is based on the 1999 International Workshop for a Classification of Periodontal Diseases and Conditions [7]. However, it is well recognized among the scientific and clinical community that the deeper the periodontal probing or pocket, the greater the concentration of bacterial burden and the less effective the scaling and root planning. Mechanical debridement or scaling of subgingival probings >3 mm is the most commonly used anti-infective therapy in the treatment of periodontal diseases [8,9]. Cobb [9] calculated the mean probing depth reduction and gain of clinical attachment that can be achieved with subgingival scaling and root planning, and they concluded that probing depth reduction usually was greater at sites with larger initial probing depths. However, with an initial pocket depth of ≥5 mm, clinicians have been shown to inadequately debride roots 65% of the time [8].

Most studies conclude that the optimum time of administration of the local agent is right after the scaling and root planing. Because there might be an optimum access for close instrumentation determined by the probing depth, these agents should be used for sites with probing depth >3 mm and with at least a moderate form of periodontitis and should be used as adjuncts to scaling and root planning because the use of a local drug delivery system alone without the mechanical debridement is not sufficient to provide an optimum outcome.

D. An extensive amount of data has been generated in the last decade justifying the use of local delivery adjunctive chemotherapeutics for the treatment of periodontitis. The introduction of a prototype fiberlike device to deliver drugs to the periodontal pocket was first introduced by Goodson and coworkers in 1983 [10]. Systematic reviews report on the efficacy of most available agents. In a review by Hanes and Purvis that consisted of a meta-analysis completed on 19 prospective studies that included scaling and root planing (SRP) and local sustained-release agents compared with SRP alone, a significant adjunctive probing depth reduction or attachment level gain was observed for minocycline, chlorhexidine chip, doxycycline gel, and tetracycline fibers when compared with SRP alone.

However, findings from the meta-analysis indicate that the average amount of pocket depth (PD) reduction achieved by the addition of sustained-release antimicrobials to SRP is quite small, although highly statistically significant. With this amount of additional PD reduction, it is necessary to consider clinically if is worth the extra time and expense required to insert the antimicrobial system. Although irrigants or rinses are not discussed in this chapter, this systematic review found no evidence for adjunctive effect on reduction of probing depth and bleeding on probing of therapist-delivered chlorhexidine irrigation during SRP compared with SRP alone [3]. A separate review performed by Bonito and coworkers found that among the locally administered adjunctive antimicrobials, the most positive results occurred for tetracycline, minocycline, metronidazole, and chlorhexidine. Adjunctive local therapy generally reduced PD levels. Differences between treatment and SRP-only groups in the baseline to follow-up period typically favored treatment groups but usually only modestly (e.g., from about 0.1 mm to nearly 0.5 mm) even when the differences were statistically significant. They evaluated a total of 50 published studies that were appropriate for analysis from 599 algorithm-identified articles [11].

It should be noted that these systematic reviews produce an average that is a summary statistic that combines negative, neutral, and positive effects into one number; this average could potentially mask individual significant results that may be clinically important to the patient [3].

E. The primary goal is to remove soft and hardened microbial deposits from the pathologically exposed root surfaces. The immediate effect of scaling and root planing is an enormous disruption of the subgingival biofilm, and curettes and ultrasonics can remove up to 90% of the subgingival plaque [12].

Thus scaling and root planing is strongly recommended prior to the time of insertion of any of the local agents to obtain the maximum benefit.

The following techniques correspond to the ones suggested by the manufacturers based on the clinical research presented and approved for the specific use by the Food and Drug Administration.

Actisite

Each Actisite fiber is 23 cm (9 inches) long and individually packaged. Remove the fiber from package and insert it into the periodontal pocket until the pocket is filled. An instrument such as a cord packer should be used to condense the fiber into the pocket. The length of fiber used will vary with pocket depth and contour. The fiber should be placed to closely approximate the pocket anatomy and should be in contact with the base of the pocket. An appropriate cyanoacrylate adhesive should be used to help secure the fiber in the pocket.

When placed within a periodontal pocket, Actisite fibers provide continuous release of tetracycline for 10 days. At the end of 10 days of treatment, all fibers must be removed. Fibers lost before 7 days

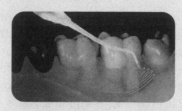

Figure 9: Placement of Actisite.

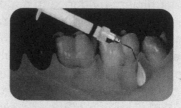

Figure 10: Placement of Atridox.

should be replaced. Fibers should not be used in an acutely abscessed periodontal pocket (Figure 9).

Atridox

Atridox® is removed from the refrigerator 15 minutes before use. Assemble "syringe A" that contains liquid polymer (red stripe) with "syringe B" that contains doxycycline hyclate powder. Mix the contents of both syringes, pushing the contents back and forth about 100 times, about 1.5 minutes. The final contents must be in syringe A (indicated by red stripe) when finished. Attach a blunt cannula and bend it to resemble a periodontal probe. Insert the cannula tip into the periodontal pocket near the base. Express product into pocket until gel reaches the top of the gingival margin. Slowly withdraw the cannula coronally as the pocket begins to fill. Consider using a moistened dental hand instrument to hold product in place and to pack it lightly.

Considerations: Atridox is most retentive in posterior interproximal sites, deeper sites, and furcations. It is least retentive in shallow pockets and single-rooted teeth, in which case you should overflow Atridox, pack it into the embrasure, and cover with periodontal dressing. For least retentive sites, overflow ATRIDOX and pack it into the embrasure and cover with periodontal dressing. It is not necessary to remove Atridox from the pocket because it will absorb completely (Figure 10).

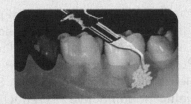

Figure 11: Placement of Arestin.

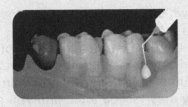

Figure 12: Placement of Elyzol.

Arestin

Arestin is packaged in a specially designed unit-dose cartridge that is inserted into a cartridge handle for product administration. Each cartridge contains enough for one periodontal pocket. It does not require preparation before administration because it is already premixed, premeasured, and does not require refrigeration.

Insert the cartridge into the handle while exerting slight pressure and twist it until you feel and hear the cartridge "lock" into place. If you need to reach difficult-to-access areas, gently bend the tip, leaving the blue cap on. Bending the tip after removal of the blue cap may cause the integral plunger to rupture the cartridge wall. Place the cartridge tip into the periodontal pocket, parallel to the long axis of the tooth. Be sure not to force the tip into the base of the pocket. Gently press the thumb ring to express the Arestin powder while withdrawing the cartridge tip away from the base of the pocket. If you feel any resistance during delivery, withdraw the device further. Once delivery is complete, retract the thumb ring and remove the cartridge with your free hand. Discard the cartridge appropriately and sterilize the handle before reuse. Arestin does not need to be removed because it is completely bioresorbable (Figure 11).

Elyzol

Elyzol comes packed in a carton containing single-use applicator and a blunt needle. The applicator is preloaded with a cartridge containing the gel. Remove the protective cover at the base of the needle. Attach the needle to the applicator. Remove the upper protective cover from the needle and bend to the preferred angle.

Slowly pump up the pressure in the applicator by depressing the blue lever until flowing gel is visible at the tip of the needle. Release the lever

and carefully move the needle down to the bottom of the pocket. Now press the lever down to its lowest position and keep it depressed until gel is visible at the gingival margin. Release the lever and repeat this procedure for all teeth to be treated.

When application is completed, dispose of the needle and the applicator including any remaining gel. Repeat the treatment with Elyzol 25% Dental Gel 1 week later (Figure 12).

F. The following patient recommendations correspond to the ones suggested by the product manufacturers.

Actisite

The most frequently reported adverse reactions in the pivotal clinical trials were discomfort on fiber placement (10%) and local erythema following removal. When Actisite fiber is in place, patients should avoid actions that may dislodge the fiber.

Instruct them not to chew hard, crusty, or sticky foods. Do not brush or floss near any treated areas (continue to clean other teeth). Do not engage in any other hygienic practices that could potentially dislodge the fibers. Do not probe at the treated area with tongue or fingers. Notify the dentist promptly if the fiber is dislodged or falls out before the scheduled recall visit, or if pain or swelling or other problems occur.

Atridox

The most common side effects may include headache; common cold; gum discomfort, pain, or soreness. Instruct the patient to contact a dentist professional about any unusual discomfort. Do not brush or floss the treated area for 7 days. Your dentist may prescribe or recommend an oral rinse to use during the 7 days following Atridox application, which is the length time when you cannot brush or floss.

Do not be alarmed if small amounts of Atridox are dislodged. Atridox is harmless if swallowed.

As your gums heal and swelling begins to subside, they may recede a bit, and you may notice some "white material" at the gum line; it is the Atridox your dentist applied, and most of it will dissolve and be absorbed within 28 days.

After 7 days, brush and floss as your dental professional recommends.

Arestin

The most frequent dental treatment-emergent adverse experiences were inflammation of the gums.

After treatment, you should avoid touching areas of your gums that your dental professional has treated. Arestin does not require bandages and won't leak or fall out. You should also wait 12 hours after treatment before brushing your teeth in the affected area, and avoid eating hard, crunchy, or sticky foods for 1 week.

You should also postpone the use of dental floss, dental tape, toothpicks, or any other devices that clean between your teeth and the affected area for at least 10 days.

Some mild to moderate sensitivity is expected during the first week after SRP and administration of Arestin.

Notify your dental professional promptly if pain, swelling, or other problems occur.

Elyzol

The most frequent side effects are local and occur directly in connection with the application, such as bitter taste and temporary local tenderness. Headache has been reported.

You may eat and drink normally. Normal dental hygiene can be observed, but dental floss, interdental brushes, and toothpicks should not be used on the day following the application.

G. The most recognized clinical parameters to measure success of a periodontal treatment reported in the literature are periodontal probing depth, clinical attachment level, and bleeding on probing. On a systematic review of the literature, Hanes and Purvis [3] concluded that SRP and sustained-release agents compared with SRP alone indicated significant adjunctive PD reduction or CAL gain for all the antibiotics discussed in this chapter. However, improvement could vary from patient to patient and from site to site in the same mouth. Thus it is strongly recommended to perform a full periodontal evaluation between 1 and 3 months after treatment. Most studies in the literature agree that if the periodontal probing is ≥5mm, further periodontal therapy might be needed.

Success in the treatment of periodontal disease is relative because although a periodontal site could have been reduced below the 5-mm threshold, close monitoring through a full periodontal evaluation every 3 months is strongly recommended.

H. Rescue therapy refers to an intervention treatment that is usually performed after an optimal periodontal therapy has been carried on a specific patient with poor short- or long-term success or recurrence. In a long-term follow-up study conducted by Haffajee and coworkers, it was found that the combination of local and systemic antibiotic therapy, used in conjunction with SRP on "refractory" periodontitis patients, a statistical significant reductions of already low levels of highly pathogenic microbial species as well as improvements in probing depth reductions and CAL gain was observed [13]. Thus it is suggested to consider a combination therapy approach for the treatment of recurrent lesions >5mm that include local and systemic antibiotics among other treatments.

All the recommendations made in this chapter should be considered cautiously and with the understanding that results will vary from patient to patient and from site to site.

Case 3

Systemic Antibiotics

CASE STORY

A 42-year-old Hispanic Caucasian male presented with a chief complaint of pain and bleeding associated with his gums. At the time of his first examination he had not received any periodontal treatment and reported having his lower first molars extracted more than 5 years before. The patient claimed that the reason the teeth were extracted was due to "pain," but he could not describe whether the cause for the pain was due to caries, periodontal problems, or endodontic infections.

LEARNING GOALS AND OBJECTIVES

- To be able to list the theoretical advantages in the use of systemic antibiotics in the treatment of periodontal infections
- To be able to identify periodontal cases that could benefit from the adjunctive use of systemic antibiotics
- To be able to list the main antibiotics used in the treatment of periodontal diseases, the criteria used in their selection, and which ones are currently the drugs of choice for these infections
- To know what clinical benefits can be anticipated with the adjunctive use of systemic antibiotics in comparison with mechanical therapy
- To understand the main risks associated with the use of systemic antibiotics
- To know at which stage of the periodontal treatment antibiotics should be prescribed

Medical History

The patient reported a history of high blood pressure that he manages with diet and exercise; otherwise his medical history was unremarkable. At the time of his first appointment he was not taking any medication besides an occasional aspirin for headaches.

Review of Systems

- Vital signs
  - Blood pressure: 140/80 mm Hg
  - Pulse rate: 75 beats/minute (regular)

Social History

The patient was married with two children. He drank alcohol socially, had never smoked, and had not used recreational drugs. His father had diabetes; his mother died of breast cancer 10 years ago. His attitude was very positive and he considered his treatment a priority.

Extraoral Examination

His extraoral examination was unremarkable: skin, head, neck, temporomandibular joint, and muscles were all within normal limits.

Intraoral Examination

The oral cancer screening was negative. There were no dental caries present at the time of examination. The gingival examination revealed generalized severe erythema, with rolled margins and swollen papilla with an edematous consistency and absent stippling (Figure 1). Spontaneous bleeding was present; exudation upon pressure was also present. There was an adequate amount of attached tissue around most teeth. Gingival recession was present at several sites (see periodontal chart in Figure 2 for details). Supra- and subgingival calculus could be detected on several teeth, particularly on the buccal surface of upper molars and lingual surfaces of lower incisors. Teeth #11, 19, and 30 were missing. Due to the absence of the lower first molars, teeth #3 and 14 had supererupted, and the lower second molars had tipped mesially. The absence of #11 resulted in the mesialization of the upper left posterior teeth. There was generalized plaque accumulation. A few amalgam restorations of adequate quality were present in the posterior teeth. Saliva was of normal flow and consistency.

The periodontal chart presented in Figure 2 includes the following periodontal parameters: (1) probing pocket depth (PD) in millimeters; (2) measurement from the cementoenamel junction (CEJ) to the gingival margin (GM) in millimeters (gingival recession was recorded as a negative value); (3) clinical attachment level (CAL), which was calculated by subtracting the CEJ-GM distance from the PD; and (4) presence (1) or absence (0) of bleeding on probing (BOP). Each clinical parameter was measured at six sites per tooth excluding third molars. Probing values were colored in blue, green, or red to highlight shallow (<4mm); intermediate (4–6mm); and deep pockets (>6mm), respectively. BOP was detected in 81% of sites, and the mean values for PD and CAL were 4.4mm and 4.3mm, respectively.

Occlusion

There were no signs of trauma from occlusion, no interferences, and no significant mobility. Despite the migration of certain teeth due to absence of #11, 19, and 30, there were no major occlusal discrepancies. The patient denied any sign or symptoms associated with his temporomandibular joint such as crepitus, clicking, or pain.

Radiographic Examination

A full-mouth set of radiographs (Figure 2) was exposed. There was generalized moderate to severe horizontal bone loss. Subgingival decay was evident on radiographic examination. Composite restorations were evident on teeth #1, 2, 12, 13, 14, 18, 21, and 31. There were images compatible with composite restorations on teeth #7, 8, and 9.

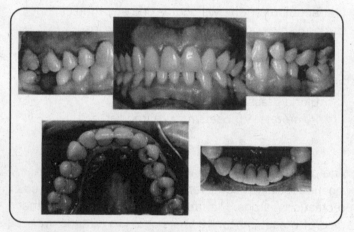

Figure 1: Clinical presentation of the case at initial visit. Courtesy of Dr. Eduardo Sampaio and Dr. Marcelo Faveri.

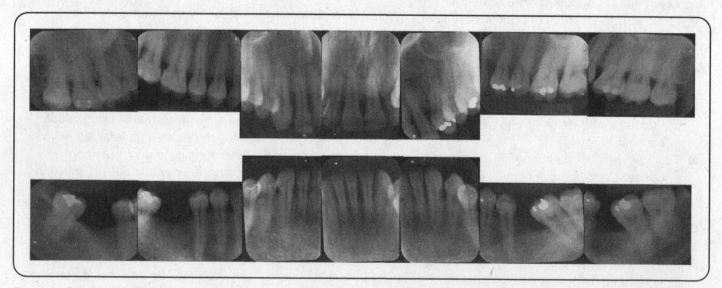

Figure 2: Full-mouth periapical radiographs of the case at initial visit. Courtesy of Dr. Eduardo Sampaio and Dr. Marcelo Faveri.

Diagnosis

The case was diagnosed as severe generalized chronic periodontitis [1].

Treatment Plan

The treatment plan for this case consisted primarily of four to six sessions of scaling and root planing (SRP) accompanied by oral hygiene instructions with the concomitant use of adjunctive systemic antibiotics: amoxicillin 500 mg three times a day (tid) plus metronidazole 250 mg tid for 7 days. The antibiotic combination was prescribed immediately after the completion of the SRP sessions. A reassessment of the case was planned for 3 months after the completion of this initial phase when the need for additional therapy would be decided.

Treatment

After the patient's initial examination, radiographs, and charting (Figures 1–3), a comprehensive treatment planning was presented and agreed upon. The first session involved full-mouth gross scaling and oral hygiene instructions on the proper toothbrushing technique and use of dental floss. Due to the presence of large amounts of subgingival calculus, the patient required six sessions of subgingival SRP under local anesthesia (one sextant of the mouth was instrumented per session). During this active phase of anti-infective therapy, previously instrumented sextants were constantly reexamined for the detection of residual supra- and subgingival calculus and, whenever detected, residual calculus was removed. Every SRP session was accompanied by reinforcement of the oral hygiene instructions. At the end of his last SRP session, amoxicillin 500 mg tid plus metronidazole 250 mg tid were prescribed for 7 days. The patients reported completing the antibiotic regimen without any adverse event.

Three months after the last SRP session, the subject was reexamined (Figures 4 and 5), residual pockets ≥4 mm received additional SRP, a full-mouth prophylaxis was performed, and oral hygiene instructions were reinforced. Mean PD and CAL were reduced to 2.8 mm and 3.5 mm, respectively, and there was a reduction in BOP from 81% to 9%. At that time no additional periodontal therapy was deemed necessary. The patient was placed in a recall system for supportive periodontal therapy every 3 months. Figures 6 and 7 illustrate the clinical presentation and the periodontal parameters 1 year after completion of periodontal therapy. The case remained stable with a mean PD of 2.9 mm, mean CAL of 3.5 mm, and only 5% of sites with BOP.

Visit: Initial Exam

Buccal (maxillary)

Tooth	2	3	4	5	6	7	8	9	10	11	12	13	14	15
PD	3 4 5	5 4 6	5 3 5	4 6 5	6 3 6	7 2 6	6 3 6	4 2 7	7 2 7	- - -	8 4 8	7 3 6	6 3 5	6 3 6
CEJ-GM	0 -2 -1	-1 -2 1	1 -1 1	1 -1 1	1 1 0	1 1 0	1 1 0	1 1 0	1 1 0	- - -	1 -1 1	1 0 0	0 -1 -1	0 -1 0
CAL	3 6 6	6 6 5	4 4 4	3 7 4	5 3 5	6 2 5	5 3 5	3 2 6	6 2 6	- - -	7 5 7	6 3 6	6 4 6	6 4 6
BOP	1 1 1	1 1 1	1 1 0	0 1 1	1 1 1	1 1 1	1 1 1	1 1 1	1 1 1	- - -	1 1 1	1 1 0	1 1 0	1 1 1

Palatal

Tooth	2	3	4	5	6	7	8	9	10	11	12	13	14	15
PD	8 3 6	6 3 5	5 3 6	5 2 7	6 3 7	6 4 5	5 3 5	4 4 5	5 5 7	- - -	7 3 7	7 3 5	6 3 6	6 3 6
CEJ-GM	0 1 1	1 -1 1	1 1 0	1 1 0	1 1 1	1 1 1	1 1 1	1 1 1	1 1 1	- - -	1 1 1	1 1 1	1 1 1	1 1 0
CAL	8 2 5	5 4 4	4 2 5	4 2 6	5 3 6	5 3 4	4 2 4	3 3 4	4 4 6	- - -	6 2 6	6 2 4	5 2 5	5 2 6
BOP	1 1 1	1 1 1	1 1 1	1 1 1	1 1 1	1 1 1	1 1 1	1 1 1	1 1 1	- - -	1 1 1	1 1 1	1 1 0	1 1 0

Buccal (mandibular)

Tooth	31	30	29	28	27	26	25	24	23	22	21	20	19	18
PD	5 3 4	- - -	3 2 3	3 2 4	4 3 5	5 3 5	5 2 4	4 2 6	6 2 5	6 2 6	4 3 3	3 3 3	- - -	8 2 3
CEJ-GM	0 0 0	- - -	0 0 0	0 0 1	1 0 1	1 0 0	0 -1 0	0 0 0	0 0 0	0 0 0	0 0 0	0 0 -1	- - -	0 0 0
CAL	5 3 4	- - -	3 2 3	3 2 3	3 3 4	4 3 5	5 3 4	4 2 6	6 2 5	6 2 6	4 3 3	3 3 4	- - -	8 2 3
BOP	1 1 1	- - -	0 0 0	0 0 0	1 1 1	1 1 1	1 1 0	1 0 1	1 0 1	1 0 1	1 0 0	0 0 0	- - -	1 0 0

Lingual

Tooth	31	30	29	28	27	26	25	24	23	22	21	20	19	18
PD	6 4 4	- - -	3 3 4	4 3 4	3 2 4	3 3 3	3 3 5	5 3 5	5 2 3	3 3 6	4 4 5	3 3 3	- - -	10 3 4
CEJ-GM	1 0 0	- - -	0 0 0	0 0 0	0 0 0	0 0 0	-1 -1 -2	-2 -2 -2	-2 -2 -2	-2 0 1	1 0 0	0 0 -1	- - -	0 0 0
CAL	5 4 4	- - -	3 3 4	4 3 4	3 2 4	3 3 3	4 4 7	7 5 7	7 4 5	5 3 5	3 4 5	3 3 4	- - -	10 3 4
BOP	1 1 1	- - -	1 0 1	1 0 1	0 0 1	1 1 1	1 1 1	1 1 1	1 1 1	1 1 0	1 0 0	0 0 1	- - -	1 0 1

Figure 3: Periodontal chart, initial visit. Courtesy of Dr. Eduardo Sampaio and Dr. Marcelo Faveri.

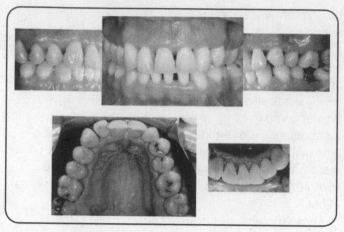

Figure 4: Clinical presentation of the case 3 months posttherapy. Courtesy of Dr. Eduardo Sampaio and Dr. Marcelo Faveri.

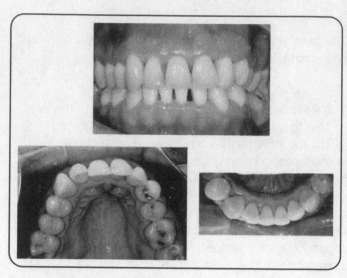

Figure 6: Clinical presentation of the case 1 year posttherapy. Courtesy of Dr. Eduardo Sampaio and Dr. Marcelo Faveri.

Visit: 3 months post-therapy

Surface: **Buccal**

Tooth	2	3	4	5	6	7	8	9	10	11	12	13	14	15
PD	3 3 4	4 2 3	3 2 3	2 3 2	3 2 3	3 3 3	3 3 3	3 3 3	3 2 3	- - -	3 2 3	3 2 3	3 3 3	3 3 4
CEJ-GM	0 -2 -1	-1 -2 0	0 -1 0	-1 -1 -1	0 0 -2	-1 -1 -2	-2 -1 0	-1 0 -2	-3 0 -2	- - -	0 -2 -1	0 0 0	0 -1 -2	-1 -1 0
CAL	3 5 5	5 4 3	3 3 3	3 4 3	3 2 5	4 4 5	5 4 3	4 3 5	6 2 5	- - -	3 4 4	3 2 3	3 4 5	4 4 4
BOP	1 0 0	0 0 0	0 0 0	0 0 0	0 0 0	0 0 0	0 0 0	0 0 0	0 0 0	- - -	0 0 0	0 0 0	0 0 0	0 0 0

Surface: **Palatal**

Tooth	2	3	4	5	6	7	8	9	10	11	12	13	14	15
PD	4 3 4	3 3 3	3 3 3	3 2 2	3 2 3	3 2 3	3 3 3	3 3 3	3 3 3	- - -	4 3 3	4 3 3	4 3 3	4 3 4
CEJ-GM	0 0 0	0 -1 0	0 0 0	0 0 -1	-1 0 -2	-3 -1 -3	-1 0 0	0 0 -2	-3 0 -2	- - -	0 0 0	0 0 0	0 0 -1	-1 0 0
CAL	4 3 4	3 4 3	3 3 3	3 2 3	4 2 5	6 3 6	4 3 4	3 3 5	6 3 5	- - -	4 3 3	4 3 3	4 3 4	5 3 4
BOP	1 0 0	1 0 0	0 0 1	0 0 0	0 0 0	0 0 0	0 1 1	0 0 0	0 0 0	- - -	0 0 0	0 0 0	1 0 0	1 0 0

Surface: **Buccal**

Tooth	31	30	29	28	27	26	25	24	23	22	21	20	19	18
PD	4 3 3	- - -	3 2 2	3 2 3	3 2 3	3 2 3	2 2 2	2 2 3	3 3 3	3 2 3	2 3 2	2 2 2	- - -	5 3 3
CEJ-GM	1 0 0	- - -	-1 0 0	0 0 0	0 0 0	0 0 -1	-2 -1 -1	-1 0 -2	-2 -1 -1	-2 0 0	0 -1 0	0 0 -1	- - -	-2 0 0
CAL	3 3 3	- - -	4 2 2	3 2 3	3 2 3	3 2 4	4 3 3	3 2 5	5 4 4	5 2 3	2 3 3	2 2 3	- - -	7 3 3
BOP	0 0 0	- - -	0 0 0	0 0 0	0 0 0	0 0 0	0 0 0	0 0 0	0 0 0	0 0 0	0 0 0	0 0 0	- - -	0 0 0

Surface: **Lingual**

Tooth	31	30	29	28	27	26	25	24	23	22	21	20	19	18
PD	4 3 3	- - -	3 2 3	3 2 3	3 2 3	2 1 2	2 2 3	2 3 2	3 2 3	2 3 3	3 3 3	3 3 2	- - -	5 3 4
CEJ-GM	0 0 0	- - -	0 -1 0	0 0 0	0 0 0	0 -1 -1	-1 -1 -2	-2 -2 -2	-2 -2 -2	-2 -1 -1	-1 0 0	0 -1 -1	- - -	1 0 0
CAL	4 3 3	- - -	3 3 3	3 2 3	3 2 3	2 2 3	3 3 5	5 4 5	4 4 5	5 3 4	3 3 3	3 4 3	- - -	4 3 4
BOP	0 0 1	- - -	0 0 1	1 0 0	0 0 0	0 0 0	0 0 0	0 0 0	0 0 0	0 0 0	0 0 0	0 0 0	- - -	1 0 1

Figure 5: Periodontal chart, 3 months after therapy. Courtesy of Dr. Eduardo Sampaio and Dr. Marcelo Faveri.

Discussion

Because periodontal diseases are mixed infections, they should benefit from the use of systemic antibiotics. In fact, systemic antibiotic therapy offers several theoretical advantages over SRP alone: (1) systemic antibiotics can achieve local concentrations at difficult-to-reach areas such as in the depth of infrabony defects and furcations; (2) antibiotics achieve local levels that are distributed throughout the oral cavity, reaching all potential reservoirs for periodontal pathogens, including periodontal pockets of all depths and other intraoral surfaces; (3) antibiotics enter the periodontal pocket through its epithelial lining, where bacteria actively involved in tissue destruction are

Visit: 1 year post-therapy

Surface	Buccal													
Tooth	2	3	4	5	6	7	8	9	10	11	12	13	14	15
PD	3 3 4	4 3 3	3 2 3	2 3 3	3 2 3	3 3 2	4 3 3	3 3 3	3 3 4	- - -	4 2 3	4 2 3	3 3 3	3 3 4
CEJ-GM	-1 -1 -1	-1 -1 -1	0 -1 0	-1 -1 -1	0 0 -1	-1 0 -1	-1 0 0	0 0 -1	-2 -1 0	- - -	-1 -2 0	0 0 0	0 0 -1	-2 -1 0
CAL	4 4 5	5 4 4	3 3 3	3 4 4	3 2 4	4 4 2	5 4 3	3 3 3	3 4 5	4 4	5 4 3	4 2 3	3 3 4	5 4 4
BOP	0 0 1	0 0 1	0 0 0	0 0 0	0 0 0	0 0 0	0 0 0	0 0 0	0 0 0	- - -	0 0 0	0 0 0	0 0 0	0 0 0

Surface	Palatal													
Tooth	2	3	4	5	6	7	8	9	10	11	12	13	14	15
PD	3 3 4	3 3 3	3 3 3	3 2 3	3 2 3	3 2 3	3 3 3	3 3 3	3 3 3	- - -	3 3 3	3 3 3	3 3 3	4 3 4
CEJ-GM	0 0 0	0 -1 0	0 0 0	0 0 0	0 -1 -1	0 -1 -3	-1 -2 -1	0 0 0	0 -2 -3	0 -2	0 0 0	0 0 0	0 0 0	-1 -1 0
CAL	3 3 4	3 4 3	3 3 3	3 3 2	4 4 2	4 6 3	5 4 3	3 3 3	3 5 6	3 5	3 3 3	3 3 3	3 3 4	5 3 4
BOP	0 0 1	0 0 0	0 0 0	0 0 1	0 0 0	0 0 0	0 0 0	0 0 0	0 0 0	- - -	0 0 0	0 0 0	0 0 1	0 0 0

Surface	Buccal													
Tooth	31	30	29	28	27	26	25	24	23	22	21	20	19	18
PD	3 3 3	- - -	3 2 3	3 2 3	3 2 3	3 2 3	3 2 3	3 3 3	3 3 3	3 2 3	2 2 2	2 2 2	- - -	5 3 3
CEJ-GM	0 0 0	- - -	0 0 0	0 0 0	0 -1 0	0 0 -1	-1 0 -1	0 0 -1	-1 -1 0	0 0 0	0 -1 0	0 0 0	- - -	-2 0 0
CAL	3 3 3	- - -	3 2 3	3 2 3	3 3 3	3 3 2	4 4 2	3 3 4	4 4 3	3 2 3	2 3 2	2 2 2	- - -	7 3 3
BOP	0 0 0	- - -	0 0 1	0 0 0	0 0 0	0 0 0	0 0 0	0 0 0	0 0 0	0 0 0	0 0 0	0 0 0	- - -	0 0 0

Surface	Lingual													
Tooth	31	30	29	28	27	26	25	24	23	22	21	20	19	18
PD	3 3 3	- - -	3 2 3	3 2 3	3 3 3	3 3 2	3 3 2	3 2 3	3 2 3	3 3 4	3 3 3	4 3 2	- - -	5 2 4
CEJ-GM	0 0 0	- - -	0 -1 0	0 0 0	0 0 0	0 -1 -1	-1 -1 -2	-2 -2 -2	-2 -2 -2	-2 -1 -1	-1 0 0	0 -1 -1	- - -	0 0 0
CAL	3 3 3	- - -	3 3 3	3 2 3	3 3 3	3 3 4	4 4 3	5 4 5	5 4 5	5 4 5	4 3 3	4 4 3	- - -	5 2 4
BOP	0 0 1	- - -	0 0 0	0 0 0	0 0 0	0 0 0	0 0 0	0 0 0	0 0 0	0 0 0	0 0 0	0 0 0	- - -	0 0 1

Figure 7: Periodontal chart, 1 year after periodontal therapy. Courtesy of Dr. Eduardo Sampaio and Dr. Marcelo Faveri.

more likely to be located; and (4) antibiotics may reach microorganisms inside the connective tissues and epithelial cells. However, despite their potential benefits, the use of systemic antibiotics can have side effects, and common risks associated with their use include toxicity, superinfection, allergic reactions, drug interactions, and bacterial resistance. In addition, their efficacy depends on the compliance of the patient with the prescribed regimen [2]. Therefore, when considering the use of systemic antibiotics in periodontal therapy, the first question the clinician must ask is if he or she can offer any additional benefit to what can be obtained with traditional mechanical therapy. That implies that the decision for using these agents has to be based on solid evidence from randomized clinical trials demonstrating a clinical outcome superior to the one obtained with SRP alone.

Evidence is accumulating that the use of systemic antibiotics as an adjunct to mechanical therapy can result in additional clinical benefits beyond what can be accomplished solely with SRP [3,4]. Particularly for aggressive periodontitis, the adjunctive use of systemic antibiotics to mechanical therapy can result in statistically significant greater changes in periodontal clinical parameters compared with SRP only such as greater mean PD reduction, increased gains in mean CAL, and higher reduction in the percentage of sites with BOP [3]. Although early reports suggested that

the clinical benefits obtained with systemic antibiotics in cases of chronic periodontitis were somewhat inferior to the ones obtained in aggressive forms of the disease [3], several recent articles have reported clinically relevant improvements with the adjunctive use of antibiotics in moderate to severe chronic periodontitis, particularly in generalized cases [5–12]. However, at times, the clinical relevance of these differences has been questioned due to their small magnitude. For instance, a recent meta-analysis indicated that adjunctive systemic antibiotics resulted in greater mean full-mouth attachment level gain of 0.3–0.4 mm 6 months after therapy [3]. These figures might seem clinically irrelevant. Nevertheless, if one considers data reported by Rosling et al [13] describing a mean full-mouth attachment loss in subjects in supportive periodontal therapy of 0.042–0.067 mm, an attachment level gain of 0.3 mm would be equivalent to reversing 4–7 years of disease progression. Even when the data from randomized clinical trials were analyzed taking into account information relevant to treatment planning decisions, such as the number of residual deep sites (i.e., PD ≥5 mm), the use of adjunctive systemic antibiotics still demonstrated clinical superiority to SRP alone. For instance, Guerrero et al [14] reported a decrease in the prevalence of sites with PD ≥5 mm of 74% for the systemic antibiotics group compared with 54% ($p < 0.01$) for the

SRP-only group. The use of adjunctive systemic antibiotics has also been associated with a lower rate of disease progression [10,14]. For instance, in the Guerrero et al study [14], disease progression occurred in 1.5% and 3.3% of the sites in the antibiotics and control groups, respectively. Further, there are data suggesting that the gains obtained with a single regimen of systemic antibiotics associated with mechanical therapy might last for up to 2 years even in the absence of subgingival SRP during maintenance [10,15].

It has been well recognized by clinicians and periodontal researchers that certain patients do not respond well to traditional periodontal therapy and continue to show disease progression despite adequate treatment and proper plaque control [16]. These "refractory cases" form a heterogeneous population and the condition is rare, making the conduct of properly powered randomized clinical trials difficult. In any case, reports of case series or small-scale clinical trials seem to indicate that these cases can also be controlled with the adjunctive use of systemic antibiotics [17–23]. However, because these subjects often have a history of several attempts to control their disease with systemic antibiotics, the choice of antibiotics to be used in these cases is complicated by the possibility of a previous selection for resistant species. Therefore, it has been recommended that in refractory periodontitis antimicrobial susceptibility testing be performed before the appropriate antibiotic can be selected [24,25]. Systemic antibiotics have been recommended to treat necrotizing ulcerative gingivitis (NUG) [26,27] due to the presence of large numbers of bacteria within the tissues in such conditions [28]. It has since become apparent that this condition responds well to local mechanical therapy [29]. Systemic antibiotics for NUG should be reserved for cases where there are signs of systemic dissemination of the infection [24,30]. When NUG progresses to include attachment loss, it is referred to as necrotizing ulcerative periodontitis (NUP). Necrotizing periodontal diseases are commonly associated with HIV/AIDS and other pathologies where the immune system is compromised. In the presence of immunosuppression, systemic antibiotics should be used to control these infections; a short course of 3 days of metronidazole has been recommended [31]. Periodontal abscesses are treated primarily with local drainage, and the use of systemic antibiotics is conditional to signs of systemic spreading of the infection [24,32]. In summary, data from randomized

clinical trials support the use of systemic antibiotics in the treatment of moderate to severe chronic and aggressive periodontitis. Cases of refractory periodontal disease and acute forms of periodontal diseases resulting in systemic symptoms such as fever and/or malaise or associated with immunosuppression might also require the use of systemic antibiotics. In addition, emerging literature suggests that smokers might also benefit from the use of these agents in the treatment of their periodontal condition [11].

Once the periodontist has opted for the adjunctive use of systemic antibiotics to treat a case he or she is still faced with several questions: (1) choice of antibiotic(s) to be used, (2) dose and dosage of the antibiotic(s), and (3) timing of drug administration in reference to mechanical therapy. None of these questions is well defined in the literature, and there is no consensus regarding any of these issues. When deciding which antibiotic(s) to select, the clinician is often advised to consider information regarding (1) in vitro activity against periodontopathogens (minimum inhibitory concentration [MIC]), (2) if a concentration greater than the MIC is reached within the subgingival environment (i.e., gingival crevicular fluid levels), (3) how long the dose should be kept to affect the microbiota, and (4) local and systemic adverse effects associated with the drug in guiding their decision [33]. Parameters such as these have been used in the selection of agents for the treatment of periodontal infections. The main antibiotics used so far in the treatment of periodontitis have been tetracycline, minocycline, doxycycline, clindamycin, spiramycin, metronidazole, amoxicillin with clavulanic acid, and the combination of amoxicillin and metronidazole [34]. The reader should refer to the appropriate literature to get familiar with the properties of these agents and the risks associated with their use; Walker et al and Roberts are suggested [35,36]. Although these considerations were essential in guiding the choice of antibiotics to be used in the treatment of periodontal infections, they were not particularly helpful in predicting the clinical outcome of their use. In fact, due to pharmacologic considerations [33] and the biofilm effect [37], it is almost impossible to predict based on in vitro data the clinical effects of systemic antibiotics. Therefore, clinicians should base their decision primarily on the results from randomized clinical trials.

Unfortunately, very few randomized clinical trials have compared different antibiotics side by side, and one cannot make any definitive statement regarding the clinical superiority of an agent or combination of agents [3]. However, there is some evidence indicating that the use of a combination of amoxicillin and metronidazole is superior to either antibiotic alone and to other antibiotics in the treatment of periodontitis [12,38]. Further, data are accumulating indicating that the use of this combination as an adjunct to SRP is superior to SRP alone in generalized aggressive periodontitis [14,38–41] and moderate to severe forms of chronic periodontitis [5–12]. In fact, every published study comparing the adjunctive use of systemic amoxicillin and metronidazole with mechanical therapy alone reported a significant clinical benefit associated with the use of this combination [5–12,14,38,40–48]. Therefore, they should be the first drugs of choice in the treatment of periodontal infections. Periodontists should refrain from using last-generation antibiotics until clinical trials have demonstrated their superiority not only to mechanical therapy alone but also to drugs currently in use that have already demonstrated efficacy. This is important not only because the clinician needs evidence of the clinical effectiveness of the new drug but also due to the phenomenon of cross-resistance. If a microorganism develops resistance to a last-generation antibiotics, it might become resistant to the entire class of antibiotics to which the new generation drug belongs [49].

The literature shows no consistency regarding the choice, dose (the quantity of antibiotic to be administered at one time), dosage (the frequency and quantity of antibiotic administered to a patient), and duration of the course of antibiotics. The different regimens were somewhat arbitrarily defined, and no scientific basis for their choice was presented in the research, making a final decision on which one to choose difficult. In addition, most clinical trials did not report on the incidence of adverse events associated with the use of antibiotics, making it impossible to estimate if a longer course resulted in a higher incidence of adverse events. The only way of finding the best regimen for this combination of antibiotics would be through a randomized clinical trial assessing not only the impact of different regimens on periodontal parameters but also on the incidence of adverse effects. In the absence of this information, the clinician should opt for a conservative approach and use the lowest dosage and shortest duration reported in the literature with a consistent additional benefit over SRP alone. In addition, a short duration of

antibiotic therapy reduces the risk for selection of resistant microorganisms [50]. We suggest 375–500 mg of amoxicillin and 250 mg of metronidazole tid for 7 days.

The timing of antibiotic administration is also an important consideration. Based on the biofilm effect of increased resistance to antimicrobials, clinicians have been instructed to initiate systemic antibiotic therapy once mechanical therapy is completed. The mechanical disruption of the biofilm would favor the antimicrobial effects of the antibiotics by decreasing the bacterial load and disrupting the glycocalyx, which decreases the antibiotic diffusion into the biofilm structure [37]. Although this recommendation makes biologic sense, data from studies using systemic antibiotics as a single therapy (i.e., without concomitant or prior mechanical treatment) have suggested that the subgingival biofilm can be significantly altered by systemic antibiotic administration even in the absence of mechanical therapy, resulting in beneficial clinical changes on the periodontium [6]. In fact, a few clinical trials demonstrating a superior clinical outcome with the adjunctive use of systemic amoxicillin and metronidazole have started the drug regimen concomitantly with the first SRP session, and the antibiotic regimen was completed before all quadrants were debrided [11,41].

The American Academy of Periodontology (AAP) recommended in a position paper that systemic antibiotic therapy should be reserved for patients with unresolved and/or progressing sites after conventional mechanical periodontal treatment [24]. That implies that a reexamination of the outcome of mechanical therapy should be obtained before any decision on the use of systemic antibiotics. That would delay the use of antibiotics up to 3 months after initial therapy. A recent study has demonstrated that adjunctive systemic antibiotics result in improved clinical outcomes when administered immediately after mechanical therapy rather than 3 months after therapy [39]. Two cohorts of generalized aggressive periodontitis subjects ($n = 17$ for each group) were analyzed retrospectively; the group that received systemic amoxicillin/metronidazole immediately after SRP had greater improvements in mean PD and CAL compared with the late antibiotic therapy in deep sites (PD >6 mm). Similarly, Griffiths et al [46] reported that when systemically amoxicillin/metronidazole was administered to a placebo group from a previous randomized clinical trial 6 months after therapy, 67% of the pockets ≥5 mm converted to ≤4 mm, whereas in the original test group that received antibiotics at initial therapy, 83% of pockets showed this level of improvement. It is possible that delaying the beginning of antibiotic therapy might result in a return of the subgingival biofilm to its original complexity, diminishing the benefits offered by a recent mechanical disruption of its structure. In addition, these 3 months of healing might decrease the amount of antibiotics being delivered to the site due to a decrease in gingival crevicular fluid flow and an enhanced epithelial barrier. Therefore, systemic antibiotic therapy should start during the initial therapy either after the first session of SRP or immediately after the completion of the final SRP and not be delayed until after reexamination of the case as an alternative retreatment.

As discussed previously, the use of systemic antibiotics is not without risks. Bacterial resistance is probably the single most important reason clinicians should refrain from the indiscriminate use of systemic antibiotics to treat periodontal infections [51]. However, concerns regarding antibiotic resistance should not preclude clinicians from using systemic antibiotics to treat periodontal diseases when indicated. There are guidelines in the medical literature to the prudent use of antibiotics to minimize the risk of antibiotic resistance. These include (1) using of antibiotics only when patient outcome can be improved, (2) using narrow-spectrum antibiotics whenever possible, (3) saving last-generation antibiotics for serious life-threatening infections; and (4) stopping antibiotic therapy as soon as possible [49]. Periodontists can easily abide by these guidelines while still offering their patients the clinical benefits of the adjunctive use of systemic antibiotics.

Another important tenet of the use of antibiotics is that it should be used only to either treat an existing infection (therapeutic use) or to prevent the establishment of infection when a sterile body part is to be exposed to microorganisms (prophylactic use; e.g., surgical procedure) [49]. When used for prophylaxis a short course of antibiotics should be prescribed, typically only enough to last the duration of the surgical procedure, and the administration should begin before surgery (2 hours prior to the procedure), so that adequate systemic levels of the antibiotic (two to eight times above MIC) are present at the time of surgical incision [52]. The practice of prescribing antibiotics to be used immediately after a surgical procedure should be avoided at all costs because it is neither therapeutic (there should be no infection at this time) nor prophylactic since the surgical wound is already closed. Most importantly this would bring no benefit to the patient, infringing on the guidelines on the prudent use of antibiotics. The prophylactic use of antibiotics during periodontal surgeries is not recommended due to the extremely low incidence of postsurgical infections [53,54]. This is mainly a consequence of drainage at the gingival margin. In essence, during healing, the periodontal tissues can be considered an "open wound." The same degree of drainage and, therefore, protection against postsurgical infections is not present in closed procedures such as sinus lifts or bone augmentations prior to implant placement. In these circumstances, prophylactic systemic antibiotics might be recommended. The insertion of endosseous dental implants also fits the recommendations for antibiotic prophylaxis in the medical literature [55], and a few studies have suggested that preoperative antibiotics might decrease the number of early implant failures [56]. In accordance with sound principles for the use of prophylactic antibiotics, the prevalence of infectious complications and success rates after implant surgery were similar with a single preoperative dose of antibiotic compared with long-term prophylactic antibiotic regimens [57,58].

In summary, despite the lack of data on important issues regarding the use of systemic antibiotics as adjuncts in periodontal therapy, there is enough documentation of their additional clinical benefits to warrant their use in clinical practice. The following general guidelines to the use of adjunctive systemic antibiotics to treat periodontal infections are recommended: (1) it should be restricted to severe generalized cases (chronic or aggressive); mild to moderate and localized forms of periodontitis are probably better addressed with local mechanical therapy; (2) amoxicillin (375–500 mg tid) and metronidazole (250 mg tid) in combination are the drugs of choice unless the patient has a history of allergy or intolerance to either drug; (3) in the presence of refractory disease, an in vitro susceptibility test is recommended prior to deciding which antibiotic(s) to prescribe, particularly if the patient has a history of previous administrations of systemic antibiotics to treat the periodontal disease; and (4) smokers might also benefit from the adjunctive use of systemic antibiotics.

Self-Study Questions

A. In which cases should the periodontist consider the use of adjunctive systemic antibiotics?

B. What should be the antibiotic regimen of choice to treat periodontal infections, and what are the alternatives in case of a history of allergy or intolerance to the antibiotic(s) of choice?

C. When during the periodontal treatment should you prescribe systemic antibiotics to obtain the greatest clinical benefit?

D. What are the general recommendations to be followed when using systemic antibiotics to minimize the risk of bacterial resistance?

E. What are the additional clinical benefits that one can expect from the adjunctive use of systemic antibiotics?

Answers located at the end of the chapter.

References

1. Armitage GC. Development of a classification system for periodontal diseases and conditions. Ann Periodontol 1999;4:1–6.
2. Guerrero A, Echeverria JJ, et al. Incomplete adherence to an adjunctive systemic antibiotic regimen decreases clinical outcomes in generalized aggressive periodontitis patients: a pilot retrospective study. J Clin Periodontol 2007;34:897–902.
3. Haffajee AD, Socransky SS, et al. Systemic anti-infective periodontal therapy. A systematic review. Ann Periodontol 2003;8:115–181.
4. Herrera D, Sanz M, et al. A systematic review on the effect of systemic antimicrobials as an adjunct to scaling and root planing in periodontitis patients. J Clin Periodontol 2002;29(Suppl 3):136–159; discussion 160–162.
5. Berglundh T, Krok L, et al. The use of metronidazole and amoxicillin in the treatment of advanced periodontal disease. A prospective, controlled clinical trial. J Clin Periodontol 1998;25:354–362.
6. Lopez NJ, Socransky SS, et al. Effects of metronidazole plus amoxicillin as the only therapy on the microbiological and clinical parameters of untreated chronic periodontitis. J Clin Periodontol 2006;33:648–660.
7. Winkel EG, Van Winkelhoff AJ, et al. Amoxicillin plus metronidazole in the treatment of adult periodontitis patients. A double-blind placebo-controlled study. J Clin Periodontol 2001;28:296–305.
8. Cionca N, Giannopoulou C, et al. Amoxicillin and metronidazole as an adjunct to full-mouth scaling and root planing of chronic periodontitis. J Periodontol 2009;80:364–371.
9. Ribeiro Edel P, Bittencourt S, et al. Full-mouth ultrasonic debridement associated with amoxicillin and metronidazole in the treatment of severe chronic periodontitis. J Periodontol 2009;80:1254–1264.
10. Ehmke B, Moter A, et al. Adjunctive antimicrobial therapy of periodontitis: long-term effects on disease progression and oral colonization. J Periodontol 2005;76:749–759.
11. Matarazzo F, Figueiredo LC, et al. Clinical and microbiological benefits of systemic metronidazole and amoxicillin in the treatment of smokers with chronic periodontitis: a randomized placebo-controlled study. J Clin Periodontol 2008;35:885–896.
12. Rooney J, Wade WG, et al. Adjunctive effects to non-surgical periodontal therapy of systemic metronidazole and amoxicillin alone and combined. A placebo controlled study. J Clin Periodontol 2002;29:342–350.
13. Rosling B, Serine G, et al. Longitudinal periodontal tissue alterations during supportive therapy. Findings from subjects with normal and high susceptibility to periodontal disease. J Clin Periodontol 2001;28:241–249.
14. Guerrero A, Griffiths GS, et al. Adjunctive benefits of systemic amoxicillin and metronidazole in non-surgical treatment of generalized aggressive periodontitis: a randomized placebo-controlled clinical trial. J Clin Periodontol 2005;32:1096–1107.
15. Haffajee AD, Tales RP, et al. The effect of periodontal therapy on the composition of the subgingival microbiota. Periodontol 2000 2006;42:219–258.
16. Korenman KS. Refractory periodontitis: critical questions in clinical management. J Clin Periodontol 1996;23:293–298.
17. Magnusson I, Clark WB, et al. Effect of non-surgical periodontal therapy combined with adjunctive antibiotics in subjects with "refractory" periodontal disease. (I). Clinical results. J Clin Periodontol 1989;16:647–653.

18. Collins JG, Offenbach S, et al. Effects of a combination therapy to eliminate *Porphyromonas gingivalis* in refractory periodontitis. J Periodontol 1993;64:998–1007.

19. Gordon J, Walker C, et al. Efficacy of clindamycin hydrochloride in refractory periodontitis: 24-month results. J Periodontol 1990;61:686–691.

20. Gordon J, Walker C, et al. Efficacy of clindamycin hydrochloride in refractory periodontitis. 12-month results. J Periodontol 1985;56:75–80.

21. Walker C, Gordon J. The effect of clindamycin on the microbiota associated with refractory periodontitis. J Periodontol 1990;61:692–698.

22. Winkel EG, Van Winkelhoff AJ, et al. Effects of metronidazole in patients with "refractory" periodontitis associated with *Bacteroides forsythus*. J Clin Periodontol 1997;24:573–579.

23. Haffajee AD, Uzel NG, et al. Clinical and microbiological changes associated with the use of combined antimicrobial therapies to treat "refractory" periodontitis. J Clin Periodontol 2004;31:869–877.

24. Slots J. Systemic antibiotics in periodontics. J Periodontol 2004;75:1553–1565.

25. Shaddox LM, Walker C. Microbial testing in periodontics: value, limitations and future directions. Periodontol 2000 2009;50:25–38.

26. Duckworth R, Waterhouse JP, et al. Acute ulcerative gingivitis. A double-blind controlled clinical trial of metronidazole. Br Dent J 1966;120:599–602.

27. Elmslie RD. Treatment of acute ulcerative gingivitis. A clinical trial using chewing gums containing metronidazole or penicillin. Br Dent J 1967;122:307–308.

28. Loesche WJ, Syed SA, et al. The bacteriology of acute necrotizing ulcerative gingivitis. J Periodontol 1982;53:223–230.

29. Parameter on acute periodontal diseases. American Academy of Periodontology. J Periodontol 2000;71(5 Suppl):863–866.

30. Holroyd SV. Antibiotics in the practice of periodontics. J Periodontology 1971;42:584–589.

31. Ryder MI. An update on HIV and periodontal disease. J Periodontology 2002;73:1071–1078.

32. Dahlin G. Microbiology and treatment of dental abscesses and periodontal-endodontic lesions. Periodontol 2000 2002;28:206–239.

33. van Winkelhoff AJ, Rams TE, et al. Systemic antibiotic therapy in periodontics. Periodontol 2000 1996;10:45–78.

34. Slots J, Ting M. Systemic antibiotics in the treatment of periodontal disease. Periodontol 2000 2002;28:106–176.

35. Walker CB, Karpinia K, et al. Chemotherapeutics: antibiotics and other antimicrobials. Periodontol 2000 2004;36:146–165.

36. Roberts MC. Antibiotic toxicity, interactions and resistance development. Periodontol 2000 2002;28:280–297.

37. Socransky SS, Haffajee AD. Dental biofilms: difficult therapeutic targets. Periodontol 2000 2002;28:12–55.

38. Xajigeorgiou C, Sakellari D, et al. Clinical and microbiological effects of different antimicrobials on generalized aggressive periodontitis. J Clin Periodontol 2006;33:254–264.

39. Kaner D, Christan C, et al. Timing affects the clinical outcome of adjunctive systemic antibiotic therapy for generalized aggressive periodontitis. J Periodontol 2007;78:1201–1208.

40. Yek EC, Cintan S, et al. Efficacy of amoxicillin and metronidazole combination for the management of generalized aggressive periodontitis. J Periodontol 2010;81:964–974.

41. Mestnik MJ, Feres M, et al. Short-term benefits of the adjunctive use of metronidazole plus amoxicillin in the microbial profile and in the clinical parameters of subjects with generalized aggressive periodontitis. J Clin Periodontol 2010;37:353–365.

42. Flemmig TF, Milian E, et al. Differential clinical treatment outcome after systemic metronidazole and amoxicillin in patients harboring *Actinobacillus actinomycetemcomitans* and/or *Porphyromonas gingivalis*. J Clin Periodontol 1998;25:380–387.

43. Lopez NJ, Gamonal JA, et al. Repeated metronidazole and amoxicillin treatment of periodontitis. A follow-up study. J Periodontol 2000;71:79–89.

44. Moeintaghavi A, Talebi-ardakani MR, et al. Adjunctive effects of systemic amoxicillin and metronidazole with scaling and root planing: a randomized, placebo controlled clinical trial. J Contemp Dent Pract 2007;8:51–59.

45. Winkel EG, van Winkelhoff AJ, et al. Additional clinical and microbiological effects of amoxicillin and metronidazole after initial periodontal therapy. J Clin Periodontol 1998;25:857–864.

46. Griffiths GS, Ayob R, et al. Amoxicillin and metronidazole as an adjunctive treatment in generalized aggressive periodontitis at initial therapy or re-treatment: a randomized controlled clinical trial. J Clin Periodontol 2011;38:43–49.

47. Lopez NJ, Gamonal JA. Effects of metronidazole plus amoxicillin in progressive untreated adult periodontitis: results of a single 1-week course after 2 and 4 months. J Periodontol 1998;69:1291–1298.

48. Flemmig TF, Milian E, et al. Differential effects of systemic metronidazole and amoxicillin on *Actinobacillus actinomycetemcomitans* and *Porphyromonas gingivalis* in intraoral habitats. J Clin Periodontol 1998;25:1–10.

49. Collignon PJ. 11: Antibiotic resistance. Med J Aust 2002;177:325–329.

50. Pallasch TJ. Pharmacokinetic principles of antimicrobial therapy. Periodontol 2000 1996;10:5–11.

51. Pallasch TJ. Antibiotic resistance. Dent Clin North Am 2003;47:623–639.

52. Classen DC, Evans RS, et al. The timing of prophylactic administration of antibiotics and the risk of surgical-wound infection. N Engl J Med 1992;326:281–286.

53. Callis S, Lemmer J, et al. Antibiotic prophylaxis in periodontal surgery. A retrospective study. J Dent Assoc S Afr 1996;51:806–809.

54. Powell CA, Mealey BL, et al. Post-surgical infections: prevalence associated with various periodontal surgical procedures. J Periodontol 2005;76:329–333.

55. Paluzzi RG. Antimicrobial prophylaxis for surgery. Med Clin North Am 1993;77:427–441.

56. Esposito M, Grusovin MG, et al. The efficacy of antibiotic prophylaxis at placement of dental implants: a Cochrane systematic review of randomised controlled clinical trials. Eur J Oral Implantol 2008;1:95–103.

57. Binahmed A, Stoykewych A, et al. Single preoperative dose versus long-term prophylactic antibiotic regimens in dental implant surgery. Int J Oral Maxillofac Implants 2005;20:115–117.

58. Kashani H, Dahlin C, et al. Influence of different prophylactic antibiotic regimens on implant survival rate: a retrospective clinical study. Clin Implant Dent Relat Res 2005;7:32–35.

TAKE-HOME POINTS

A. The use of systemic antibiotics is formally recommended by the AAP for aggressive periodontitis cases; refractory cases, and acute forms of periodontal diseases with systemic symptoms [24]. Several authors have discouraged the use of systemic antibiotics to treat chronic periodontitis on the grounds that this form of periodontal infection responds well to mechanical therapy. It has been suggested that systemic antibiotics should be reserved for cases of chronic periodontitis with a poor response to SRP as a retreatment option. However, studies reviewed in the discussion section clearly demonstrated that moderate to severe cases of chronic periodontitis also benefit from the use of adjunctive antibiotics. In addition, a few studies demonstrated that the clinical improvements were greater if the antibiotics were administered during the initial therapy rather than after reevaluation of the results obtained with the mechanical treatment.

B. Ideally, one would like to match the antibiotic therapy to clinical and, microbiological characteristics of the patient that would indicate which subject would respond better to which antibiotic. Unfortunately, this is not the state of the art of systemic antibiotic use in periodontal therapy. The most reliable evidence available comes from randomized clinical trials. Based on these studies, a combination of amoxicillin and metronidazole is the first choice to treat aggressive and chronic periodontal infections. Several regimens have been used in different studies, and in the absence of clear evidence of superiority of one over the other; the prudent use of these drugs would be to opt for the lowest doses and the shortest duration that have resulted in additional clinical benefits over SRP alone. Based on this criterion, the following regimen is suggested: amoxicillin 375–500 mg tid and metronidazole 250 mg tid for 7 days. In case of a history of allergy to penicillin, the recommendation would be to replace amoxicillin with ciprofloxacin [24]. Alternatively, metronidazole as a single therapy has also demonstrated beneficial results in several clinical trials. In case of intolerance to metronidazole and an allergy to penicillin, an alternative would be the use of azithromycin. Patients should be told about the risk of allergies and any other potential side effects (e.g., patients cannot drink any alcohol when they are taking metronidazole).

C. The AAP recommends the use of systemic antibiotics in chronic periodontitis only in cases that did not respond to conventional mechanical therapy, therefore, as a retreatment option [24]. However, since these guidelines were issued, well-conducted randomized clinical trials have demonstrated greater clinical improvements in moderate to severe cases of chronic periodontitis when systemic antibiotics were used as adjuncts to the mechanical therapy during the active phase of the treatment (prior to a reevaluation of the case). In addition, recent studies have suggested that delaying the administration of antibiotics to a retreatment phase of the therapy might mitigate their clinical benefit.

Therefore, they should be administered during the active phase of the mechanical therapy. To completely avoid interference by the biofilm structure, some authors have recommended starting immediately after the last SRP session.

D. The prudent use of systemic antibiotics to minimize the risk of bacterial resistance should involve 1) the use of antibiotics only when patient outcome can be improved, (2) the use of narrow-spectrum antibiotics whenever possible, (3) saving last-generation antibiotics for serious life-threatening infections, and (4) stopping antibiotic therapy as soon as possible. When used prophylactically a short course of antibiotics should be prescribed, typically only enough to last the duration of the surgical procedure, and the administration should begin prior to surgery (2 hours before the procedure), so that adequate systemic levels of the antibiotic (two to eight times above MIC) are present at the time of surgical incision.

E. Additional clinical benefits associated with the use of systemic antibiotics as adjuncts to mechanical therapy reported in the literature include (1) greater reduction in mean PD and gains in mean CAL, (2) fewer residual deep pockets (≥5 mm), (3) slower rate of disease progression during follow-up, and (4) clinical gains can be maintained for at least 2 years after a single course of systemic antibiotics.

3

Resective Periodontal Therapy

Clinical Cases in Periodontics, First Edition. Nadeem Karimbux.
© 2012 John Wiley & Sons, Inc. Published 2012 by John Wiley & Sons, Inc.

Case 1

Gingivectomy

CASE STORY

A 16-year-old Caucasian male presented with a chief complaint of: "My gums are puffy and bleed on flossing." After 2 years of orthodontic therapy, treatment had been discontinued 2 months before due to nonresolvable gingival enlargement (Figure 1). The patient had been informed of his gingival overgrowth, and oral hygiene instructions had been reinforced. The patient had no significant gingival inflammation and/or enlargement before the start of orthodontic treatment. He stated that the gingival enlargement developed gradually during orthodontic treatment (Figures 2 and 3).

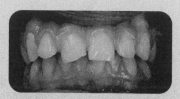
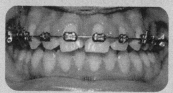

Figure 2: Clinical example of plaque-induced gingivitis with gingival enlargement: frontal occlusal views before orthodontic presentation (top) and during the orthodontic treatment (bottom).

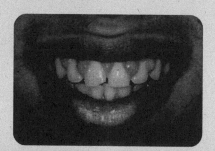

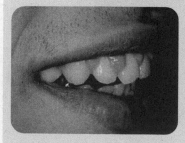
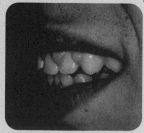

Figure 1: Clinical presentation after removal of orthodontic appliances: smile frontal and side views.

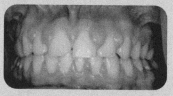

Figure 3: Clinical presentation 2 months after removal of orthodontic appliances: intraoral frontal view in occlusion.

LEARNING GOALS AND OBJECTIVES
- To learn the indications for gingivectomy
- To understand the surgical technique for gingivectomy

Medical History

The patient reported no significant medical problems and no known allergies. He did not have a family history of gingival overgrowth or a history of chronic or current medication.

Dental History

The patient reported that orthodontic treatment began 2 years ago to align his teeth. Slowly during this time, his gums became "puffy," and despite his best efforts at oral hygiene no improvement had been achieved. Therefore, 2 months ago, the orthodontic brackets were removed and the patient was referred to the Department of Periodontology for consultation and appropriate treatment. The patient was currently wearing a retainer. He denied a history of tooth extraction, restorations, or endodontic treatment. The anatomic crown of tooth #8 was previously chipped due to trauma.

Social History

The patient was a sophomore in high school and denied smoking and drinking alcohol.

Oral Hygiene

The patient used a manual toothbrush that was replaced every 3 months and reported tooth brushing and flossing in the morning only. He also used Listerine mouth rinse once a day.

Extraoral and Intraoral Examinations

- There were no significant findings. The patient had no masses or swelling, and the temporomandibular joint was within normal limits.
- With the exception of the gingiva, the soft tissues of the mouth appeared normal.
- A periodontal examination revealed localized mild marginal erythema, localized rolled margins, swollen papillae, bleeding on probing, no recession or mobility, probing depths ranging from 2 to 5 mm, and keratinized gingiva ranging from 3 to 8 mm (Figures 3 and 4).
- The hard tissue examination found no active decay and no dental restorations. Tooth #8 was reported as fractured.

Occlusion

Class I angle occlusion was present after orthodontic treatment.

Radiographic Examination

The full-mouth set of radiographs demonstrated crestal bone levels to be within normal limits (Figure 5 shows the patient's anterior periapical X-rays).

Diagnosis

After reviewing the history, clinical, and radiographic examinations, the patient was diagnosed with plaque-induced gingivitis resulting in gingival overgrowth.

Treatment Plan

The treatment plan for this patient included prophylaxis, improved oral hygiene, and surgical correction (with gingivectomy/gingivoplasty) of the gingival contour and periodontal maintenance.

Treatment

Treatment for this patient included oral hygiene instructions and supra- and subgingival scaling followed by reevaluation at 4 weeks. During the reevaluation appointment, an improvement in oral hygiene technique was noted. However, the gingival enlargement persisted. Therefore, surgical excision of excessive soft tissue was performed via external bevel gingivectomy technique (B). Following the administration of local anesthesia, bleeding points corresponding to the apical extent of the pocket depth were created on the external gingiva using a periodontal probe (Figure 6). Using #15C blades, a coronally directed external bevel incision was made starting slightly apical to the bleeding points and coronal to the mucogingival junction. The inner portion of the blade should contact the teeth at the base of the pocket at a position corresponding to the bleeding point. The incision line should be a straight-line incision that begins and ends in the gingival sulcus mesially and distally to the gingival area removed. The detached gingiva was removed with a scaler, and rotary diamond burs were used to reshape the gingival margin to normal physiologic contours, as shown in Figures 6 and 7. This reshaping of the gingival is referred to as gingivoplasty (A). Oral hygiene instructions were reinforced, and the patient was asked not to brush the wounded areas until the next appointment in 2 weeks and was given a prescription for Peridex rinse and ibuprofen 600 mg for pain control.

The patient was evaluated 2 weeks post-gingivectomy to assess the healing (Figure 8). Oral hygiene was reinforced, instructing on brushing the area of surgery.

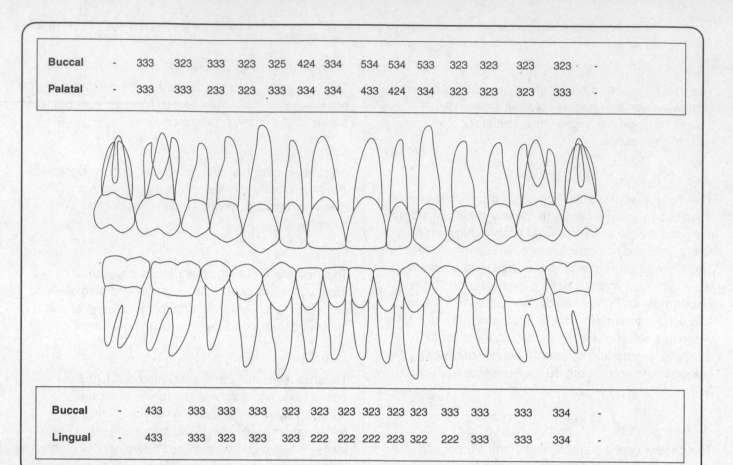

Buccal	-	333	323	333	323	325	424	334	534	534	533	323	323	323	323	-
Palatal	-	333	333	233	323	333	334	334	433	424	334	323	323	323	333	-

Buccal	-	433	333	333	333	323	323	323	323	323	323	333	333	333	334	-
Lingual	-	433	333	323	323	323	222	222	222	223	322	222	333	333	334	-

Figure 4: Probing pocket depth measurements.

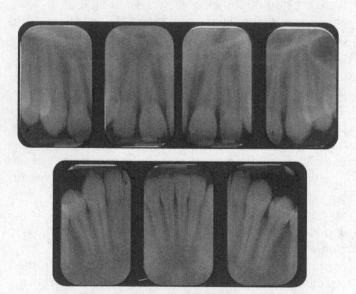

Figure 5: Periapical radiographs depicting interproximal bone levels.

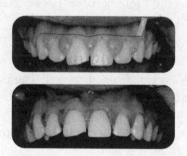

Figure 6: External bevel gingivectomy in anterior maxillary region; gingival marking for the external bevel incision (top) and immediately after gingivectomy (bottom).

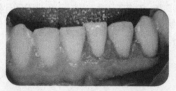

Figure 7: External bevel gingivectomy in anterior mandibular region: immediate post-gingivectomy.

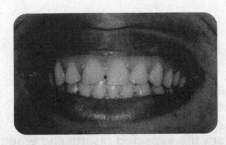

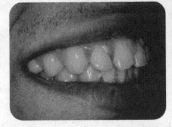
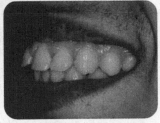

Figure 8: Two-week post-gingivectomy: full smile frontal and side views.

Discussion

Patients undergoing orthodontic treatment may experience various oral clinical manifestations such as sensitivity, increased caries risk, and gingival enlargement [2,3]. Gingival enlargement associated with orthodontic therapy can begin as dental plaque–induced gingivitis followed by gingival overgrowth. The enlargement is usually associated with an inflammatory response triggered by the corrosion of the orthodontic appliances. The most likely component of the brackets creating this response is nickel. Therefore, the condition is frequently classified as nickel allergic contact stomatitis [1]. A recent study by Gursoy et al [2] describes the appearance of orthodontic treatment–induced gingival overgrowth as a specific fibrous and thickened gingiva, different from fragile gingiva with marginal gingival redness that is seen in allergic or inflammatory gingival lesions. The histologic analysis of orthodontic-induced gingival enlargement tissues demonstrated an increase in epithelial thickness and a significant increase in epithelial cell proliferation in response to low-dose nickel concentrations, and the in vitro results are suggestive of the continuing low-dose nickel release to epithelium as the initiating factor of gingival overgrowth induced by orthodontic treatment [2]). Complete resolution of gingival enlargement developed during orthodontic treatment may not appear even 3–12 months after the removal of the fixed appliances, as reported by Kouraki et al [3].

Therefore, because in the present case the gingival enlargement persisted 4 months after removal of orthodontic appliances and phase 1 therapy, including professional dental cleaning and reinforcement of home care dental hygiene, the surgical excision of excessive gingiva was planned and performed.

External bevel gingivectomy was performed using #15C blades and final reshaping of gingival contours using diamond burs. The postoperative follow-up showed excellent healing as well as a significant improvement in the aesthetic appearance that improved local access for proper oral hygiene. Similar results were described by Benoist et al [4] in two cases of gingival enlargement treated with gingivectomy in young Senegalese women undergoing orthodontic treatment with fixed appliances, with improvement in morphologic conditions of gingiva allowing better plaque control. The same authors emphasized that periodic evaluation of the child and adolescent during orthodontic therapy is required for healthy periodontium and that collaboration between orthodontist and periodontist is one of the most important keys to successful treatment.

Laser gingivectomy has been also pursued for the removal of excessive gingiva in the case of orthodontic treatment-associated gingival enlargement. In a study by Gama et al [5], the effect of the use of the CO_2 laser on the treatment of gingival hyperplasia in orthodontic patients wearing fixed appliances was reported. This study concluded that the use of the CO_2 laser was effective in the treatment of gingival hyperplasia. Additionally, the use of the Nd:YAG and diode laser in the surgical management of soft tissues related to orthodontic treatment, including recontouring of gingival overgrowth, was described in a study by Fornaini et al [6]. The laser-assisted surgery was particularly beneficial due to reported reduced bleeding during surgery with consequent reduced operating time and rapid postoperative hemostasis, thus eliminating the need for sutures, as well as improved postoperative comfort and healing, which make this technique particularly useful for very young patients [6].

In a comparative study of the histologic effects of scalpel, CO_2 laser, electrosurgery, and constant-voltage electrosurgery, incisions were evaluated for mucosal incisions and excisions on a swine model [7]. The results of this study show that the speed of incisions and excisions was fastest with the scalpel and electrosurgery unit, the amount of bleeding was least for electrosurgery and CO_2 laser, and the histologic damage was least with a scalpel, followed by constant-voltage electrosurgery.

Self-Study Questions

A. What is gingivectomy/ gingivoplasty? What are the indications and contraindications for gingivectomy/gingivoplasty?

B. What are the surgical techniques for doing gingivectomy/gingivoplasty?

C. What is the oral hygiene protocol after gingivectomy?

D. What are the expected results and wound healing after gingivectomy?

Answers located at the end of the chapter.

ACKNOWLEDGMENT

The authors thank Dr. Athbi Alquareer, orthodontic resident at Harvard School of Dental Medicine, for referral and collaboration on the case presented in this chapter.

References

1. Holmstrup P. Non-plaque induced gingival lesions. Ann Periodontol 1999;4:20–29.
2. Gursoy UK, Sokucu O, et al. The role of nickel accumulation and epithelial cell proliferation in orthodontic treatment-induced gingival overgrowth. Eur J Orthod 2007;29:555–558.
3. Kouraki E, Bissada NF, et al. Gingival enlargement and resolution during and after orthodontic treatment. N Y State Dent J 2005;71:34–37.
4. Benoist HM, Ngom PI, et al. Gingival hypertrophy during orthodontic treatment: contribution of external bevel gingivectomy. Case report. Odontostomatol Trop 2007; 30(120):42–6.
5. Gama SK, De Araújo TM, et al. 2007 Use of the CO(2) laser on orthodontic patients suffering from gingival hyperplasia. Photomed Laser Surg 2007;25:214–219.
6. Fornaini C, Rocca JP, et al. Nd:YAG and diode laser in the surgical management of soft tissues related to orthodontic treatment. Photomed Laser Surg 2007;25:381–392.
7. Liboon J, Funkhouser W, et al. A comparison of mucosal incisions made by scalpel, CO₂ laser, electrocautery, and constant-voltage electrocautery. Otolaryngol Head Neck Surg 1997;116:379–385.
8. Robicsek S. Ueber das Wesen und Entstehen der Alveolar-Pyorrhoe und deren Behandlung. 1884. The 3rd Annual Report of the Australian Dental Association (reviewed in J Periodontol 1965;36:265).
9. Grant DA, Stern IB, et al. Periodontics in the Tradition of Orban and Gotlieb. 5th ed. St. Louis, MO: Mosby.
10. Goldman HM. Gingivectomy. Oral Surg Oral Med Oral Pathol 1951;4:1136–1157.
11. Mavrogiannis M, Ellis JS, et al. The management of drug-induced gingival overgrowth [review]. J Clin Periodontol 2006;33:434–439.
12. Engler WO, Ramfjord SP, et al. Healing following simple gingivectomy. A tritiated thymidine radiographic study. I. Epithelialization. J Periodontol 1966;37:298–308.
13. Ramfjord SP, Engler SP, et al. A radiographic study of healing following simple gingivectomy. II. The connective tissue. J Peridontol 1966;37:179–189.
14. Listgarten M. Ultrastructure of the dento-gingival junction after gingivectomy. J Periodontal Res 1972;7:151–160.
15. Stahl SS, Witkin G, et al. Gingival healing II. Clinical and histologic repair sequences following gingivectomy. J Periodontol 1968;39:109–118.

TAKE-HOME POINTS

A. The gingivectomy procedure was first recognized by Robicsek [8] (straight incision technique) as an alternative surgical approach to subgingival scaling for pocket therapy. Grant et al later on [9] defined gingivectomy as "the excision of the soft tissue wall of a pathologic periodontal pocket" to eliminate the pocket and restore a physiologic gingival contour.

Gingivoplasty represents reshaping of the gingiva to a so-called physiologic form. Indications for gingivectomy/gingivoplasty are the following:

1. To eliminate gingival pockets – suprabony pockets – that persist after completion of oral hygiene instructions, scaling and root planning, and other disease control measures (Figures 3, 6, and 7)
2. To reduce gingival enlargements resulting from medications or genetic factors (Figure 9)
3. To create clinical crown length for restorative or endodontic purposes when ostectomy is not required (Figure 10)
4. To eliminate soft tissue craters resulting from disease or subsequent to other surgical procedures (Figure 11)
5. To create aesthetic gingival form in cases of delayed passive eruption

Contraindications to the performance of gingivectomy are as follows:

1. Acute inflamed gingiva
2. Inadequate oral hygiene
3. Inadequate keratinized gingiva: pocket depth is located apical to the mucogingival junction
4. Presence of interdental osseous craters and infrabony defects
5. Inadequate depth of vestibule
6. Presence of large exostoses and osseous ledges
7. When removal of the soft tissue would lead to an undesirable aesthetic compromise
8. In case of increased rate of caries that jeopardizes maintenance of dentition

B. Gingivectomy can be performed using the classical external bevel gingivectomy (as described by Goldman in 1951 [10]), internal bevel gingivectomy technique, or distal wedge procedures as well as by the use of electrosurgery, lasers, or chemical gingivectomy. Gingivoplasty can also be performed by using rotary instruments with appropriately shaped coarse diamond stones in addition to using the edge of a round-bladed gingivectomy knife.

External bevel gingivectomy (shown in Figure 6 for a case of dental plaque-induced gingivitis after orthodontic treatment and in Figure 9 for a case of phenytoin-induced gingival enlargement; the clinical case was previously detailed in Chapter 1, Case 4) consists of several steps:

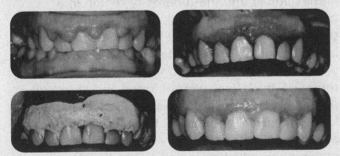

Figure 9: Clinical example of external bevel gingivectomy for phenytoin-induced gingival overgrowth. Frontal view in occlusion before gingivectomy (top left); external bevel gingivectomy in the anterior maxilla (top right); periodontal dressing applied at the end of gingivectomy (bottom left); 1 week after maxillary gingivectomy, after periodontal dressing removal (bottom right).

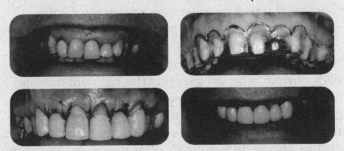

Figure 10: Clinical example of gingivectomy for restorative and aesthetic reasons. Smile at the initial presentation (top left); gingival marking using a vacuum-form template prior to gingivectomy (top right); delivery of temporary prosthesis at the end of gingivectomy (bottom left); smile at delivery of the final restoration #6–11, 5 months post-gingivectomy (bottom right).

- Pocket marking (placement of a series of bleeding points on the outside of the gingiva that correspond to apical extent of the pocket using either the periodontal probe or a mechanical device such as the Crane-Kaplan or Goldman-Fox pocket marker; usually three points are marked per tooth: mid-radicular area, mesial, and distal line angles)
- A primary coronally directed external bevel incision, of about 45 degrees, is next made using an appropriate surgical knife: broad-blade or round-blade gingivectomy knife such as the Goldman-Fox #/8, or Kirkland #5K /16K, or #5/15C blade that starts slightly apical to the "dotted line" created by the bleeding points but always coronal to the mucogingival junction with an internal end point corresponding to the base of the pocket as indicated by the bleeding points
- A secondary interdental incision is made to sever the interproximal portion of the soft tissue pocket using a triangular narrow-blade knife such as the Goldman-Fox 8 or #1 or the Orban #/ 2
- Removal of the excised soft tissue using a Prichard curette or any sharp universal curette provides a surface that is smooth and free of tags
- The exposed root surfaces are examined and instrumented to ensure proper and complete removal of calculus
- After debridement, refinement by gingivoplasty of the margins of the gingiva is performed if needed by means of knives or rotary diamond burs
- Periodontal dressing can be placed over the incised area during the initial period of healing (10–14 days) (Figure 9)

Internal bevel gingivectomy generally begins with a scalloped internal bevel incision placed several millimeters apical to the free gingival margin, following a scalloped contour associated with normal gingival margin. The gingival marking for the incision line can be performed by using a previously vacuum-form template representing the final gingival margins fabricated on the patient's cast as shown in Figure 10 prior to gingivectomy to create clinical crown length for restorative and aesthetic purposes.

In the case of internal bevel gingivectomy, a mucoperiosteal flap is produced that can then be positioned and sutured to cover the alveolar bone

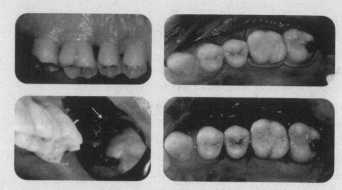

Figure 11: Clinical example of an inverse bevel distal wedge. Palatal preoperative view (top left); outline of the initial scalloped incision and extended into the tuberosity region in a triangular shape (top right); osseous defect from the distal view after removal of the collar of tissue and distal wedge and thorough debridement (bottom left); the flaps positioned and sutured to gain primary closure (bottom right).

(Figure 10, bottom left). This procedure is most frequently referred to as a partial-thickness flap procedure, rather than a true gingivectomy.

The inverse bevel distal wedge technique is usually associated with buccal and palatal inverse bevel access incisions and flap reflection for pocket reduction. Figure 11 is an example of the distal wedge (Mohawk) procedure distal of the second maxillary molar, presenting a preoperative palatal view of the enlarged tuberosity region with excessive probing depth (top left). The procedure included an initial scalloped incision apically to the gingival margin and coronal to mucogingival junction made around the first and second molars and extended into the tuberosity region in a triangular shape (top right). The palatal view shows the underlying bony defect with no distal furcation involvement. Once the distal triangular-shaped wedge was dissected from the underlying bone and removed, thick flaps were thinned and thorough debridement in the area was completed (bottom left). The buccal and palatal flaps are positioned and sutured apically using vertical mattress sutures obtaining a reduction in soft tissue height in the tuberosity region in addition to the palatal and buccal areas of the first and second molars (bottom right). Often this procedure is combined with osteotomy/ostectomy procedures, detailed in Chapter 3, Case 3.

Electrosurgery (reviewed in [11]) and chemical gingivectomy are currently outdated procedures due to delayed healing [7] and poor accuracy in reshaping of gingival tissue, as well as damage to the healthy adjacent hard and soft tissues.

Laser-assisted surgery has been introduced for the treatment of soft tissue, including removal and recontouring of gingiva in case of persistent gingival enlargement of various etiologies. Various types of lasers such as the ND:YAG laser and the CO_2 laser have been used for a variety of intraoral soft tissue procedures, and the overall benefits of laser treatment include reduced bleeding during surgery with consequent reduced operating time and rapid postoperative hemostasis, no need for sutures, and improved postoperative comfort and healing [6,11].

C. The critical period for a complete healing of a gingivectomy wound is between 2 and 5 weeks after the surgery; therefore meticulous oral hygiene is essential for the establishment of a physiologic gingival sulcus [12].

D. The sequence of wound healing process after gingivectomy has been studied by various methods, in both animal models as well as humans. The initial study by Engler et al [12] looking at the epithelialization post-gingivectomy in rhesus monkeys using tritiated thymidine radiography found that migrating epithelial cells start to cover the wound between 12 and 24 hours after surgical excision. Complete healing of the sulcus aspect of the gingivectomy takes 4 to 5 weeks, although the surface appears to be healed after 2 weeks.

Moreover, the same group [13] published a follow-up paper describing the connective tissue aspect of healing and regeneration following simple gingivectomy in three monkeys with histologic and radioautographic techniques. Their results show that connective tissue proliferation is initiated 1–2 days after the surgery and reaches a peak 3–4 days after the surgery. However, functional arrangement and collagenous maturation of the gingival connective tissue fibers as well as the establishment of a physiologic restoration of a gingival crevice, with a sealing normal epithelial attachment that depends on a firm gingival tone, both require 3–5 weeks following gingivectomy.

Similarly, Listgarten [14], using an electron microscopic examination of the dento-gingival junction after gingivectomy in monkeys, found that epithelial reattachment against morphologically normal and superficially altered cementum may occur in ≤12 days after surgical excision.

Another study [15] investigating the clinical and histologic gingival healing in humans following gingivectomy reported that complete surface epithelization of the gingivectomy wound appears within 7–14 days after surgery; still active connective tissue repair was seen 28 days after gingivectomy, the last time point examined after the surgery.

Case 2

Preprosthetic Hard Tissue and Soft Tissue Crown Lengthening

CASE STORY

The patient was a 29-year-old male who had been referred to the Department of Periodontology for an evaluation of the anterior mandibular sextant based on a history of trauma. He had been accidentally hit in the anterior mandible with a racket while playing squash; #24 was extracted subsequently to the accident. His chief complaint was to save and restore as many teeth as possible. Figures 1–4 illustrate the clinical situation at the first periodontal examination.

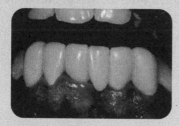

Figure 1: Preoperative condition with the temporary fixed partial denture, facial view.

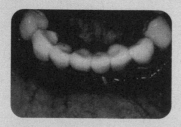

Figure 2: Preoperative condition with the temporary fixed partial denture, occlusal view.

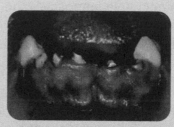

Figure 3: Preoperative condition without the temporary fixed partial denture, facial view.

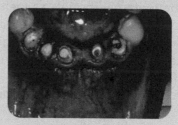

Figure 4: Preoperative condition without the temporary fixed partial denture, occlusal view.

LEARNING GOALS AND OBJECTIVES
■ To identify the indications for crown lengthening
■ To understand the prosthetic needs and periodontal requirements to restore altered teeth
■ To understand key considerations at the time of surgery

Medical History

The patient was healthy and received a medical examination every year. He did not take medications and did not report any allergies or any medical problems.

Review of Systems

- Vital signs
  - Blood pressure: 123/68 mm Hg
  - Pulse rate: 62 beats/minute (regular)

Social History

The patient drank alcohol occasionally. He did not smoke and did not use recreational drugs.

Extraoral Examination

No significant findings were found (Figure 5). The patient had no masses or swelling and the temporomandibular joints were within normal limits.

Intraoral Examination

- The soft tissues of the mouth appeared normal. The oral cancer screen was negative.
- The gingival examination revealed a thick and flat periodontium with generalized mild marginal erythema, rolled margins, and blunted papillae in the mandibular anterior sextant (Figures 1 and 3).
- A hard tissue examination was completed. There was a small amount of sound tooth structure available for the prosthetic restoration of teeth #22, 23, 25, 26, and 27 (Figures 3 and 4).
- The edentulous ridge (site #24) had deformities in the buccolingual and apico/coronal directions (Seibert class 3).

Occlusion

Findings included canine and molar angle class 1, group function on lateral excursion, and incisal guidance in protrusion.

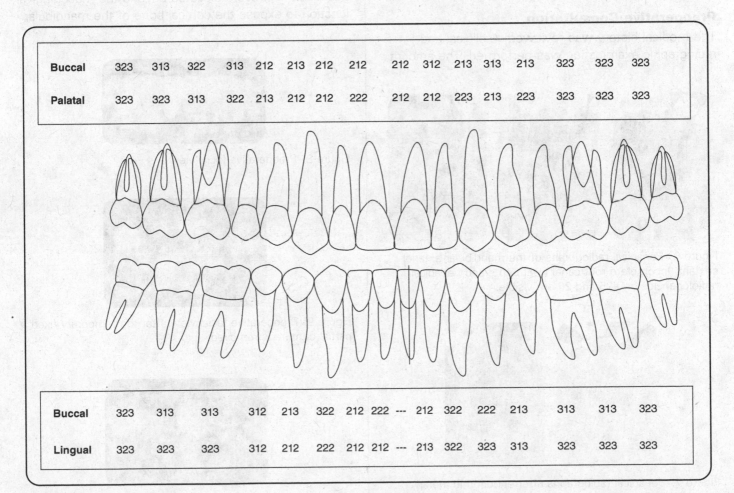

| Buccal | 323 | 313 | 322 | 313 | 212 | 213 | 212 | 212 | 212 | 312 | 213 | 313 | 213 | 323 | 323 | 323 |
| Palatal | 323 | 323 | 313 | 322 | 213 | 212 | 212 | 222 | 212 | 212 | 223 | 213 | 223 | 323 | 323 | 323 |

| Buccal | 323 | 313 | 313 | 312 | 213 | 322 | 212 | 222 | --- | 212 | 322 | 222 | 213 | 313 | 313 | 323 |
| Lingual | 323 | 323 | 323 | 312 | 212 | 222 | 212 | 212 | --- | 213 | 322 | 323 | 313 | 323 | 323 | 323 |

Figure 5: Periodontal charting.

Radiographic Examination

Incomplete root canal treatments on teeth #22, 23, 25, 26, and 27 and periapical radiolucencies on #25 & 26 were observed on the periapical radiographs. There was no horizontal bone loss, the lamina dura was visible and continuous, and bone trabeculations appeared normal (Figure 6).

Treatment Plan

Periodontal, prosthodontic, and endodontic evaluations were performed to assess the restorability of the teeth. The multidisciplinary team deemed the teeth restorable with an endodontic retreatment for teeth #22, 23, 25, 26, and 27, crown lengthening, cast post and core, PFM crowns #22, 27, and a fixed partial denture (FPD) #23-X-25-26.

Treatment

The patient received oral hygiene instructions and a prophylaxis. The endodontic retreatments were performed (Figure 7), and a temporary FPD #22-23-X-25-26-27 was fabricated (Figure 8).

Preoperative Consultation

The medical history was reviewed. A clinical and radiographic examination was performed. The amount of sound tooth structure present in the mandibular anterior sextant supragingivally was inadequate, and there was a lack of ferrule (Figure 3); the restorative margins were subgingival in some areas and were impinging on the biologic width (Figure 4). Upon radiographic examinations (Figure 6), the periodontal support for the incisors and canines was sufficient and could tolerate 3 mm of ostectomy.

The consent form addressing benefits and risks associated with the procedure was reviewed with the patient. Preoperative prescriptions were delivered to the patient: Ibuprofen 600 mg (every 4–6 hours for pain as needed) and Peridex 0.12% (bid).

Crown Lengthening Procedure

Bilateral mental nerve blocks and local infiltrations were achieved with lidocaine 2% (epinephrine 1/100,000). The temporary FPD was removed (Figures 8 and 9). A submarginal incision was performed around #22, 23, 25, 26, and 27 (Figure 10) to achieve 2–3 mm of gingivectomy (Figure 11). Buccal and lingual full-thickness flaps were elevated beyond the mucogingival junction to expose the cortical bone of the mandibular

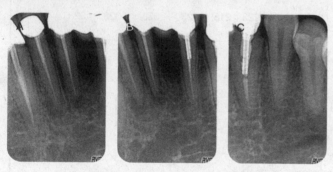

Figure 6: Periapical radiographs of the mandibular anterior sextant. Incomplete root canal treatments and periapical radiolucencies on #25 and 26 are visible.

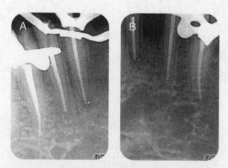

Figure 7: Periapical radiographs after endodontic therapy. Courtesy Dr. Fiza Singh.

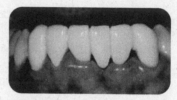

Figure 8: Preoperative facial view.

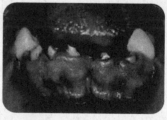

Figure 9: Preoperative facial view after the temporary fixed partial denture is removed.

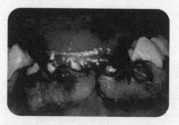

Figure 10: Submarginal incisions.

anterior sextant (Figure 12). Ostectomy was carried out to expose at least 4 mm of sound tooth structure above the crestal bone and allow for 2 mm of biologic width and at least 1.5 mm of ferrule. Osteoplasty allowed the removal of widow's peaks, ledges, and bony irregularities (Figure 13). Odontoplasty was performed as needed when the embrasure space was too narrow (Figures 14 and 15). The buccal and lingual flaps were apically positioned and stabilized with vertical mattress sutures (Figure 16). The temporary

FPD was cemented back (Figure 17). Postoperative instructions including oral hygiene instructions were delivered and an ice pack was placed against the patient's lip.

The patient was seen for a postoperative consultation 7 days and 21 days after the procedure. The prosthetic margins were refined 8 weeks after surgery, cast post and core (Figures 18 and 19) and final restorations (Figure 20) were cemented 3 weeks later.

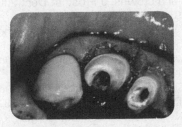

Figure 11: Gingivectomy.

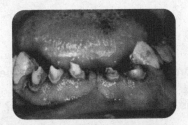

Figure 12: A full-thickness flap is elevated and cortical bone is exposed.

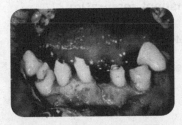

Figure 13: Ostectomy and osteoplasty allow a greater exposure of sound tooth structure.

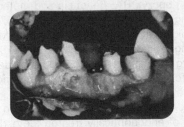

Figure 14: The embrasure between #21 and 22 is narrow.

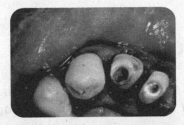

Figure 15: Odontoplasty of the distal surface of #22 is performed to open the embrasure between #21 and 22.

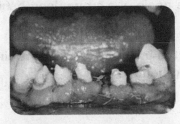

Figure 16: The flaps are apically positioned and stabilized with vertical mattress sutures.

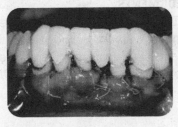

Figure 17: The temporary FPD is cemented back.

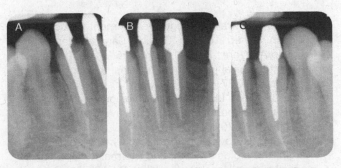

Figure 18: Periapical radiographs after cementation of the final cast post and core. Courtesy Dr. Priyank Taneja.

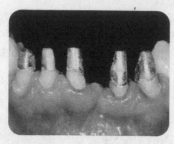

Figure 19: Final cast post and core. Courtesy Dr. Priyank Taneja.

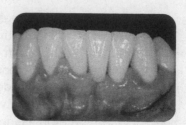

Figure 20: Permanent FPD.

Self-Study Questions

A. What are the components of the attachment apparatus of a tooth? What does "biologic width" mean?

B. What is the definition of crown lengthening? What are the goals of a crown lengthening procedure?

C. What are the indications and contraindications of crown lengthening?

D. How do you perform a crown lengthening?

E. How does a crown lengthening heal?

F. How does the gingival contour reestablish? How long after crown lengthening should a tooth receive permanent restoration?

Answers located at the end of the chapter.

ACKNOWLEDGMENTS

Thanks to Dr. Priyank Taneja, Department of Prosthodontics, Harvard School of Dental Medicine, and Dr. Fiza Singh, Department of Endodontics, Harvard School of Dental Medicine.

References

1. Ten Cate AR. Oral Histology Development, Structure and Function. 3rd ed. Toronto, Ontario, Canada: Mosby, 1989.
2. Gargiulo A, Wentz F, et al. Dimensions and relations of the dentogingival junction in humans. J Periodontol 1961;32:261–267.
3. Ingber JS, Rose LF, et al. The "biologic width" – a concept in periodontics and restorative dentistry. Alpha Omegan 1977;70:62–65.
4. Nevins M, Skurow HM. The intracrevicular restorative margin, the biologic width, and the maintenance of the gingival margin. Int J Periodontics Restorative Dent 1984;3:31–49.
5. Rose LF, Mealey BL, et al. Periodontics: Medicine, Surgery, and Implants. St. Louis, MO: Mosby, 2004. pp424–464.
6. Palomo F, Kopczyk RA. Rationale and methods for crown lengthening. J Am Dent Assoc 1978;96:257–260.
7. Assif D. Pilo R, et al. Restoring teeth following crown lengthening procedures. J Prosthet Dent 1991;65:624.
8. Wagenberg B. Eskow R, et al. Exposing adequate tooth structure for restorative dentistry. Int J Periodontics Restorative Dent 1989;9:323–331.
9. Sorensen JA, Engelman MJ. Ferrule design and fracture resistance of endodontically treated teeth. J Prosthet Dent 1990;63:529–536.
10. Gegauff AG. Effect of the crown lengthening and ferrule placement on static load failure of cemented cast post-cores and crowns. J Prosthet Dent 2000; 84:169–179.
11. Coslet JG, Vanarsdall R, et al. Diagnosis and classification of delayed passive eruption of the dentogingival junction in the adult. Alpha Omegan 1977;70;24–28.
12. Allen EP. Surgical crown lengthening for function and esthetics. Dent Clin North Am 1993;37:163–179.
13. Friedman N. Periodontal osseous surgery: osteoplasty and ostectomy. J Periodontology 1955:26: 257.

14. Ochsenbein C. A primer for osseous surgery. Int J Periodontics Restorative Dent 1986;6:8–47.

15. Ivey DW, Calhoun RN, et al. Orthodontic extrusion: its use in restorative dentistry. J Prosthet Dent 1980; 43;401.

16. Lanning SK, Waldrop TC, et al. Surgical crown lengthening: evaluation of the biological width. J Periodontol 2003;74:468–474.

17. Caton JG, Zander HA. The attachment between tooth and gingival tissues after periodic root planing and soft tissue curettage. J Periodontol 1979;50:462–466

18. Waerhaug J. Healing of the dento-epithelial junction following subgingival plaque control. II. As observed on extracted teeth. J Periodontol 1978;49:119–134.

19. Van Der Velden U. Regeneration of the interdental soft tissues following denudation procedures. J Clin Periodontol 1982;9:455–459.

20. Carnevale G, Sterrantino S, et al. Soft and hard tissue wound healing following tooth preparation to the alveolar crest. Int J Periodontics Restorative Dent 1983;3:37–53.

21. Oakley E, Rhyu IC, et al. Formation of the biologic width following crown lengthening in nonhuman primate. Int J Periodontics Restorative Dent 1999; 19:529–541.

22. Schluger S. Osseous resection – a basic principle in periodontal surgery. Oral Surg Oral Med Oral Pathol 1949;2:316–325.

23. Levine H, Stahl S. Repair following periodontal flap surgery with the retention of gingival fibers. J Periodontol 1972;43:W-103.

24. Lindhe J, Socransky SS, et al. Dimensional alteration of the periodontal tissues following therapy. Int J Periodontics Restorative Dent 1987;7:9–21.

25. Kaldahl WB, Kalkwarf KL, et al. Long-term evaluation of periodontal therapy: I. Response to 4 therapeutic modalities. J Periodontol 1996;67:93–102.

26. Pontoriero R, Carnevale J. Surgical crown lengthening: A 12-month clinical wound healing study. J Periodontol 2001;72:841–848.

27. Bragger U, Lauchenauer D: Surgical lengthening of the crown. J Clin Periodontol 1992;19:58–63.

28. Listgarten MA. Periodontal tissue repair over surgically exposed dentin and cementum surfaces [abstract 473]. Int Ass Dent Res, 49th General Meeting, 1971.

TAKE-HOME POINTS

A. The attachment apparatus of a human tooth [1] (Figure 21) is composed of these elements:
1. An epithelial attachment that attaches the enamel surface with hemidesmosomes
2. A connective tissue attachment made of type 1 collagen fibers and Sharpey fibers inserting into the cementum at a 90° angle
3. Alveolar bone covered by bundle bone in its inner surface and periosteum on it outer surface
4. A periodontal ligament with type 1 and 3 collagen fiber bundles and Sharpey fibers inserted in the alveolar bone and the cementum
5. Cementum overlaying dentin on the root surface. Gargiulo and coworkers [2] found a great consistency in the distance located between the bone alveolar crest and the bottom of the sulcus in human dentitions. They called this area of the attachment apparatus of the tooth the dentogingival junction, made of an epithelial attachment coronally and a connective tissue attachment apically. Their study determined an average dimension of 0.97 mm for the epithelial attachment and 1.07 mm for the connective tissue attachment. The combined dimension of these two structures was called thereafter "biologic width" [3] and averages 2.04 mm according to the findings of Gargiulo et al [2]. Nevins and Skurow [4] include the space occupied by the gingival sulcus (at least 1 mm) in addition to the epithelial and connective tissue attachment space and therefore estimate that biologic width measures a minimum of 3 mm.

B. The goals of the crown lengthening procedure include increasing the dimension of the clinical crown, maintaining or recreating favorable periodontal conditions, establishing appropriate biologic width, creating adequate ferrule effect for anterior teeth, and aid in the overall delivery of

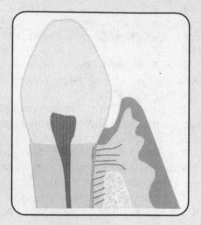

Figure 21: The attachment apparatus of a human tooth.

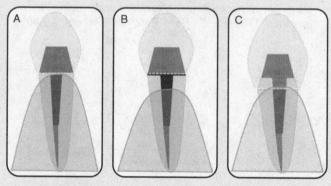

Figure 22: (A) Initial situation: inadequate prosthetic margin, lack of prosthetic retention. (B) A crown lengthening is performed; some sound tooth structure is exposed. (C) Final situation: The prosthetic margin is moved apically, adequate retention is provided, and the biologic width is preserved

prosthetic restorations. There are two types of crown lengthening: functional and aesthetic.

Functional crown lengthening is indicated when the clinical crown is too short to provide sufficient retention for an overlying crown [5] (Figure 22A). In the absence of crown lengthening, the restorative margin will impinge on the biologic width and produce an inflammatory response, resulting in loss of bone and connective tissue attachment as well as apical migration of the epithelial attachment. The goal of the crown lengthening procedure is to expose more sound tooth structure when wear, caries, or fracture have altered tooth integrity [3,4,6] (Figure 22B). As a result, the prosthetic margin can be placed supragingivally or intrasulcularly, enhancing the quality of the

restoration and facilitating access for oral hygiene (Figure 22C). To achieve this objective, a space of at least 3 mm must be created between the preparation margin and the alveolar bony crest; 2 mm are devoted to the reestablishment of the biologic width, and 1 mm of intrasulcular tooth structure is available for crown retention. Many authors advocate the exposure of further tooth surface (4–5 mm) to provide more retention for the restoration [7,8]. In addition, it has been described that the presence of ≥2 mm of tooth structure available for the prosthetic crown to encircle is beneficial to the structural integrity of the tooth. This so-called ferrule effect improves fracture resistance of endodontically treated anterior teeth [9,10] (Figure 22C).

This ferrule effect is needed for anterior teeth that have an extra component that make the tooth a two-piece unit instead of a one piece, such as a core or a post and a core. This 2 mm of solid tooth structure beneath the core will help direct the forces of occlusion toward the periodontal ligament and reduce the stress on the post or core interface, thus preventing the cement fatigue of the restoration and the dislodgment over time (Figure 22A–C)

Aesthetic crown lengthening has a cosmetic goal. It is performed in the following situations:
1. Short clinical crowns. In that situation, the periodontium and the skeletal bases are normal. The tooth is shorter because of attrition. Sometimes the tooth keeps on erupting as wear reduces its length. Therefore, the width of keratinized tissue continuously increases and results in an excessive gingival display that can be corrected by aesthetic crown lengthening [5]. However, if eruption does not happen in conjunction of attrition, a loss of vertical dimension will occur. In that situation, a restorative treatment restoring the vertical dimension will be indicated and a crown lengthening of a functional rather than an aesthetic nature will be required.
2. Excessive gingival display in the aesthetic area (also called "gummy smile"). It can be caused by delayed passive eruption when the attachment apparatus fails to establish properly around the tooth [11]. The clinical crown can appear too short because of an excess of

keratinized gingiva when the attachment apparatus is positioned too coronally on the anatomic crown or when the two phenomena are combined.

Gingival enlargement induced by medications (such as calcium channel blockers, phenytoin, and cyclosporine among others) or orthodontic treatment can be surgically managed once the etiology is corrected (replacement of the medication, removal of braces). These situations are managed most of the time with gingivectomy without bone recontouring, the goal of which is both aesthetic and functional. Excessive gingival display caused by hereditary gingival fibromatosis and vertical maxillary excess can also be treated with aesthetic crown lengthening, although it might not be sufficient to entirely treat the problem. For instance, vertical maxillary excess most of the time requires orthognathic surgery in addition to crown lengthening.

C. Crown lengthening is indicated in the following situations [1,2]:
1. Caries extending under the gingival line. Crown lengthening will provide better access to remove caries and will simplify the restoration (i.e., having a dry field for bonding, having an intrasulcular or supragingival prosthetic margin).
2. Tooth fracture. The amount of tooth structure left might be nonsufficient for retention of the restorative material or the crown.
3. Existing restoration impinging on the biologic width. The violation of biologic width generates chronic inflammation that leads to periodontal ligament destruction. Space must be recreated for the establishment of the epithelial and connective tissue attachment and crown retention.
4. Lack of available tooth structure for prosthetic retention or lack of ferrule effect.
5. Improved aesthetic in the presence of short clinical crowns or excessive gingival display. There is not necessarily a functional need.

Crown lengthening is contraindicated in the following situations [12]:
1. Nonrestorable tooth.
2. Unfavorable crown-to-root ratio. This would compromise the long-term prognosis

of the tooth and increase the risk of tooth fracture (blunted roots, history of apicoectomies).
3. Root proximity. It mainly concerns the interproximal space between the first and second maxillary molar where the distobuccal root of the first molar can be closely located to the mesiobuccal root of the second molar. A thin amount of interproximal bone makes ostectomy nonfeasible and increases the chance of damaging the integrity of both roots.
4. Exposure of the furcation for multirooted teeth. If the ostectomy generates a furcation involvement, the long-term prognosis of the tooth is compromised. An alternative approach such as root resection or tooth hemisection should be considered.
5. Improper oral hygiene and lack of patient cooperation.

D. Crown lengthening can be performed in two different ways:
1. Surgical crown lengthening:
   a. A preoperative consultation is performed to review the patient's past medical history, detect contraindications to surgery, and determine the restorability of the tooth. Clinical and radiographic findings will allow the practitioner to determine the amount of crown lengthening needed. The tooth should ideally be prepared and have a temporary restoration to better evaluate the final prosthetic margin (Figure 23A). Premedication (antibiotics, sedative, analgesic medication) should be prescribed as needed.
   b. Surgical procedure: The temporary restoration is removed and the excess of cement washed away. An intrasulcular or submarginal incision is performed to the crestal bone (submarginal incision is preferred in the presence of adequate amount of keratinized tissue). A vertical releasing incision might be considered to enhance surgical access. Then a full-thickness flap is elevated to expose the cortical bone; soft tissue tags are removed if present (Figure 23B). The distance from the crestal bone to the prosthetic margin is measured to determine where and how much ostectomy is needed (removal of the

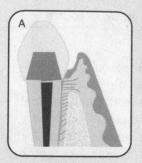 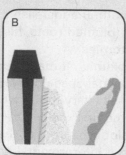 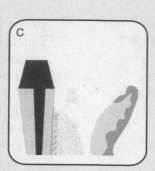 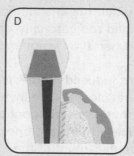 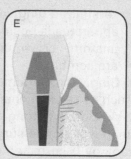

Figure 23: (A) Preoperative situation: inadequate prosthetic margin, lack of prosthetic retention. (B) A full thickness flap is elevated, cortical bone is exposed. (C) Ostectomy is performed to expose adequate sound tooth structure. (D) The flap is apically repositioned. (E) Final restoration. The epithelial and connective tissue attachment is reestablished. The prosthetic margin stands on sound tooth structure with adequate retention.

supporting bone next to a tooth). Ostectomy is performed with an end-cutting bur or bone chisels so that the desired amount of tooth structure is exposed (see question B) (Figure 23C). One should make sure that a positive architecture (buccal and/or lingual margin of bone apical to the proximal margin of bone) is maintained or reestablished to prevent pocket formation [13,14]. An osteoplasty (removal of nonsupporting bone) is most of the time needed to remove "widow's peaks" and recreate a bony contour favorable to a healthy gingival architecture. Exposed root surfaces should be scaled and root planed. The flap is eventually apically positioned or repositioned at the level of the new bone crest and sutured with vertical mattress sutures that will prevent the movement of the flap on a mesiodistal or apico/coronal direction. The temporary crown is cemented back on the tooth (Figure 23D). A surgical dressing (such as Coe-Pak) can be placed over the surgical site.

c. Postoperative care: Postoperative instructions (including oral hygiene instructions) are delivered to the patient and an ice pack is placed adjacent to the surgical site. Pain medications (ibuprofen or acetaminophen) and a 0.12% Chlorhexidine mouthwash are prescribed. Antibiotics can also be prescribed, although they are not mandatory for a healthy patient. The patient should be seen for a postoperative visit and suture removal at 7 to 10 days postsurgery and before the final prosthetic restoration (Figure 23E).

2. Orthodontic extrusion [15]: A bracket is bonded on the crown and vertical forces are applied to force the eruption of the tooth until the appropriate amount of supragingival tooth structure is exposed. This technique is mainly used in the maxillary anterior sextant to preserve the gingival contour.

E. Evidence has shown that biologic width reestablishes after crown lengthening in about 6 months [16]. However, the biologic mechanisms involved in the recreation of epithelial and connective tissue attachment after a periodontal flap surgery is still not completely understood. There is large consensus regarding reestablishment of the epithelial attachment: a long junctional epithelium will form along the root-planed surface to the apical level of root planing [17,18]. Reestablishment of the connective tissue attachment is more controversial. Some authors believe it reforms coronal to the apical level of root planing [19], whereas some others consider it recreates apical to the apical level of root planing by crestal resorption of the alveolar bone [20,21]. This divergence in opinion explains why some authors expose more tooth structure above the crestal bone than others.

In any situation, general principles of osseous resective surgery should be applied to prevent pocket formation [13,22]. Recreation of a positive architecture and a scalloped bony contour without ledges, notches, and peaks will allow appropriate soft tissue healing. Widows' peaks should be removed carefully, and the root surface should be root-planed thoroughly to prevent too coronal an attachment apparatus reattachment [23] that might require retreatment [21].

F. It has been described that the gingival margin tends to move coronally over a year after a flap procedure with bone recontouring [24,25] and crown lengthening [19] to eventually stabilize in this position [25]. Pontoriero et al [26] described in a human study a 3-mm coronal displacement of the gingival margin after 1 year, with most of the coronal displacement occurring within the first month of healing (about 2mm). Gingival displacement is influenced by multiple parameters including gingival biotype and the magnitude of ostectomy performed [16]. Bragger et al [27] do not observe the coronal displacement of the gingival margin over time in most cases and report that the gingival margin position remains stable from 6 weeks to 6 months.

As a consequence, a healing period of time should be respected before final prosthetic restoration to allow the gingival contour to reestablish and stabilize. The final restoration should not be performed sooner than 6 weeks postsurgery to allow stabilization of the gingival margin [27] and to obtain the repair of the attachment apparatus [28]. In certain situations, such as the presence of a thin gingival biotype or an aesthetic area, more time might be needed to observe the gingival margin stabilization and proceed with the permanent restoration [26,27].

Case 3

Flap Osseous Surgery

CASE STORY

The patient was a 34-year-old female who presented to the Department of Endodontics for assessment of a painful tooth. Following examination a periodontal consult was requested. Before this appointment she had been seen regularly for hygiene appointments at a community dental clinic (Figure 1).

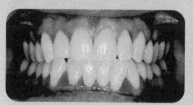 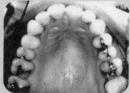

Figure 1: Initial photographs.

LEARNING GOALS AND OBJECTIVES

■ To diagnose severe periodontal disease and identify the indications for flap osseous surgery (FOS) as opposed to other surgical techniques

■ To identify preoperatively any conditions that may compromise the final outcome of this procedure

■ To be introduced to a surgical technique used to perform FOS.

Medical History

The patient was in good health. She indicated that as a child she had been diagnosed with a heart murmur. A recent examination by her physician had revealed that the murmur was no longer audible; thus no antibiotic prophylaxis was required. A mild allergic reaction to penicillin recently indicated sensitivity to this drug class. She suffered from seasonal allergies and a mild form of asthma for which she did not take any medication. For several months she had been dealing with mild to moderate anxiety.

Review of Systems

- Vital signs
  - Blood pressure: 128/75 mm Hg
  - Pulse rate: 70 beats/minute (regular)

Social History

The patient did not drink alcohol or use recreational drugs. She exercised regularly and was a nonsmoker.

Extraoral Examination

No major significant findings were discovered. The patient had no masses or swelling, and the health of the temporomandibular joints was within normal limits. Mild tenderness of the left masseter and temporalis muscles were recorded (Figure 2).

Intraoral Examination

- The soft tissues of the mouth including tongue and floor of the mouth appeared normal. The oral cancer screen was negative.
- The gingival examination revealed generalized mild to moderate marginal erythema with areas of severe

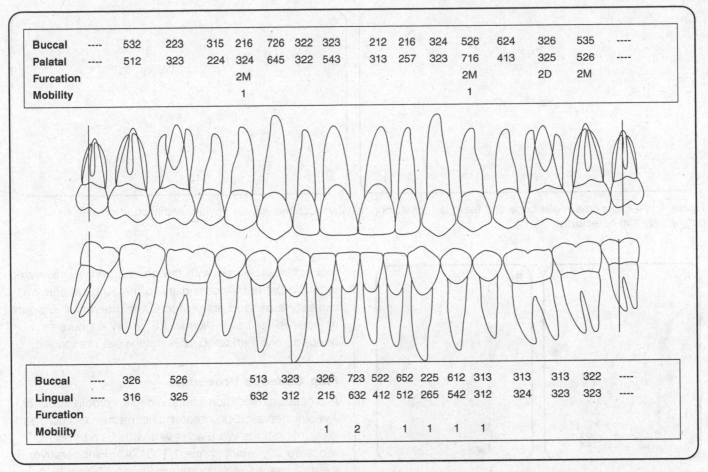

Buccal	----	532	223	315	216	726	322	323	212	216	324	526	624	326	535	----
Palatal	----	512	323	224	324	645	322	543	313	257	323	716	413	325	526	----
Furcation					2M							2M		2D	2M	
Mobility						1							1			

Buccal	----	326	526	513	323	326	723	522	652	225	612	313	313	313	322	----
Lingual	----	316	325	632	312	215	632	412	512	265	542	312	324	323	323	----
Furcation																
Mobility						1	2		1	1	1	1				

Figure 2: Probing pocket depth measurements (following phase 1 therapy).

inflammation. Bleeding on probing was generalized and significant.
- A hard tissue examination was negative for caries.
- A mild generalized discomfort on percussion of the teeth was noted.

Occlusion

The patient's occlusion was considered class I with no occlusal interferences evident. Crowding of the mandibular anterior teeth was recorded. Mutually protected occlusion was evident on examination (Figure 3).

Treatment Plan

Recommendations were made to the patient to follow up with her primary care physician regarding her anxiety. Our concern was not only for her mental well-being but also for her clenching and poor oral hygiene that could be a result of this condition. A

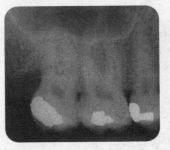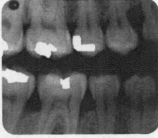

Figure 3: Preoperative radiographic evaluation (periapical and bite wing in the maxillary right quadrant).

transitional night guard was provided to the patient and was ultimately replaced with a permanent one following treatment. Endodontic consultations were required to establish a comprehensive treatment plan. Full-mouth radiographs and plaque accumulation analysis (disclosing solution) were performed.

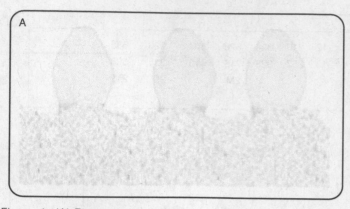

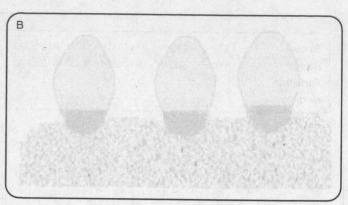

Figure 4: (A) Exposed alveolar bone and teeth demonstrating negative architecture. (B) Positive architecture created by osteoplasty and ostectomy.

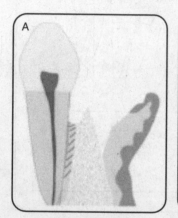

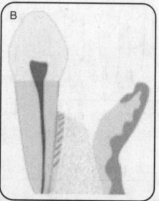

Figure 5: (A) Exposed alveolar bone demonstrating sharp, irregular peaks. (B) smoothing of the irregular bone structure to provide an environment that promotes pocket reduction.

The final treatment plan included extensive periodontal surgical treatment as well as protecting the teeth and periodontium from occlusal trauma (Figures 4 and 5).

Treatment

This patient received oral hygiene instruction and two complete scaling and root planning sessions before surgical therapy. A transitional occlusal protective appliance (acrylic) was provided. The patient was reevaluated to determine the effectiveness of phase 1 therapy and to see if she demonstrated good oral hygiene practices. Pocket depths were recorded following phase 1 therapy. Surgical therapy then began.

Preoperative Consultation

The medical history was reviewed. Her blood pressure was monitored. The consent form addressing benefits and risks associated with the procedure was reviewed with the patient. Accessibility to the surgical site was clinically assessed. Ibuprofen 600 mg (every 4–6 hours as needed for pain), Vicodin ES (every 6 hours as needed), and Peridex 0.12% (bid) were prescribed.

Flap Osseous Procedure

A procedural sedation and analgesia, middle superior alveolar nerve block, greater palatine nerve block, and local infiltrations were achieved with 5 mg Valium, lidocaine 2% (epinephrine 1/100,000). Preoperative view of tissues is illustrated in Figure 6A and B. A submarginal incision was made in a scalloped fashion in all interproximal regions (Figure 6C and D). A full-thickness flap in the maxillary right quadrant was elevated buccal and palatal from mesial of tooth #6 to distal of #2 (Figure 6E and F). The teeth in this region were thoroughly scaled and root planed. Complete degranulation of all bony defects followed. A rotary finishing burr was used to reduce the concavity of the furcation on mesial tooth #5 and conservatively recontour surrounding bone to produce a positive architecture (Figures 6G–J). A distal wedge procedure was performed on tooth #2 (Figure 6K). The surgical site was thoroughly rinsed with sterile saline and the flap was reapproximated and then sutured (Figure 6L). External vertical mattress sutures were placed to apical position the tissue. Healing was uneventful thereafter.

Discussion

FOS is a predictable procedure to reduce pocket depths and provide a healthy "positive" architecture to the surrounding bone and tissue so the patient now can access these sites for cleaning.

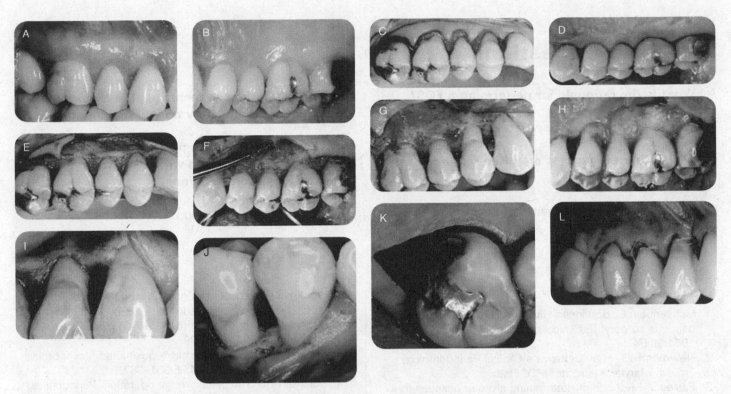

Figure 6: Intraoral surgical photos.

Healthy "positive" architecture can be defined as follows: when alveolar bone is consistently more coronal on the interproximal surfaces than on the facial and lingual surface and there exists a smooth, flowing alveolar bone anatomy such that the interproximal surfaces are flat leading to a spillway buccally and lingually. This technique is most appropriate for patients with early to moderate bone loss (2–3 mm) with moderate-length root trunks [1] that have bony defects with one or two walls. Patients with deep intrabony defects are not candidates for FOS. To achieve this positive architecture in these situations, so much bone would have to be removed that the survival of the teeth could be compromised [2]. The surgery was uneventful. The patient was seen for postoperative visits at 1 week to remove the sutures and at 6 weeks. She did not complain of significant postoperative tooth sensitivity that may occur due to the exposure of root cementum. Following 3 months

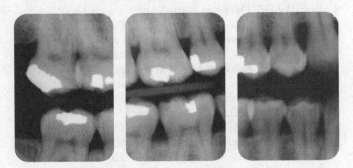

Figure 7: Postoperative periapical radiographs following 6 months of healing.

of healing, a permanent acrylic night guard was provided for the patient.

After 6 months, periapical and bite-wing radiographs were taken to assess this region (Figure 7). Because regenerative periodontal procedures were performed elsewhere, the radiographs allowed us to assess these areas as well (i.e., opposing arch).

Self-Study Questions

A. What is the rationale for performing a FOS?

B. What techniques are used?

C. What other procedures are often required at the time of the FOS?

D. What are the determinants of success of FOS?

E. What alterations in technique are required due to unique anatomy? How do you manage these?

F. What are the possible postoperative complications associated with FOS? How do you manage these complications?

Answers located at the end of the chapter.

References

1. Ochsenbein C, Bohannan HM. The palatal approach to osseous surgery. II. Clinical application. J Periodontol 1964;35:54.
2. Newman MG, et al. Carranza's Clinical Periodontology. 3rd ed. Maryland Heights, MO: Elsevier.
3. Easley J. Methods of determining alveolar osseous form. J Periodontol 1967;38:112.
4. Kaldahl WB, Kalkwarf KL, et al. Long-term evaluation of periodontal therapy. I. Response to four therapeutic modalities. J Periodontol 1996;67:93.
5. Selipsky HS. Osseous surgery: how much need we compromise? Dent Clin North Am 1976;20:79.
6. Tibbetts L, Ochsenbein C, et al. The lingual approach to osseous surgery, J Periodontol 1976;20:61.
7. Kaldahl WB, Kalkwarf KL, et al. Evaluation of four modalities of periodontal therapy: mean probing depth, probing attachment level and recession changes, J Periodontol 1988;59:783.
8. Knowles J, Burgett F, et al. Results of periodontal treatment related to pocket depth and attachment level: eight years. J Periodontol 1979;50:225.
9. Schluger S. Osseous resection – a basic principle in periodontal surgery. Oral Surg 1949;2:316–325.
10. Goldman H, Cohen D. The intrabony pocket: classification and treatment. J Periodontol 1958; 29:272–291.
11. Friedman N. Periodontal osseous surgery: osteoplasty and osteoectomy, J Periodontol 1955;26:257.
12. Nabers CL. Repositioning the attached gingiva. J Periodontol 1954;25:38–39.
13. Donnenfeld OW. The apically repositioned flap: a clinical study. J Periodontol 1964;35:381–387.
14. Robinson RE. The distal wedge operation. Periodontics 1966;4:256–264.
15. Nyman S, Lindhe J, et al. Periodontal surgery in plaque-infected dentitions. J Clin Periodontol 1977;4:240–249.
16. Froum SJ, Coran M, et al. Periodontal healing following open debridement flap procedures. I. Clinical assessment of soft tissue and osseous repair. J Periodontol 1982;53:8–14.
17. Black GV. Surgical treatment of pockets. In: Black AD, ed. Special Dental Pathology. 3rd ed. Chicago, IL: Medico Dental, 1917.
18. Garguilo AW, Wentz FM, et al. Dimensions and relations of the dentogingival junction in humans. J Periodontol 1961;32:261.
19. Ochsenbein C, Bohannan HM. The palatal approach to osseous surgery. I. Rationale. J Periodontol 1963;34:60–68.
20. Sachs HA, Farnoush A, et al. Current status of periodontal dressings. J Periodontol 1984;55:689–696.

TAKE-HOME POINTS

A. Inflammatory periodontal disease if left untreated will lead to destruction of the tooth-supporting bone. The deformities are rarely uniform and can vary in severity and location from one tooth to the next. As can be appreciated from the images, the soft tissue architecture does not necessarily have to follow the bone architecture. Bone loss can be classified as "horizontal," "vertical," and/or a combination of both. The severity, morphology, and position of the defect will determine the technique of FOS and whether or not regenerative therapy (guided tissue regeneration) should be considered.

Ultimately this loss of bone leads to deep pockets, which then become a harbor for pathogenic bacteria that the patient is unable to access. It has been also suggested that the change in the normal anatomy of the alveolar bone predispose patients to the recurrence of pocket depth postsurgically [3]. To achieve the desired result of pocket depth reduction, this technique is usually combined with apical flap repositioning.

In summary, FOS provides pocket depth reduction, access for surgeons to clean diseased areas, and a positive bone and soft tissue architecture that enhances the ability of the site to be cleaned [4–6]. The literature fully supports the fact that FOS is the most predictable pocket reduction technique [4,7,8].

B. Schluger first introduced the original technique that outlines the surgical principles of FOS in 1949 [9]. Prior to this, gingivectomy was the preferred surgical method of dealing with deep pockets.

Goldman and Cohen first classified types of infrabony osseous defects according to the number of remaining walls: three, two, or one osseous walls and combinations thereof [10]. In combination defects they determined that the apical parts may have more walls than coronal parts. This classification now allows us to communicate the severity of the infrabony defect and assign the most successful treatment for each category. Variations of this technique have been introduced since then and include lingual ramping of the bone

in the posterior mandible [6] and palatal ramping in the posterior maxilla [1].

Bone manipulation in FOS involves osteoplasty and ostectomy [11]. Osteoplasty refers to reshaping the bone without removing tooth-supporting bone. Ostectomy includes the removal of tooth-supporting bone. One or both of these procedures may be required for optimal outcomes.

The technique of osseous recontouring involves four basic steps: vertical grooving, radicular blending, flattening of interdental bone, and ostectomy [2].

1. Vertical grooving is the first step of the resective process. It provides continuity from the interproximal surface onto the radicular surface. This step is usually performed with rotary instruments, such as round carbide burs or diamonds.
2. Radicular blending, the second step of the osseous reshaping technique, is an attempt to gradualize the bone over the entire radicular surface. This provides a smooth, blended surface for good flap adaptation.
3. Flattening of the interdental bone is indicated when interproximal bone levels vary horizontally.
4. The final step is ostectomy. Bone removal is minimal but necessary to provide a sound regular base for the gingival tissue to follow. This step involves the removal of small bony discrepancies on the gingival line angles of teeth (widow's peaks).

Following osseous recontouring the open flaps should be thoroughly rinsed with sterile saline and the flaps apically repositioned [12,13] (Figure 17).

Healing of the surgical site is usually uneventful. Normally the flaps attach to the underlying bone in 14–21 days [2]. Maturation and remodeling can continue for up to 6 months. The literature supports the idea that 6 weeks of healing should pass before beginning dental restorations [2].

C. Depending on the severity of the bone defect and the amount of remaining keratinized gingiva, a scalloped submarginal incision is made to remove the excess gingival tissue and thus prevent pocket reformation. Usually this is required on the palatal aspects of maxillary teeth where apical repositioning is not possible.

Excess connective tissue is often removed from this region as well to facilitate closer adaptation of the tissues to the tooth.

A third procedure often required in this region is the distal wedge [14]. The objectives of this treatment are to obtain access the bone, to preserve and use attached gingival tissue, to eliminate the pocket by wound closure, to decrease the healing period, and to minimize periodontal pocket recurrence of any proximal periodontal pocket (Figure 16). The three classical distal wedge operations include the triangular, the square, and the linear. Each has its own indication but essentially differs on the quantity of attached gingival that is removed [14].

If it has been determined that the vertical defect is too severe for treatment with FOS, other treatment modalities may have to be added to the procedure to facilitate ideal treatment. One may want to consider a regenerative procedure or a resective procedure, such as gross total resection, root resection, or hemisection procedure, if a particular root is not salvageable or furcation involvement is severe. If the bone loss is too severe, extraction of the tooth may be the only option.

D. Some determinants promoting success have been reported in the literature, as follows:

1. Absence of medical conditions (including systemic diseases, bisphosphonate therapy, irradiation, and smoking. The patient should be referred to a physician if there is any significant medical condition reported during the preoperative examination.
2. Appropriate patient and site selection are essential for predicable long-term success of FOS. Thorough debridement of granulation tissue as well as appropriate handling of the hard and soft tissue is critical.
3. Even if all the surgical principles are closely adhered to, if the patient is not competent with oral hygiene practices, this treatment is likely to fail. A study by Nyman et al covered postoperative results of treatment following five methods of surgical pocket elimination in

patients that were not recalled for maintenance [15]. In patients who were unable to meet the requirements for proper oral hygiene, treatment of periodontitis failed irrespective of the surgical technique used for pocket elimination. Other studies looking at the role plaque control plays in the predictability of FOS support these finding [16].

E. However, more than any other surgical technique, osseous resective surgery is performed at the expense of bony tissue and attachment levels [2,17,18]. If excessive bone is removed to facilitate a positive architecture, no remediation for this error exists. The patient may then experience significant root sensitivity and mobility. As mentioned earlier, studies demonstrate that we do not have to obtain ideal architecture of the bone if it means compromising adjacent teeth extensively [5,19]. Furthermore, if the furcation is exposed, the likelihood of further progression of periodontal disease is assured.

If the surgery involves aesthetic regions, FOS may have to be modified to a palatal approach or the patient may have to be treated conservatively with scaling and root planning. If not, permanent disfigurement of the gingival architecture may be lost due to the appearance of "black triangles" that are difficult if not impossible to correct.

Poor suturing technique such that the tissue is not apically repositioned may lead to excessive pocket depth again. The only solution to this would be a gingivectomy if the bony architecture has not changed. Some practitioners place a surgical dressing over the surgical site to maintain apical pressure on the tissue [20].

One of the most common complaints following FOS is root sensitivity and tooth mobility. Root sensitivity generally can be treated with over-the-counter toothpastes that contain desensitizers or in office application of fluoride pastes. Rarely is endodontic treatment necessary to deal with this issue. As far as tooth mobility is concerned, studies demonstrate that within 1 year of the surgery the mobility of these teeth return to their presurgical levels [5].

Food accumulation in the now open embrasures may also be an issue. The patient needs to be instructed on the use of alternative hygiene devices such as the proxy brush to effectively cleanse interproximally.

F. Postoperative complications:
1. Infection
2. Bleeding
3. Nerve paresthesia, dysesthesia
   Management of postoperative complications:
1. Infections: Antibiotics such as penicillin, amoxicillin, clindamycin, azithromycin, or metronidazole can be used. If the infection cannot be controlled with antibiotics, referral to the appropriate specialist is necessary. To reduce the chances of postoperative infections, it is important to rinse under the flaps with sterile saline to remove debris that has accumulated.

2. Instruct the patient to apply pressure to the area and then reassess. If this is not successful, arrangements should be made to see the patient as soon as possible.

3. Damage to the mental nerve is possible when FOS is performed in the mandible. If the surgeon had not exposed the nerve, stretching of the tissue and the nerve in this region is the most likely cause. Follow the patient closely until paresthesia has diminished. At each follow-up appointment a diagram should be made that indicates the regions that have regained feeling.

Case 4

Root Resection

CASE STORY

A 65-year-old Caucasian male had been referred by his general dentist with a chief complaint of: "pain and bleeding of my gums in the upper right back area with deep pockets." He noted there was bleeding when flossing as well as swelling and pain in this region.

LEARNING GOALS AND OBJECTIVES

■ To gain an understanding of the underlying and contributing etiologic factors resulting in furcation involvement

■ To understand a differential treatment plan and identify teeth suitable for root resection therapy

Medical History

There were no contributing medical problems, and the patient had no known allergies. Upon further questioning the patient reported that he was not taking any prescription medications or naturopathic remedies/supplements.

Review of Systems

- Vital signs
  - Blood pressure: 124/76 mm Hg
  - Pulse rate: 68 beats/minute (regular)
  - Respiration: 14 breaths/minute
  - Temperature: 37°C

Social History

The patient drank alcohol "socially" (i.e., at parties and/or one to two drinks on the weekend). The patient had never been a smoker and did not use any tobacco products. The patient did not use recreational or illicit street drugs. He was a retired nurse who presently volunteered at a local hospital.

Extraoral Examination

The patient was obese (body mass index: 32), and he did not exhibit any skeletal discrepancies or deformation of extremities. There were no visible or palpable nodal involvements throughout the head and neck region. The patient displayed a unilateral functional clicking of the right temporomandibular joint but no crepitation or tenderness of the masticatory muscles.

Intraoral Examination

All soft tissues of the mouth including mucosal surfaces, oropharynx, tongue surfaces, and floor of the mouth appeared to be within normal limits. The gingiva displayed mild to moderate inflammation and generalized slight/moderate marginal erythema. The patient did not report any tactile sensitivity, discomfort with percussion, or apical palpation tenderness. The patient explained that he has been experiencing sensitivity to hot and cold in the upper left region. Observation of plaque control techniques revealed inadequate brushing and flossing. Figures 1 and 2 offer an overview.

Occlusion

There were no occlusal discrepancies or interferences in working and nonworking excursions. The patient did not report habitual bruxing or clenching, either diurnal or nocturnal, although he displayed mild generalized attrition and wear facets.

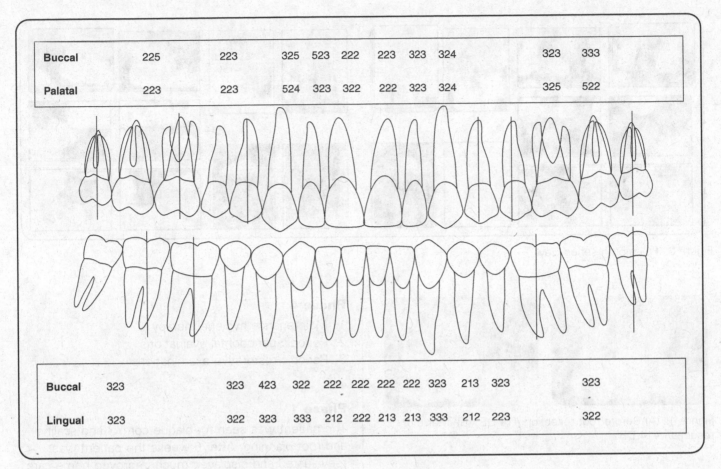

Buccal	225	223	325	523	222	223	323	324		323	333
Palatal	223	223	524	323	322	222	323	324		325	522

Buccal	323		323	423	322	222	222	222	222	323	213	323	323
Lingual	323		322	323	333	212	222	213	213	333	212	223	322

Figure 1: Periodontal charting.

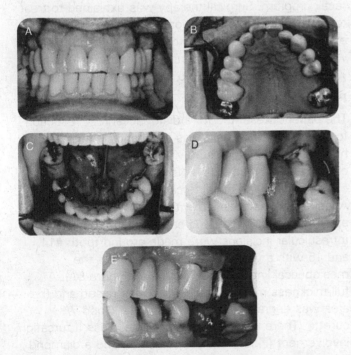

Figure 2: Intraoral initial visit. (A) frontal view; (B) maxillary view; (C) mandibular view; (D) right lateral; (E) left lateral.

Radiographic Examination

Figures 3 and 4 show part of the radiographic examination.

Diagnosis

Per the American Academy of Periodontology, the diagnosis was generalized moderate chronic periodontitis associated with mucogingival defects and occlusal trauma.

Treatment Plan

Additional consultations were as follows:

1. Consultation with the patient's general dentist regarding general restorative needs and specifically the restoration of tooth #14 following root resection therapy
2. Endodontic evaluation of tooth #14 to confirm the integrity of the existing root canal therapy

Phase 1

The first phase consisted of plaque control instruction, scaling and root planning of maxillary right sextant

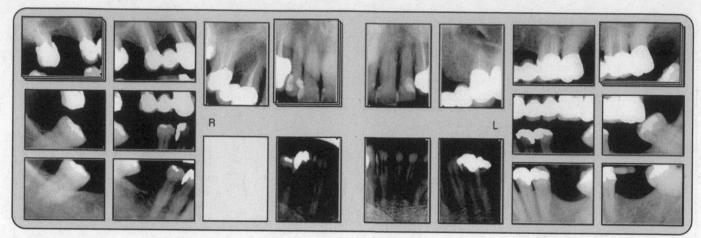

Figure 3: Full-mouth series view.

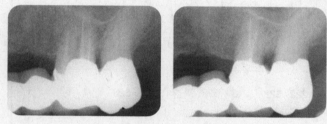

Figure 4: (A) Before root resection #14 DB, (B) after root resection #14 DB.

(#6M, #7D) and maxillary left sextant (#14D, #15M), and generalized supragingival scaling and polishing (two or more visits).

Reevaluation included the following:

1. Place the patient on an appropriate periodontal maintenance schedule pending periodontal status following localized scaling and root planning.
2. Consider surgical pocket reducing intervention if localized areas do not respond adequately to scaling and root planning (i.e., persistent deep pockets).

Phase 2

Perform flap #14 with the following treatment options:

1. Distobuccal root resection of tooth #14
2. Extraction of tooth #14 with ridge preservation and subsequent implant placement .
3. Gingival curettage and local delivery antibiotic therapy

Phase 3

The third phase would consist of possible crown recontouring or placement of a new crown to accommodate resection and allow for adequate home care by the patient and sealing of the root canal orifice.

Phase 4

1. Maintenance hygiene therapy
2. Periodic periodontal evaluations
3. Periodic restorative examinations

Treatment

Phase 1

The patient was seen for plaque control and scaling and root planning. After 6 weeks the patient was reevaluated and displayed much improved home care techniques and significantly reduced gingival inflammation. The patient will be placed on a 6-month recall program. Surgical therapy was explained to treat tooth #14 including the options of root sectioning or extraction. A consent form for surgery for tooth #14 was obtained. The postoperative surgical instructions were explained and given to the patient.

Phase 2

The patient presented for a distobuccal root resection for tooth #14, and there was no change in his medical history. His blood pressure was 135/85 mm Hg, and clinical examination with a Nabers probe revealed a class II buccal and distal furcation on tooth #14. Anesthesia was obtained with lidocaine 2% (1:100,000 epinephrine) by buccal and palatal infiltration. Intrasulcular incisions were made around teeth #14 and 15 with a vertical releasing incision at the mesiobuccal line angle of tooth #14 (Figure 5A). A full-thickness mucoperiosteal flap was raised and the area was degranulated with a Younger-Good 7/8 curette. There was a buccal and distal class II furcation involvement (Figure 5B) on tooth #14, and a diamond bur was used to section the distobuccal root at the fornices of the buccal and distal furcations (Figures 5C

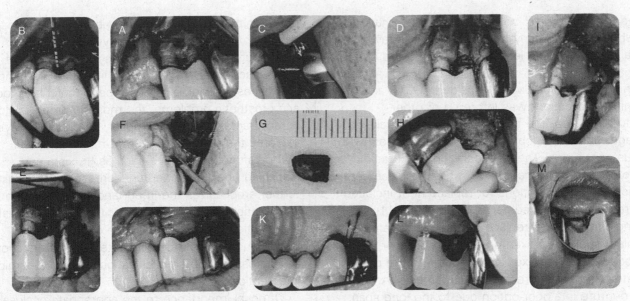

Figure 5: Root resection #14 DB.

and D). After removing a portion of the buccal bony plate, the distobuccal root was removed with an elevator (Figures 5E–G). Scaling and root planning was performed to remove residual granulation tissue, and osteoplasty was done to assure adequate gingival contour to provide access for hygiene. A complete gutta percha seal was evident at the root canal orifice. Due to the thickness of the palatal mucosa, the underlying connective tissue was thinned. Mineralized freeze-dried bone allograft (FDBA) was placed in the socket, and a collagen membrane covered the graft. (Figures 5H and I) The flaps were coapted with 5-0 chromic gut, single interrupted and vertical mattress sutures. Primary closure could not be achieved (Figures 5J and K). Postoperative instructions were again reviewed, and the patient appeared to have a good understanding of them. Prescriptions included 0.12% chlorhexidine gluconate to be rinsed 0.5 oz bid, 800 mg ibuprofen every 6 hours for the first 3 days and then as needed for comfort.

The patient presented for a postoperative appointment following root resection of tooth #14 (Figure 5L). There was no change in the patient's medical or dental history. The patient reported slight pain and swelling for the first few days following the procedure. The patient did not report bleeding, fever, or lymphadenopathy following surgery. The surgical site appeared to be healing normally with minimal inflammation and absence of suppuration. The sutures were removed and the area cleansed with 0.12% chlorhexidine. After an endodontic consultation, it was advised to remove a portion of the exposed gutta percha and replace it with a restorative material (Glass Ionomer: Fuji 2) to accomplish a better seal (Figure 5M).

Discussion

After a comprehensive intraoral examination and subsequent classification of class II buccal and distal furcation invasions of tooth #14, consideration was given to the appropriate therapy and the long-term prognosis of the tooth. The presence of a class II furcation involvement presents a distinct barrier for good oral hygiene with normal home care techniques for the patient and must be treated surgically in an effort to allow for maintenance. It has consistently been shown that if teeth with interproximal furcation involvements are not treated definitively, the patient's teeth are eventually lost despite the patient's best efforts at home care [1–3].

In spite of the numerous advances in guided tissue regeneration (GTR), limited evidence supports predictable regenerative treatment of class II furcation involvements in maxillary molars with respect to various clinical parameters such as clinical attachment gain and reduced probing depth following therapy [4,5]. Few cases show complete resolution of class II furcations. Improvement to a grade I furcation is more common at best. Although a number of studies have been successful in showing that class II furcations are amenable to GTR, most are lacking in sample size and a strong level of evidence [6–8].

In addition, interproximal furcation defects have been shown to be poorly responsive to an array of surgical modalities and less than those located on the buccal aspect [7].

In this case, in addition to considering GTR and root sectioning, the patient was informed of other procedures to treat the tooth, which included closed curettage, open flap debridement, or flap surgery with osseous contouring. The consideration of extraction with no tooth replacement or with tooth replacement was discussed. The options for replacement included either removable or fixed partial prostheses (11-x-x-x-x-15), single implants to replace teeth #12, 13, and 14 or an implant-supported fixed prosthesis (12-x-14). All of the procedures were explained in detail to the patient. The patient declined a removable prosthesis. A fixed partial denture is a poor option due to the long span and periodontally compromised abutment teeth. Both single implants and implant-supported prosthesis would require ridge augmentation and sinus elevation. The patient's choice was to retain the tooth and have root resective therapy performed. The fact that root canal therapy had already been completed and there was an inability to predictably improve such defects with GTR, a more predictable approach was that of root resection. Root sectioning therapy is a procedure to remove one of the roots from a multirooted tooth, usually molars. It is undertaken to create a soft tissue morphology that will allow the patient and clinician complete access for plaque removal. Although root resective therapy can be performed on both maxillary and mandibular molars, greater longevity and lower failure rates have been associated with the maxillary molars [9,10]. When selecting which root is to be amputated, a number of factors play into the decision and are discussed later in this case. Ultimately, the root to be sectioned is the root showing the least support to the tooth, the greatest attachment loss and providing the best access for plaque control. In the maxilla, the distobuccal root is the most common, and it is usually the root with the least attachment [11].

It has also been shown that when performing a root resection, having the endodontic therapy completed in advance is favorable as in the given case. A so-called nonvital approach is preferable and has been advocated in the literature [12]. If the decision is made to proceed with therapy while the tooth is vital, root canal therapy should be completed within a 2-week window to increase the chance of success [13]. Many times the decision to resect a root is made following flap reflection and degranulation. This affords the best opportunity for the operator to visualize and palpate the extent of the furcation involvement.

Although there are many reasons for failure of root resected teeth cited in the literature including root caries, endodontic failure, periodontal breakdown, and prosthetic problems, the most common etiology is root fracture [9,14]. Moreover, studies that have explored the origin of such root fractures reveal that parafunctional habits such as bruxism and clenching often remained unaddressed. This finding further emphasizes the importance of a thorough examination of the patient's occlusion at the initial examination. During the disease control phase, interferences should be eliminated and habits should be addressed with an occlusal guard before surgical intervention.

Of equal importance to the appropriate occlusal adjustment at the outset of therapy is the manner in which the root resected tooth is restored prosthetically [15]. The prosthodontic literature has endorsed the need for full coronal coverage of these teeth due to the predisposition of endodontically treated root-resected teeth to fracture due to a lack of natural tooth support. The unique anatomy following such therapy calls for placement of an appropriately designed crown or the recontouring of an existing crown, as was the case with tooth #14. If possible reducing the occlusal table buccolingually and reducing cusp steepness is preferable on a root-sectioned tooth. An adequate emergence profile will allow for access for the patient's plaque removal techniques. Fractures of root canal–treated teeth relate to the weakening of the tooth as a result of root canal and/or after preparation.

If in this case exploratory flap surgery had revealed caries on the palatal root, grade II mobility following resection, a mesiobuccal root dehiscence, a deep grade II or a III furcation involvement with the distobuccal and palatal roots or other compromising findings, the decision to remove the tooth in an atraumatic fashion would have been undertaken. The patient had been informed of this possibility in advance of therapy. The patient was aware that in the event the tooth was nontreatable, the alternative plan in this circumstance would involve a ridge preservation procedure, involving allograft and barrier membrane, in an effort to minimize future bone resorption, the possibility of a sinus elevation, and the placement of an implant in the future [16] (see Chapter 4).

Although placement of implants have become a popular approach to replace questionable teeth, a number of studies have observed equal rates of success in root-resected teeth when compared with similar sites replaced by implant therapy [10]. Such studies stress the importance of appropriate case selection and technique in ensuring the high degree of success achieved for both modalities. In this case, the tooth was stable, the furcation invasion was confined primarily to the distobuccal root of tooth #14, and there was little or no furcation involvement of the mesial and palatal root. In addition, root canal therapy had previously been done and was determined to be successful. Although there was a full crown on the tooth before root sectioning, it could be modified by recontouring and was not an aesthetic problem for the patient. Thus the decision to retain the tooth and do a root resection took into consideration all of the parameters just described. It was also a better financial option for the patient than if the tooth were removed, guided bone regeneration (GBR) done, and an implant placed and restored. In addition, because GBR was done to regenerate bone in the socket of the distofacial root, should an implant need to be placed in the future, the bone volume would not be compromised as a result of the root section.

Self-Study Questions

A. What is the difference between root resection, root amputation, and hemisection?

B. How do we classify furcation involvements?

C. What are the indications and contraindications for root resections?

D. What is the difference between vital and nonvital resection (i.e., what comes first, the surgery or the endodontic therapy)?

E. How do we select the root that is to be removed and why?

F. Is root resection a predictable therapeutic modality?

G. How does root resection compare with extraction and implant therapy as a treatment option?

H. What is the relationship between periodontal disease, obesity, and systemic disease?

I. Why is it important to seal the canal orifice with a permanent restorative material?

Answers located at the end of the chapter.

References

1. Goldman MJ, Ross IF, et al. Effect of periodontal therapy on patients maintained for 15 years or longer. A retrospective study. J Periodontol 1986;57:347–353.
2. Hirschfeld L, Wasserman B. A long-term survey of tooth loss in 600 treated periodontal patients. J Periodontol 1978;49:225–237.
3. McFall WT Jr. Tooth loss in 100 treated patients with periodontal disease. A long-term study. J Periodontol 1982;53:539–549.
4. Metzler DG, Seamons BC, et al. Clinical evaluation of guided tissue regeneration in the treatment of maxillary class II molar furcation invasions. J Periodontol 1991; 62:353–360.
5. Yukna RA, Yukna CN. Six-year clinical evaluation of HTR synthetic bone grafts in human grade II molar furcations. J Periodontal Res 1997;32:627–633.
6. Camello M, Nevins ML, et al. Periodontal regeneration in human class II furcations using purified recombinant human platelet-derived growth factor-BB (rhPDGF-BB) with bone allograft. Int J Periodontics Restorative Dent 2003;23:213–225.
7. Pontoriero R, Lindhe J. Guided tissue regeneration in the treatment of degree II furcations in maxillary molars. J Clin Periodontol 1995;22:756–763.
8. Rosen PS, Marks MH, et al. Regenerative therapy in the treatment of maxillary molar class II furcations: case reports. Int J Periodontics Restorative Dent 1997; 17:516–527.
9. Langer B, Stein SD, et al. An evaluation of root resections. A ten-year study. J Periodontol 1981;52:719.
10. Fugazzotto PA. A comparison of the success of root resected molars and molar position implants in function in a private practice: results of up to 15-plus years. J Periodontol 2001;72:1113–1123.
11. American Academy of Periodontology literature review.
12. Filipowicz F, Umstott P, et al. Vital root resection in maxillary molar teeth: A longitudinal study. J Endodont 1984;10:264–268.
13. Smukler H, Tagger M. Vital root amputation. A clinical and histological study J Periodontol 1976;47:324–330.
14. Carnevale G, Gianfranco D, et al. A retrospective analysis of the periodontal prosthetic treatment of molars with interradicular lesions. Int J Periodontics Restorative Dent 1991;11:189–205.
15. Gerstein KA. The role of vital root resection in periodontics. J Periodontol 1977;48:478–483.
16. Iasella JM, Greenwell H, et al. Ridge preservation with freeze-dried bone allograft and a collagen membrane compared to extraction alone for implant site development: a clinical and histologic study in humans. J Periodontol 2003;74:990–999.
17. Hamp SE, Nyman S, et al. Periodontal treatment of multirooted teeth. Results after 5 years. J Clin Periodontol 1975;2:126–135.
18. Glickman I. The treatment of bifurcation and trifurcation involvement. In: Glickman I, Clinical Periodontology. Philadelphia, PA: Saunders, 1958. pp693–704.
19. Basaraba N. Root amputation and tooth hemisection. Dent Clin N Am 1969;13:121–132.
20. Haskell EW, Stanley H, et al. A new approach to vital root resection. J Periodontol 1980;51:217–224.
21. Buhler H. Evaluation of root-resected teeth. Results after 10 years. J Periodontol 1988;59:805–810.
22. Erpenstein H. A 3 year study of hemisectioned molars. J Clin Periodontol 1983;10:1–10.
23. Green EN. Hemisection and root amputation. J Am Dent Assoc 1986;112:511–518.
24. Ross IF, Thompson RH. A long term study of root retention in the treatment of maxillary molars with furcation involvement J Periodontol 1978;49:238–244.
25. Ordovas JM, Shen J. Gene–environment interactions and susceptibility to metabolic syndrome and other chronic diseases. J Periodontol 2008;79:1508–1513.
26. Khayat A, Lee SJ, et al. Human saliva penetration of coronally unsealed obturated root canals. J Endod 1993;19:458–461.
27. Swanson K, Madison S. An evaluation of coronal microleakage in endodontically treated teeth. Part I. Time periods. J Endod 1987;13:56–59.

TAKE-HOME POINTS

A. See Table 1.

B. The furcation is defined as the point at which the roots of multirooted teeth divide into separate entities. In a healthy periodontal state the bone surrounding the teeth normally lies coronal to the furcations. When bone loss takes place as in periodontitis, the furcations can become involved to varying degrees.

A number of classifications exist but the two most common are these:

1. Hamp et al [17]
   Grade I: Horizontal loss <3 mm
   Grade II: Horizontal loss >3 mm but not encompassing the total width
   Grade III: Horizontal through-and-through
2. Glickman [18]

Grade I: Incipient; pocket is suprabony; no radiographic change

Grade II: Loss of interradicular bone and pocket formation but not extending through to the opposite side; "cul-de-sac" radiographic change may or may not be seen

Grade III: Through and through; permit complete passage of a probe

Grade IV: Through and through with gingival recession, "Tunnel"; a clearly visible furcation area

C. See Table 2.

D. A vital root resection implies that the root removal takes place before endodontic therapy, whereas nonvital resection indicates

Table 1: Differentiating Between Root Resection, Root Amputation, and Hemisection

Root Resection	Root Amputation	Hemisection
Surgical removal of all or a portion of a tooth root [11]	The removal of an entire root from a multirooted tooth [11]	The surgical separation of a multirooted tooth, usually a mandibular molar, through the furcation in such a way that a root and the associated portion of the crown may be removed [11]

Table 2: Indications and Contraindications for Root Resection [19]

Indications	Contraindications
• The patient's desire to retain the tooth • Severe bone loss affecting a single root • Class II, III, IV furcation(s) [18] where the furcas are not amenable to be treated via odontoplasty • Unfavorable root proximity with adjacent teeth • Root fracture, perforation, root caries or root resorption involving a single root • When required endodontic therapy of a particular root cannot be performed adequately • When the tooth has little or no mobility	• Medical condition not allowing surgical intervention • Insufficient alveolar bone to support remaining root (i.e., poor crown-to-root ratio) • Unfavorable anatomy • Long root trunk; fused roots • Root canal therapy not possible on remaining root following procedure • Unrestorable remaining tooth • Postoperative periodontal state compromised or not maintainable • Significant tooth mobility • Does not complement the prosthetic plan

that root canal treatment has already been undertaken.

Although literature does exist supporting the performance of root resection prior to endodontic intervention [12,13,20], most evidence advocates completion of the root canal therapy before removal of the targeted root [12]. Filipowicz et al [12] found that almost half of the teeth treated via vital root resection were nonvital at 6 months and increased to 87% nonvital at 5-year follow-up.

In spite of the increased success of resecting a root following endodontic therapy, a significant concern is the possibility that upon flap elevation the tooth is deemed unsuitable for the recommended treatment and requires extraction. A fine balance must be struck by the clinician to ensure that the tooth is amenable to root resection so as to avoid unnecessary endodontic care to the patient. If the decision to undertake vital therapy is made, it is considered prudent to have the subsequent root canal treatment done within 2 weeks [13].

E. The most commonly resected roots are the distobuccal in maxillary molars and mesial root of the mandibular molars [11].

Resection therapy is undertaken in multirooted teeth, namely the maxillary and mandibular molars. The clinician must weigh many variables when assessing not only the appropriateness of resection therapy but also which specific root should be removed. Interdisciplinary lines of communication are essential between the surgeon, endodontist, and prosthodontist to increase the efficacy of this modality of therapy. Generally the maxillary molars are the most common teeth chosen for root sectioning.

Some of the factors to consider in the decision of which root to remove are the following:
1. Removal of the root, which most completely eliminates the bone loss in the furcation, in essence reducing future periodontal complications
2. Removal of the most pathologically involved root (i.e., greatest bone defect, attachment loss, caries, etc.)
3. Removal of the root, which affords patient the greatest ability to achieve home care and successful maintenance

4. Removal of the root, which facilitates sound prosthetic rehabilitation whether it be a single crown or abutment tooth
5. Removal of the root, which might pose the greatest challenge to endodontic therapy
6. Removal of a root that is in very close proximity to a neighboring tooth, creating an interdental space that is difficult or impossible to clean or restore.

F. Historically, root resection was one of the few options that existed for teeth with significant furcation involvements and teeth with a periodontally questionable or nontreatable prognosis, which otherwise would require extraction. Many studies have examined the predictability of root sectioning therapy by comparing outcomes to similar teeth with furcation involvements where root sectioning was not done. Reports of failure rates of root resected teeth show a large range with various authors observing anywhere between 16% and 73% depending on the length of follow up [9,17,21,22]. These studies show a consistent trend for the failure rate to increase significantly in relation to the length of follow-up [9,21,23]. The less compliant patients were with recall, the more likely failure occurred. However, there are two major exceptions. One study by Carnevale [14] found a higher rate of failure between 3 and 6 years versus 7–11 years, and a recent study by Fugazzotto showed a success rate comparable with the implant success rate [10].

In contrast, a classic study [24] maintained 88% of maxillary molars with furcation invasion that did not receive root resection or osseous surgery and rather were maintained via scaling and root planing, gingivectomy, or apically positioned flaps over 5–24 years.

In addition, these same studies sought to investigate the causes behind failures of resected teeth over the long term. The variables, which have been considered to be associated with failure of teeth undergoing root resection, included periodontal disease, caries, and root fracture. Root fracture has been deemed the most common cause for the failure of such teeth. Mandibular molars also have a tendency to have a higher failure rate when compared with maxillary molars [9,17,21,22]

G. Before the advent of osseoIntegration, there were few options available to those teeth, which had been severely compromised due to periodontal disease. Such teeth commonly had furcation involvement, which was unable to be maintained by patients or periodontal maintenance and required extraction.

Although many studies indicate a significantly higher success rate for endosteal implants, a recent paper that retrospectively compared implant success with resected molars reported almost identical cumulative success rates of 97.0% and 96.8%, respectively [10]. The author attributes this high rate of success to a number of factors including comprehensive management of the patient's occlusion and a thorough and consistent maintenance hygiene program.

H. Chronic periodontal disease and obesity are conditions that produce cytokines responsible for various systemic conditions including cardiac disease, diabetes, cerebrovascular accidents, rheumatoid arthritis, and others [25]. Achieving periodontal health can reduce the host's inflammatory response and production of cytokines, which could otherwise contribute to these conditions.

I. Gutta percha does not provide an adequate seal of a root canal–treated tooth. To prevent bacterial contamination, a definitive restorative material such as amalgam or glass ionomer should be placed [26,27].

4

Regenerative Therapy

Clinical Cases in Periodontics, First Edition. Nadeem Karimbux.
© 2012 John Wiley & Sons, Inc. Published 2012 by John Wiley & Sons, Inc.

Case 1

Treatment of Furcations

Regenerative Therapy

CASE STORY

A 47-year-old Caucasian female was referred for periodontal evaluation of the maxillary posterior teeth by a dental hygienist at the office of a general dentist. She was aware of bleeding when brushing but had no other clinical symptoms. However, the hygienist was concerned by gingival distension and the deep probing depth. The patient reported that she brushed her teeth two to three times a day and flossed regularly.

LEARNING GOALS AND OBJECTIVES

- To be able to diagnose/classify furcation involvement
- To identify possible etiologic factors
- To be aware of appropriate treatments for furcation involvement

Medical History

There was no significant medical history. She was not currently taking any medication except multivitamins, and the patient had no known drug or food allergies.

Review of Systems

- Vital signs on the day of initial visit
  - Blood pressure: 128/83 mm Hg
  - Pulse: 74 beats/minutes (regular)
  - Respiratory rate: 16 breaths/minute
- No significant problems were reported.

Social History

The patient was a well-spoken certified public accountant. She denied any use of tobacco, alcohol, or recreational drugs. There were no parafunctional habits reported such as clenching, bruxism, tongue thrusting, and mouth breathing.

Extraoral Examination

This articulate patient appeared to be under no apparent distress. The extraoral examination revealed no masses, swelling, or lymphadenopathy. Her temporomandibular joints were in full range of motion and within normal limits.

Intraoral Examination

The oral mucosa including lips, tongue, and palate demonstrated no aberrations. The periodontal examination revealed generalized pink gingiva with localized marginal erythema. There was a deviated papilla, and exudate was present at tooth #14. Periodontal charting was completed (Figure 1).

Occlusion

There was a minimal discrepancy between centric relation and centric occlusion but no eccentric interferences.

Diagnosis

Review of the full-mouth radiographic survey demonstrated minimal osseous loss excluding tooth #14, giving a diagnosis of generalized mild chronic periodontitis. A vertical probing depth of 6 mm and horizontal probing depth of 5 mm were present at the site of the buccal furcation on tooth#14. The palatal root prevented further horizontal probing. The nonsurgical diagnosis of this furcation was a class II

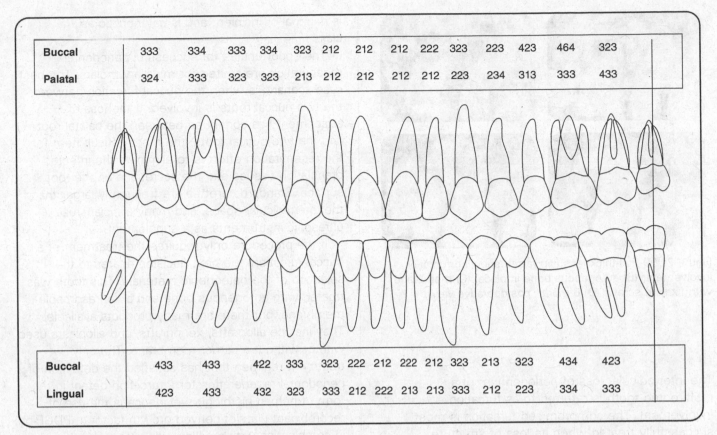

Buccal	333	334	333	334	323	212	212	212	222	323	223	423	464	323
Palatal	324	333	323	323	213	212	212	212	212	223	234	313	333	433

Buccal	433	433	422	333	323	222	212	222	212	323	213	323	434	423
Lingual	423	433	432	323	333	212	222	213	213	333	212	223	334	333

Figure 1: Periodontal charting.

furcation involvement in the buccal of #14 according to Glickman's classification.

Treatment Plan

The treatment plan was to address the generalized mild chronic periodontitis with four quadrants of root planning under local anesthesia complemented by oral hygiene instruction. Surgical intervention would be necessary to treat #14 with the hope that periodontal regeneration could be performed. It was impossible to determine mesial and distal extension of furcation involvement until the time of surgery.

Treatment

The left maxillary quadrant was anesthetized buccally and palatally around #14 with 2% Xylocaine with 1:50,000 of epinephrine. A full-thickness buccal flap was reflected using mesial and distal vertical incisions to obtain the maximum visibility. All granulation tissue was removed from the affected area, and root planning removed all accretions from the tooth. This was the appropriate time to evaluate any loss of

proximal structure between the palatal and two buccal roots. The internal proximal areas were evaluated with a #23 explorer and Kramer Nevins #4 curette, but there was no proximal extension. We therefore concluded that this problem was limited to the buccal furcation and we could treat the area to achieve periodontal regeneration. A tetracycline slurry was introduced to decontaminate the surface. The area was thoroughly washed with sterile saline. Autogenous bone was harvested with a trephine from an edentulous mandibular posterior site. The cores were ground with a bone mill and adapted to the defect. Ti-reinforced membrane (Gore, Newark, DE, USA) was fitted to cover the defect, apically tacked with a fixation screw, and sutured coronally with 4.0 Gore-Tex suture. Then flap was repositioned coronally to protect the surgical site. The area was reopened to remove the membrane at 6 months. There was clinical evidence of periodontal regeneration interradicularly and to a lesser extent on the radicular surface of the buccal roots. The patient was under observation at the periodontal office for a year and returned to the family practice (Figure 2A–D).

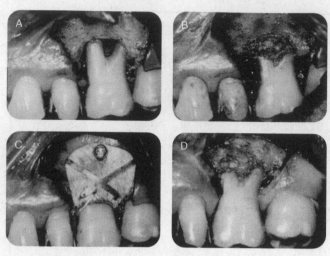

Figure 2: (A) Full-thickness flap raised showing furcation involvement; (B) autogenous bone in place; (C) membrane with fixation screw; (D) 6-month postoperative view.

Discussion

The interradicular loss of periodontium of a multirooted tooth is referred to as furcation involvement. The compromised furcation is most successfully treated when its loss of structure is minimal or incipient and is categorized as class I.

The opportunities for successful periodontal regeneration are limited for maxillary molars. The best case scenario is when the buccal furcation between the two buccal roots is involved. If the loss of attachment has continued between the palatal root and the two buccal roots, the most difficult item for the regeneration effort is to eliminate the infected granulation tissues and the accretions on the root surface. Standard curettes are frequently larger than the interradicular space, and many clinicians use ultrasonic instruments as a supplement.

If the procedure only requires the treatment of a buccal furcation, the next decision relates to the selection of the osteogenic materials. This tooth was treated with autogenous bone and a nonresorbable membrane, but there are many products available. They include allografts, xenografts, and alloplasts used with or without a barrier membrane. The only treatment regimen that has satisfied the definition of periodontal regeneration for a furcation defect in the form of human histological evidence is the use of recombinant platelet-derived growth factor (rhPDGF-bb) in combination with an allograft [1,2].

Self-Study Questions

A. How would you classify/define furcation involvement?

B. What information would you need to make a correct diagnosis of furcation involvement?

C. What etiologic and anatomic factors influence furcation involvement?

D. How would you treat different furcation involvements?

E. What are the factors that affect treatment outcome?

F. What is the long-term prognosis of treatment of furcation involvement?

G. What are possible complications from the treatment of furcation involvement?

H. What would be the maintenance protocol after the treatment of furcation involvement?

Answers located at the end of the chapter.

References

1. Camelo M, Nevins M, et al. Periodontal regeneration in human class II furcations using purified recombinant human platelet-derived growth factor-BB (rhPDGF-BB) with bone allograft. Int J Periodontics Restorative Dent 2003;23:213–225.
2. Nevins M, Camelo M, et al. Periodontal regeneration in humans using recombinant human platelet-derived growth factor-BB (rhPDGF-BB) and allogenic bone. J Periodontol 2003;74:1282–1292.
3. Glickman I. The treatment of bifurcation and trifurcation involvement. In: Clinical Periodontology. Philadelphia, PA: Saunders, 1958. pp693–704.
4. Hamp SE, Nyman S, et al. Periodontal treatment of multirooted teeth. Results after 5 years. J Clin Periodontol 1975;2:126–135.
5. Eskow RN, Kapin SH. Furcation invasions: correlating a classification system with therapeutic considerations. Part I. Examination, diagnosis, and classification. Compend Contin Educ Dent 1984;5:479–483, 487.
6. Tarnow D, Fletcher P. Classification of the vertical component of furcation involvement. J Periodontol 1984;55:283–284.
7. Ricchetti PA A furcation classification based on pulp chamber-furcation relationships and vertical radiographic bone loss. Int J Periodontics Restorative Dent 1982;2:50–59.
8. Al-Shammari KF, Kazor CE, et al. Molar root anatomy and management of furcation defects. J Clin Periodontol 2001;28:730–740.
9. Zappa U, Grosso L, et al. Clinical furcation diagnoses and interradicular bone defects. J Periodontol 1993;64:219–227.
10. Mealey BL, Neubauer MF, et al. Use of furcal bone sounding to improve accuracy of furcation diagnosis. J Periodontol 1994;65:649–657.
11. Abdallah F, Kon S, et al. The furcation problem: etiology, diagnosis, therapy, and prognosis. J West Soc Periodontol Periodontal Abstr 1987;35:129–141.
12. Larato DC. Furcation involvements: incidence and distribution. J Periodontol 1970;41:499–501.
13. Tal H. Relationship between the depths of furcal defects and alveolar bone loss. J Periodontol 1982;53:631–634.
14. Hermann DW, Gher ME Jr, et al. The potential attachment area of the maxillary first molar. J Periodontol 1983;54:431–434.
15. Bower RC Furcation morphology relative to periodontal treatment. Furcation entrance architecture. J Periodontol 1979;50:23–27.
16. Everett FG, Jump EB, et al. The intermediate bifurcational ridge: a study of the morphology of the bifurcation of the lower first molar. J Dent Res 1958;37:162–169.
17. Gutmann JL Prevalence, location, and patency of accessory canals in the furcation region of permanent molars. J Periodontol 1978;49:21–26.
18. Moskow BS, Canut PM Studies on root enamel (2). Enamel pearls. A review of their morphology, localization, nomenclature, occurrence, classification, histogenesis and incidence. J Clin Periodontol 1990;17:275–281.
19. Masters D, Hoskins SW. Projection of cerival enamel into molar furcations. J Periodontol 1964;35:49–53.
20. Pontoriero R, Lindhe J. Guided tissue regeneration in the treatment of degree II furcations in maxillary molars. J Clin Periodontol 1995;22:756–763.
21. Filipowicz F, Umstott P, et al. Vital root resection in maxillary molar teeth: a longitudinal study. J Endod 1984;10:264–268.
22. Langer B, Stein SD, et al. An evaluation of root resections. A ten-year study. J Periodontol 1981;52:719–722.
23. Newell DH. The role of the prosthodontist in restoring root-resected molars: a study of 70 molar root resections. J Prosthet Dent 1991;65:7–15.
24. Nevins M, Langer B. The successful application of osseointegrated implants to the posterior jaw: a long-term retrospective study. Int J Oral Maxillofac Implants 1993;8:428–432.
25. Bahat O, Handelsman M. Use of wide implants and double implants in the posterior jaw: a clinical report. Int J Oral Maxillofac Implants 1996;11:379–386.
26. Bowers GM, Schallhorn RG, et al. Factors influencing the outcome of regenerative therapy in mandibular Class II furcations: Part I. J Periodontol 2003;74:1255–1268.
27. Mellonig JT, Valderrama Mdel P. Histological and clinical evaluation of recombinant human platelet-derived growth factor combined with beta tricalcium phosphate for the treatment of human class III furcation defects. Int J Periodontics Restorative Dent 2009;29:169–177.
28. Karring T, Cortellini P. Regenerative therapy: furcation defects. Periodontol 2000 1999;19:115–137.
29. Pontoriero R, Nyman S, et al. The angular bony defect in the maintenance of the periodontal patient. J Clin Periodontol 1988;15:200–204.

TAKE-HOME POINTS

A.

a. Glickman's classification of furcation involvement [3]
  i. Grade I: Early furcation involvement just into the flute of the furcation is present, but the interradicular bone is intact. There is no significant destruction of bone or connective tissue in the furcation proper.
  ii. Grade II: Distinct horizontal destruction of the furcation area including interradicular bone is present. Destruction should not be extended to the other side of furcation. Vertical bone loss may or may not be present.
  iii. Grade III: Destruction of interradicular bone and connective tissue all the way through the furcation so that an instrument can be passed through the furcation. The furcation defect is not yet visible clinically.
  iv. Grade IV: Severe destruction of interradicular bone and connective tissue all the way through the furcation so that the tunnel is completely visible through the furcation defect when viewed clinically.
b. Horizontal furcation classification [4]
  i. Degree I: Horizontal loss of periodontal tissue support <3 mm.
  ii. Degree II: Horizontal loss of support >3 mm but not encompassing the total width of the furcation area.
  iii. Degree III: Horizontal "through-and-through" destruction of the periodontal tissue in the furcation.
c. Vertical furcation classification [5,6]
  In addition to the horizontal classification:
  i. Subclass A: Probeable vertical depth of 1–3 mm from the roof of the furcation apically.
  ii. Subclass B: Probeable vertical depth of 4–6 mm from the roof of the furcation apically.
  iii. Subclass C: Probeable vertical depth >7 mm from the roof of the furcation apically.
d. Horizontal and vertical furcation classification [7]
  Ricchetti's furcation classification system divides the molar into buccal, middle, and lingual/palatal thirds. The classifications are as follows:

  i. Class I: Incipient involvement; horizontal involvement just into the interradicular area.
  ii. Class Ia: Involvement into approximately the first half of the buccal or lingual third.
  iii. Class II: Horizontal involvement beyond class Ia but not into the middle third of the molar.
  iv. Class IIa: Horizontal involvement into the middle third of the molar but not beyond halfway.
  v. Class III: Horizontal involvement beyond half of the tooth width.

B. Al-Shammari et al [8]
a. Radiographs: may assist in the diagnosis of furcation defects but have a limited value if used as the sole diagnostic tool, especially in early and moderate defects.
b. Clinical examination: Clinical measurements alone also have limited value [9]. However, the combination of radiographic and clinical examinations improves detection to 65% for maxillary molars but only to 23% for mandibular molars. Probing the deepest interradicular site does not measure the true pocket depth or the attachment level of the furcation area. This indicates that the probing measurement recorded the depth of probe penetrating into the inflamed connective tissue rather than the true pocket depth.
c. Bone sounding: Bone sounding with local anesthesia may assist in the diagnosis of furcation defects by more accurately determining the underlying bony contours [10].
d. Diagnosing furcation invasion is best accomplished using a combination of radiographs, periodontal probing with a curved explorer or Nabers probe, and bone sounding (Figure 3).

C.
a. Primary factor
  i. Bacterial plaque
    1. The extension of inflammatory periodontal disease into the furcation area leads to interradicular bone resorption and formation of furcation defects [11].

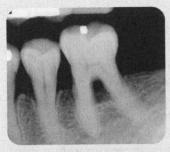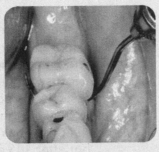

Figure 3: Mandibular furcation involvement, showing a probe entering the furcation.

ii. Age
  1. The average number of furcation involvements increases with age [12].

b. Occlusal trauma
  i. Glickman showed that the hyperfunction of rat molar makes the furcation area susceptible to attachment loss. The heavy occlusal load on molar teeth may render them susceptible to increased bone loss in the furcation areas if inflammation is present.

c. Predisposing anatomic factors:
  i. Root trunk length
    1. The distance from the cementoenamel junction (CEJ) to the entrance of the furcation varies by individual. The shorter the trunk length, the less attachment loss needs before the furcation involvement [13].
  ii. Root length
    1. Teeth with long root trunks and short roots may have lost most of their support by the time the furcation becomes affected [14].
  iii. Root form
    1. Furcation entrance diameter
      a. 81% of entrances on molars are <1mm in width, and 58% are <0.75mm, which is less than the diameter of the blade of standard curettes [15]. A small furcation entrance further complicates the proper maintenance of good hygiene.
    2. Root concavity [15]
      a. Mandibular first molars have concavities in 100% of mesial roots and 99% of distal roots. Deeper concavity is

found in the mesial root than the distal root.
      b. Maxillary first molars have concavities in 94% of mesiobuccal roots, 31% of distobuccal roots, and 17% of palatal roots. Deepest concavity is found in the mesiobuccal root.
  iv. Interradicular dimension
    1. Root proximity can be a precipitating factor. Closely proximated or fused roots can impede complete periodontal treatment or maintenance once they get involved.
  v. Anatomy of furcation
    1. The presence of bifurcational ridges, a concavity in the dome [16], and possible accessory canals [17] can complicate appropriate periodontal treatment and maintenance therapy.
  vi. Developmental anomaly
    1. Developmental anomalies are enamel pearls (EPs) and cervical enamel projection (CEPs). EPs are larger round deposits of enamel, and CEPs are flat ectopic extensions of enamel beyond the CEJ junction. EPs are seen in 1–5% of permanent molars [18]. CEPs are seen in 29% of mandibular molars and 17% of maxillary molars [19]. These anatomic structures interfere with the attachment apparatus, making furcation more vulnerable to the disease process.

d. Other factors
  i. Orthodontics
    1. Poorly planned orthodontic procedures may make teeth super-erupt, exposing furcations.
  ii. Pulpal pathology
    1. When present, especially with accessory canals, it is very likely that furcation would be involved.
  iii. Vertical root fractures
    1. Vertical root fractures are associated with rapid and localized alveolar bone loss.
  iv. Iatrogenic factors
    1. Overhanging margin of restorations near furcations can lead to furcation involvement.

D.

a. Class I

  i. Limited to the incipient lesions

    1. Scaling and root planning in conjunction with debridement

      a. Good root preparation is the key to successful therapy. Efficacy decreases with more roots involved. Presence of precipitating anatomic factors also hinders the success of therapy.

    2. Apically positioned flap in conjunction with osteoplasty/osteoectomy

      a. This provides an environment for improved oral hygiene application with the reduced pocket depth postoperatively.

b. Class II

  i. Buccal and lingual mandibular/buccal maxillary furcations

    1. Apically positioned flap in conjunction with osteoplasty/osteoectomy

      a. A shallow class II mandibular lesion with divergent roots will benefit from this procedure.

    2. Guided tissue regeneration (GTR)

      a. Combination treatment (debridement + bone graft + membrane) at buccal class II furcations results in decreased probing depth and bone gain and reduces the amount of soft tissue recession above what was accomplished by flap debridement alone. [20].

      b. Introduction of growth factor. Use of growth factors has permitted the treatment of many mandibular class III defects and maxillary class II defects with a regenerative approach. Nevins et al [2] used rhPDGF-BB with DFDBA to successfully treat human class II furcation defects.

    3. Root resection (see other chapters)

      a. Factors that influence the outcome of root resections include (1) the patency of the root canal system, (2) occlusal forces, (3) the length of the edentulous span, and (4) the length, width, and shape of the root.

      b. Root resection in conjunction with endodontic therapy is necessary because long-term survival of vital root resection is poor [21].

      c. In the short term of 3 or 4 years, this treatment has been highly successful, but after 10 years approximately a third fail. A substantial number of failures were attributed to recurrent periodontal disease, recurrent caries, root fractures, or endodontic failures [22,23].

    4. Extraction and implant (see other chapters)

      a. This treatment completely removes etiology and successfully restores the function.

      b. It is highly predictable with success rate of 99% [24]. Wide implant (diameter >5 mm) also favors successful treatments of furcation involvements [25].

  ii. Other proximal furcations

    1. Access to proximal maxillary furcation must proceed with individual defect analysis based on surgical access.

  iii. It is critical not to allow class II to become class III.

c. Class III furcation

  i. Debridement treatment

    a. Maintenance and no invasive therapy

  ii. Root resection (see other chapters)

  iii. Tunneling

    a. This treatment will convert grade III and deep grade II furcations into grade IV furcation to improve access for oral hygiene.

    b. Success is challenged with interradicular caries with limited access to repair; size of pulp chamber is 2 mm.

  iv. Extract and implant (see other chapters)

  v. Regeneration with growth factors

    a. Studies report favorable results in mandibular class II furcation; less favorable results were found in mandibular class III defects and

maxillary class II defects [20,26]. In general, class III has a less favorable outcome than class II.
  b. Histologic evidence of regeneration in class III furcation is not available yet. Mellonig et al used rhPDGF-BB with BCP for improving human class III furcation defect [27]. However, predictability remains questionable.

E. Karring and Cortellini [28]
a. Patient factors
  i.   Oral hygiene: Patient compliance
  ii. Smoking
  iii. Systemic conditions (diabetics, metabolic disorders, etc.)
b. Defect factors
  i.   Mandibular versus maxillary teeth
  ii. Location of the defect (buccal class II defects have better prognosis [29])
  iii. Vertical height of the defect (<3 mm of vertical defect: better prognosis)

c. Technique factors
  i.   Operators skill (technique sensitive)
  ii. Incomplete removal of etiologic factors
  iii. Postoperative infection control
  iv. Adjunctive systemic antibiotics (minimal benefits?)

F.
a. Depending on diagnostic skills, all of these methods have been clinically demonstrated as efficacious; none are exclusive

G.
a. The patient should be seen with periodicity of 3 months because they already have demonstrated their susceptibility to periodontal disease.
b. Successful treatment resulting in minimal probing depth will benefit both the oral hygienist and the patient.
c. Proximal brush for interproximal furcation.

Case 2

Treatment of Intrabony Defects Using Allografts

CASE STORY

The patient was a 63-year-old male who presented to the Department of Periodontology for consultation regarding several "loose teeth" in both the maxilla and mandible. His chief complaint was his missing teeth and his desire to have fixed restorations to replace them (Figure 1).

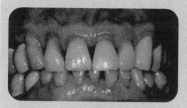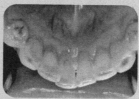

Figure 1: Intraoral photo of both maxillary and mandibular teeth in occlusion and occlusal view of maxillary arch.

LEARNING GOALS AND OBJECTIVES

■ To identify and appropriately diagnose patients requiring guided tissue regeneration (GTR)

■ To understand preoperative and postoperative issues that lead to successful GTR therapy

■ To be introduced to surgical techniques and biomaterials used to perform GTR

Medical History

The patient had been diagnosed with type 1 hypertension several years ago and had been under treatment with his physician ever since. His physician had prescribed atenolol 50 mg once daily and hydrochlorothiazide 25 mg daily. He regularly monitored his condition and had been stable since prescription treatment began. Otherwise this patient was in good health, did not have any other significant medical problems, and did not report any allergies or history of diabetes.

Review of Systems

- Vital signs
  - Blood pressure: 126/75 mm Hg
  - Pulse rate: 58 beats/minute (regular)

Social History

The patient was married with three children. He did not consume alcohol and did not smoke.

Extraoral Examination

No significant findings were noted. The patient had no masses or swelling, and the temporomandibular joints were within normal limits. Figure 2 shows pocket depth measurements after phase 1 therapy.

Intraoral Examination

- The soft tissues of the mouth including tongue appeared normal. Oral cancer screen was negative.
- The gingival examination revealed a generalized moderate marginal erythema. Several areas of boggy tissue and mobile teeth were noted.
- A hard tissue examination was completed.
- The edentulous ridge in the maxillary right quadrant had deficiencies bucco-lingually and apico-coronally (Seibert class 3).
- Minimal salivary flow of mucus consistency.

Occlusion

There was a lack of posterior support in the right quadrant and unprotected occlusion. First occlusal contacts were on anterior teeth (Figure 3).

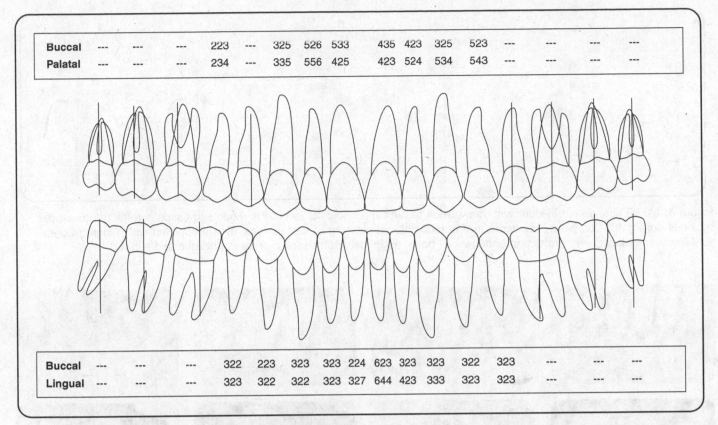

Buccal	---	---	---	223	---	325	526	533	435	423	325	523	---	---	---	---
Palatal	---	---	---	234	---	335	556	425	423	524	534	543	---	---	---	---

Buccal	---	---	---	322	223	323	323	224	623	323	323	322	323	---	---	---
Lingual	---	---	---	323	322	322	323	327	644	423	333	323	323	---	---	---

Figure 2: Probing pocket depth measurements (following phase 1 therapy).

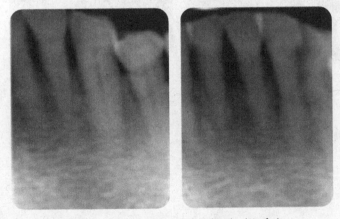

Figure 3: Radiographic evaluation (peri-apicals of the mandibular anterior teeth).

Treatment Plan

The primary care physician was contacted to obtain comprehensive information regarding the patient's cardiovascular status and to suggest alternative medication to increase salivary flow. Prosthodontic and endodontic consultations were required to establish a comprehensive treatment plan. A cone beam computed tomography scan was ordered for the maxillary and mandibular arch for potential implant placement in edentulous areas.

The final treatment plan included extensive periodontic, prosthetic, and occlusal rehabilitation with implant-supported crowns. Guided tissue regeneration (GTR) procedures involved several teeth including tooth #24. Figure 4 illustrates the steps involved in GTR surgery.

Treatment

The patient received oral hygiene instructions and three complete scaling and root planing sessions prior to surgical therapy. The patient was placed on a permanent saliva substitute program. Pocket depths shown (Figure 2) were recorded following phase 1 therapy.

Preoperative Consultation

The medical history was reviewed. His blood pressure was again monitored. The consent form addressing benefits and risks associated with the procedure was reviewed with the patient. Accessibility to the surgical site was clinically assessed. Significant (Class II) mobility of tooth #24 was noted. The following prescriptions were delivered to the patient: amoxicillin

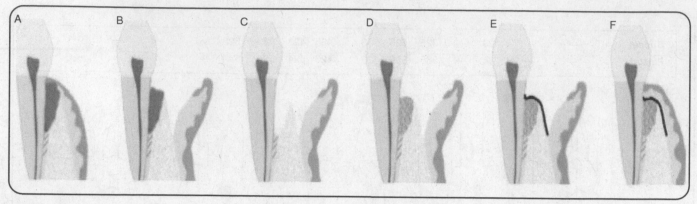

Figure 4: (A) Vertical defect evident with granulation tissue fill. (B) Sulcular incision is made and tissue is reflected to expose osseous defect. (C) Complete debridement of defect and root planning of root surface. (D) Defect filled with allograft bone. (E) Membrane placed over grafts and endogenous bone. (F) Primary soft tissue closure is obtained and sutured.

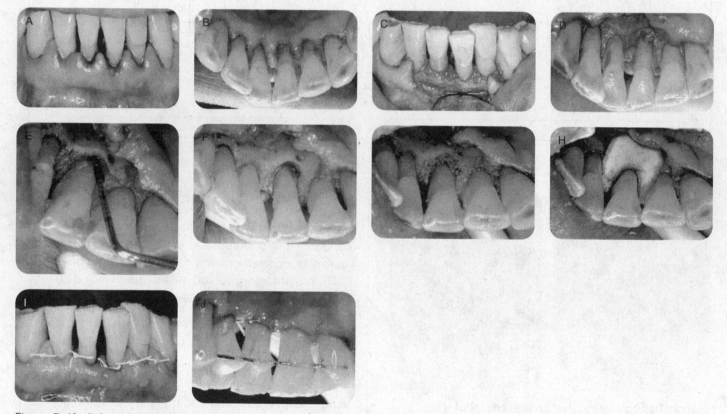

Figure 5: (A–J) Intraoral surgical photos.

500 mg (tid for 10 days starting 24 hours before the procedure), ibuprofen 600 mg (every 4–6 hours as needed for pain), and Peridex 0.12% (bid).

Guided Tissue Regeneration Procedure

Bilateral mental nerve blocks and local lingual infiltration were achieved with lidocaine 2% (epinephrine 1/100,000). A full-thickness flap was elevated buccally and lingually from distal of teeth #23 to mesial #27 to achieve access (Figure 5A–D). The teeth in this region were thoroughly scaled and root planed, and the osseous defect was completely degranulated (Figure 5E and F). A rotary finishing bur was used to remove additional debris and conservatively recontour surrounding bone. Following a thorough rinse of the teeth, rehydrated freeze-dried mineralized bone allograft (FDBA) was placed in the defect to the crest of the surrounding bone (Figure 5G). A resorbable

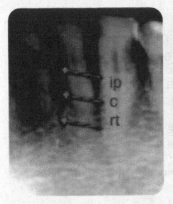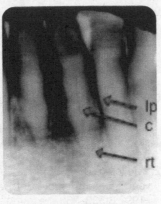

Figure 6: Periapical radiographs (A) initial; (B) following 6 months of healing.

collagen membrane was placed over the augmented site (Figure 5H) and the flap was reapproximated to achieve primary closure and then sutured (Figure 5I). The six mandibular anterior teeth were splinted together with orthodontic wire and composite resin to stabilize the mobile tooth #24 (Figure 5J). Healing was uneventful thereafter (Figure 6).

Discussion

GTR is a predictable procedure for regenerating bone adjacent to teeth that was lost due to inflammatory periodontal disease. It is important to understand the limitations of this procedure in order to achieve these results. Successful oral hygiene management as well as appropriate maintenance intervals is an essential part of the treatment. Good communication with the referring general dentist and/or hygienist is necessary in order to provide patients with optimal care.

Although we were unable to change this patient's blood pressure medication, we were able to provide saliva substitutes that will provide an additional defense against future periodontal breakdown.

The surgery was successful and uneventful. The patient was seen for postoperative visits at 2 weeks to remove the sutures and at 3 and 6 weeks for evaluation. After 6 months the fixed splint was removed from this region and periapical radiographs were taken to assess the amount of bone regenerated (Figure 5G). Tooth #24 was now only slightly mobile compared with the +2 mobility originally recorded. Final occlusal rehabilitation by the prosthodontist following additional periodontic therapy provided the patient with a stable atraumatic occlusion.

Self-Study Questions

A. What is the rationale for performing GTR as opposed to other available surgical techniques?

B. What are the techniques used in GTR therapy?

C. Which biomaterials can be used in GTR? Is there histologic evidence of bone formation?

D. What are the determinants of success in GTR?

E. Do traumatic occlusal events affect the success of treatment with GTR?

F. What are the complications associated with GTR? How do you manage these complications?

Answers located at the end of the chapter.

References

1. Melcher AH. On the repair potential of periodontal tissues. J Periodontol 1976;47:256–260.

2. Becker W, Becker BE, et al. New attachment after treatment with root isolation procedures: Report for treated class III and class II furcations and vertical osseous defects. Int J Periodontics Restorative Dent 1988;8:8–23.

3. Dahlin C, Linde A, et al. Healing of bone defects by guided tissue regeneration. Plast Reconstr Surg 1988;81:672–676.

4. Garrett JS, Crigger M, et al. Effects of citric acid on diseased root surfaces. J Periodontal Res 1978;13:155–163.

5. Stahl SS, Froum SJ, et al. Healing responses of human intraosseous lesions following the use of debridement, grafting and citric acid root treatment. II. Clinical and histologic observations: One year postsurgery. J Periodontol 1983;54:325–338.

6. Albair WB, Cobb CM, et al. Connective tissue attachment to periodontally diseased roots after citric acid demineralization. J Periodontol 1982;53:515–526.

7. Terranova VP, Franzetti LC, Hic S, et al. A biochemical approach to periodontal regeneration: tetracycline treatment of dentin promotes fibroblast adhesion and growth. J Periodontal Res 1986;21:330–337.

8. Blomlof J, Blomlof L, et al. Effect of different concentrations of EDTA on smear removal and collagen exposure in periodontitis-affected root surfaces. J Clin Periodontol 1997;24:534–537.

9. Blomlof J, Jansson L, et al. Root surface etching at neutral pH promotes periodontal healing. J Clin Periodontol 1996;23:50–55.

10. Caffesse RG, Kerry GJ, et al. Clinical evaluation of the use of citric acid and autologous fibronectin in periodontal surgery. J Periodontol 1988;59:565–569.

11. Mariotti A. Efficacy of clinical root surface modifiers in the treatment of periodontal disease. A systematic review. Ann Periodontol 2003;8:205–226.

12. Newman MG, Takei H, et al. Carranza's Clinical Periodontology. 3rd ed. Maryland Heights, MO: Elsevier/Saunders, 1995.

13. Carranza FA Sr. A technic for reattachment, J Periodontol 1954;25:272.

14. Moskow BS, Tannenbaum P. Enhanced repair and regeneration of periodontal lesions in tetracycline-treated patients: case reports. J Periodontol 1991;62:341.

15. Lindhe J, Karring T, et al. Clinical Periodontology and Implant Dentistry. 4th ed. Hoboken, NJ: Wiley-Blackwell, 2003.

16. Zellin G, Gritli-Linde A, et al. Healing of mandibular defects with different biodegradable and non-biodegradable membranes: an experimental study in rats. Biomaterials 1995;16:601.

17. Friedmann A, Strietzel FP, et al. Histological assessment of augmented jaw bone utilizing a new collagen barrier membrane compared to a standard barrier membrane to protect a granular bone substitute material. Clin Oral Implant Res 2002;13:587.

18. Sandberg E, Dahlin C, et al. Bone regeneration by the osteopromotive technique using bioabsorbable membranes: an experimental study in rats. Int J Oral Maxillofac Surg 1993;51:1106.

19. Hollinger JO, Brekke J, et al. Role of bone substitutes. Clin Orthop 1996;324:55–65.

20. Tolman DE. Reconstructive procedures with endosseous implants in grafted bone: a review of the literature. Int J Oral Maxillofac Implants 1995;10:275–294.

21. Mowlem R. Cancellous chip bone grafts: Report on 75 cases. Lancet 1944;2:746–748.

22. Mellonig JT. Autogenous and allogeneic bone grafts in periodontal therapy. Crit Rev Oral Biol Med 1992;3:333–352.

23. Mulliken JB, Glowacki J. Induced osteogenesis for repair and construction in the craniofacial region. Plast Reconstr Surg 1980;65:553–560.

24. Cammack GV II, Nevins M, Clem DS III, et al. Histologic evaluation of mineralized and demineralized freeze-dried bone allograft for ridge and sinus augmentations. Int J Periodontics Restorative Dent 2005;25:231–237.

25. Simion M, Trisi P, et al. Vertical ridge augmentation using a membrane technique associated with osseointegrated implants. Int J Periodontics Restorative Dent 1994;14:496–511.

26. Cochran DL, Douglas HB. Augmentation of osseous tissue around nonsubmerged endosseous dental implants. Int J Periodontics Restorative Dent 1993;13:506–519.

27. Becker W, Becker BE, et al. A comparison of demineralized freeze-dried bone and autologous bone to induce bone formation in human extraction sockets. J Periodontol 1994;65:1128.

28. Becker W, Schenk R, et al. Variations in bone regeneration adjacent to implants augmented with barrier membranes alone or with demineralized freeze-dried bone or autologous grafts: a study in dogs. Int J Oral Maxillofac Implants 1995;10:143.

29. Becker W, Urist MR, et al. Human demineralized freeze-dried bone: inadequate induced bone formation in athymic mice-a preliminary report. J Periodontol 1995;66:822.

30. Nabers CL, O'Leary TJ. Autogenous bone transplants in the treatment of osseous defects. J Periodontol 1965;36:5.

31. Sanders J, Sepe W, et al. Clinical evaluation of freeze-dried bone allografts in periodontal osseous defects. III. Composite freeze-dried bone allograft with and without autogenous bone, J Periodontol 1983;54:1.

32. Sepe W, Bowers G, et al. Clinical evaluation of freeze-dried bone allograft in periodontal osseous defects. Part II. J Periodontol 1978;49:9.

33. Mellonig JT. Freeze-dried bone allografts in periodontal reconstructive surgery. Dent Clin North Am 1991;35:505.

34. Mellonig JT, Bowers GM, et al. Comparison of bone graft materials. Part I. New bone formation with autografts and allografts determined by strontium-85. J Periodontol 1981;52:291.

35. Mellonig JT, Bowers GM, et al. Comparison of bone graft materials. Part II. New bone formation with autografts and allografts: a histological evaluation. J Periodontol 1981;52:297.

36. Libin BM, Ward HL, et al. Decalcified lyophilized bone allografts for use in human periodontal defects. J Periodontol 1975;46:51.

37. Pearson GE, Rosen S, et al. Preliminary observations on the usefulness of a decalcified freeze-dried cancellous bone allograft material in periodontal surgery. J Periodontol 1981;52:55.

38. Quntero G, Mellonig JT, et al. A six-month clinical evaluation of decalcified freeze-dried bone allografts in periodontal osseous defects. J Periodontol 1982;53:726.

39. Andereeg CR, Martin SJ, et al. Clinical evaluation of the use of decalcified freeze-dried bone allograft with guided tissue regeneration in the treatment of molar furcation invasions. J Periodontol 1991;62:264.

40. Schallhorn RG, McClain PK. Combined osseous composite grafting, root conditioning, and guided tissue regeneration. Int J Periodont Restor Dent 1988;8:8.

41. Magnusson I, et al. A long junctional epithelium – a locus minoris resistentiae in plaque infection. J Clin Periodontol 1983;10:333–340.

42. Cortellini P, Pini Prato G, et al. Periodontal regeneration of human infrabony defects. II. Re-entry procedures and bone measures. J Periodontol 1993;64:261–268.

43. Selvig KA, Kersten BG, et al. Surgical treatment of intrabony periodontal defects using expanded polytetrafluoroethylene barrier membranes: influence of defect configuration on healing response. J Periodontol 1993;64:730–733.

44. Cortellini P, Carnevale G, et al. Radiographic defect angle influences the outcome of GTR therapy in intrabony defects. J Dent Res 1999;78:38.

45. Anderegg CR, Metzler DG, et al. Gingiva thickness in guided tissue regeneration and associated recession at facial furcation defects. J Periodontol 1995;66: 397–402.

46. Periodontal Literature Reviews. 3rd ed. Chicago, IL: American Academy of Periodontology, 1996.

47. Flezar TJ, Knowles JW, et al. Tooth mobility and periodontal therapy. J Clin Periodontol 1980;7: 495–505.

48. Trejo PM, Weltman RL. Favorable periodontal regenerative outcomes from teeth with presurgical mobility: a retrospective study. J Periodontol 2004;75:1532–1538.

TAKE-HOME POINTS

A. Regeneration refers to our ability to recreate the original healthy periodontal apparatus that was destroyed because of disease or injury. Our goals are then to end up with a reproduction of alveolar bone, cementum, and a functional periodontal ligament. The cells responsible for this regeneration are osteoblasts, cementoblasts, and periodontal ligament cells. Fundamental to GTR therapy is the presence of a barrier membrane that prevents the infiltration of epithelial and connective tissue cells (fibroblasts) into the environment adjacent to the root surface and bone such that the three cells just mentioned have an opportunity to regenerate their respective tissues. Because epithelial cells and fibroblast proliferate at a much greater rate, it is essential that this barrier be in place. Following a period of healing of approximately 3–6 months, the barrier can then be removed if a nonresorbable membrane was used. GTR differs from other more traditional procedures such as flap osseous surgery in terms of regenerating tissue as opposed to resecting it.

B. The principles of surgical technique involved in GTR are similar to the general principles of periodontal surgery with some additional concepts as summarized here (refer to Figure 4) [1–3]:

- Isolation of the debrided periodontal defect (usually filled with bone material) with a barrier membrane such that the borders of the membrane extend 3–4 mm beyond the confines of the defect in all the directions.
- Adaptation of the membrane with sling sutures with respect to the periodontal defect so the defect is isolated from the gingival cellular components and if the membrane is resilient, to achieve the function of space maintenance during wound healing (regeneration).
- Following thorough scaling and root planning of the root surface, many surgeons prefer to use a root surface modifier to enhance attachment and stimulate connective tissue ingrowth. Examples of some surface modifiers include citric acid, tetracycline, and ethylenediaminetetraacetic acid (EDTA). Although human studies fail to support

these arguments, some animal studies provide evidence of its effectiveness. Histologically, the healing patterns do not result in significant improvement in clinical outcome compared with control sites in human studies [4–11].

- Complete coverage of the mucoperiosteal flap over the membrane.
- Optional coronal displacement of the flap is indicated to further facilitate the delay in the potential migration of the gingival cells into the wound area.

Systemic antibiotics are generally used after reconstructive periodontal therapy, although definitive information on the advisability of this measure is still lacking [12]. Case reports have shown extensive reconstruction of periodontal lesions after scaling, root planing, and curettage, with systemic and local treatment using penicillin or tetracycline, in combination with other forms of therapy [13,14].

C. GTR procedures are based on the use of a membrane to prevent epithelial and connective tissue growth into the regenerating site with or without a bone filler that primarily provides a scaffold to which cells can attach. Membranes can be classified as resorbable or nonresorbable.

- Resorbable membranes: Can be a tissue, such as connective tissue graft or allogeneic dermal matrix, but usually refers to membranes made of collagen. Synthetic resorbable membranes (polyglactin 910, polylactic acid, polyglycolic acid, polyorthoester, polyurethane, and polybutyrate) are also used.
- Nonresorbable membranes: Usually made of polytetrafluoroethylene (PTFE) or expanded PTFE (ePTFE) and can be reinforced by titanium structure to give more stability. Titanium mesh and titanium foil are also nonresorbable membranes used for GTR. Typically, nonresorbable membranes are removed after 6–12 months [15].

The primary advantage of nonresorbable membranes is stabilization of the graft. The disadvantages of a nonresorbable barrier membrane relates to its difficulty in handling and the possibility of its exposure during the healing process. Exposed membranes become contaminated with oral bacteria, which may lead to

infection of the site and result in bone loss [12]. It is important to remove these membranes at a designated time period during the healing process. If the membrane is removed too early, bone loss can also occur [12].

The advantages of a resorbable membrane are the elimination of surgical reentry for membrane removal as well as reduced complications if the membrane becomes exposed. Disadvantages of using resorbable membranes include the possibility of early degradation prior to completion of bone formation as well as the presence of inflammation brought on by this degradation process [16]. More recently, new developments including cross-linking of collagen to increase resistance to biodegradation have been developed [17]. Fortunately, the mild inflammatory reaction caused by bioresorbable membranes does not seem to interfere with osteogenesis [12]. In addition to these attributes, resorbable membranes are also user friendly. However, their lack of resiliency results in a collapse of the membrane into the defect area [18]. Resorbable membranes are best reserved for clinical indications that allow the graft material or hardware (tenting screws, plates) to maintain the space required [12].

Bone Materials
The available sources of bone materials include the following [19]:

1. Autograft: the patient's own bone
2. Allograft-processed cadaver bone from another human (FDBA), and DFDBA (demineralized freeze-dried bone allograft)
3. Alloplast: synthetic bone substitutes such as tricalcium phosphate
4. Xenograft: cadaver bone from an animal such as bovine or porcine (i.e., Bioss-Osteohealth, Shirley, NY, USA)

These products are provided in a particulate form of various sizes as well as in block form. Particulate grafts from the preceding list may also be combined [19].

The particulate autograft is still considered the gold standard for most ridge augmentation procedures primarily due to its inherent osteogenic behavior [20,21]. Blood vessels are able to penetrate the spaces between the particles compared with a block graft and thus provide for more rapid in growth of blood vessels. Larger osteoconduction surface area, more exposure of osteoinductive growth factors, and easier biologic remodeling are also advantages of the particulate graft [12].

However, autografts have limitations that include donor site morbidity, increased cost, potential resorption, size mismatch, and an inadequate volume of graft material [22,23]. Bone allografts overcome many of the shortfalls of autogenous grafts but are considered primarily osteoconductive and to some degree osteoinductive (DFDBA) in nature. The literature suggests that DFDBA may have greater osteoinductive potential because of the availability of morphogenic proteins. However, a histologic study comparing FDBA or DFDBA for ridge augmentation demonstrated regeneration of 42% new bone area with no statistical difference between the two materials [24].

Bone allograft is bone collected from a human cadaver that is commercially available from tissue banks. They are obtained from cortical or cancellous bone within 12 hours of the death of the donor, defatted, cut in pieces, washed in absolute alcohol, and flash frozen. The material may then proceed to the next steps (mineralized, FDBA) or be demineralized (DFDBA). Both products then are ground and sieved to a particle size of 250–750 μm and freeze-dried. They are then vacuum-sealed in glass vials [12].

The use of particulate allograft bone replacement substitute has been reported for numerous applications, including GTR [25,26]. From a histologic standpoint, biopsies of some studies using bone allografts indicate viable bone cells and visible osteocytes in lacunae, and a 9-month specimen showed no remaining allograft material [4]. However, there are some contradictory results using DFDBA and membrane combinations [27–29].

Several clinical studies by Mellonig, Bowers, and coworkers reported bone fill exceeding 50% in 67% of the defects grafted with FDBA and in 78% of the defects grafted with FDBA plus autogenous bone. [30–32]. FDBA, however, is considered an osteoconductive material, whereas decalcified FDBA (DFDBA) is considered an osteoinductive graft and thus potentially has greater osteogenic

potential. Several studies back up this theory [12,33–35].

In 1975, Libin et al [36] reported three patients with 4–10 mm of bone regeneration in periodontal osseous defects. Clinical studies were also done that compared cancellous DFDBA and cortical DFDBA [37,38]. The results of these studies demonstrated the superiority of cortical particulate (2.4 mm vs. 1.38 mm of bone fill).

These studies provided strong evidence that DFDBA in periodontal defects results in significant probing depth reduction, attachment level gain, and osseous regeneration. The combination of DFDBA and GTR has also proved to be very successful [39–41].

Even though there are studies that demonstrate true periodontal regeneration, this issue still remains a topic for discussion because other studies demonstrate a long junctional epithelial (LJE) attachment as opposed to a connective tissue attachment. The question arises as to whether or not LJE is as resistant to disease as connective tissue. In an animal study, Magnusson et al were able to demonstrate that LJE is not more prone to new pocket formation and reinstitution of a disease activity compared with connective tissue [41].

To enhance the quality and quantity of bone regenerated there is a growing interest in growth factors. Products that are now clinically available include recombinant platelet-derived growth factor (rhPDGF-BB): Gem 21 (Osteohealth Inc, Shirley, NY, USA), the recombinant human bone morphogen protein 2 (rhBMP-2) (Infuse Medtronics Inc, Minneapolis, MN, USA). Platelet-rich growth factors derived from the patient's own blood are compounds rich in different growth factors.

In summary, many well-controlled studies of interdental lesions show pocket depth reductions of up to 4 mm, with associated similar attachment level gains and fill of osseous defects. Reconstructive surgical treatment of furcation lesions has a more moderate result but still is superior to other surgical and nonsurgical therapies. Reports also show that these initial postsurgical gains are maintained for 3–5 years in patients who comply with normal maintenance schedules [12].

D. Success in GTR therapy relies on several factors that need to be an essential part of preoperative, perioperative, and postoperative treatment:

- Preoperative
  1. Absence of medical conditions including systemic diseases, bisphosphonate therapy, diabetes, autoimmune disease, irradiation, and smoking. The patient should be referred to a physician if there is any significant medical condition reported during the preoperative examination.
  2. The patient's oral hygiene practices and response to phase 1 therapy are important factors to consider before proceeding with treatment.
- Perioperative
  1. The depth of the infrabony lesion will determine the ultimate amount of regeneration according to well-accepted studies. Two or three wall defects were 95% filled; one wall or hemiseptal defect as 39% filled [42,43].
  2. The defect angle was also considered a determinant of success by Cortellini and colleagues. They found that if the infrabony defect angle was <25° (narrow defect) there was 1.5 mm more bone fill compared with a defect >37° (wide defect) [44].
  3. The literature supports rigorous cleaning of both the tooth surface and complete degranulation of the defect.
  4. Control of excessive mobility with splint stabilization has been shown to influence success of therapy. Refer to question F.
  5. Follow proper technique protocol as outlined in question B.
  6. Tissue thickness has also been indicated as a factor that may affect the success of this procedure [45].
- Postoperative
  The surgeon should deliver postoperative instructions emphasizing care not to disturb the surgical site with brushing, eating, and so on. It should be emphasized that the patient should not pull at the lip or tissues at the surgical site. The patient should also be instructed to take all medications that were prescribed until finished and apply ice to reduce swelling that may otherwise place excessive stretching forces on the tissue. To help prevent potential adverse events, the patient should be followed over the next 6–8 weeks.

E. According to the Periodontal Literature Review (1996), occlusal trauma can be defined as follows [46]:

- **Occlusal trauma:** An injury to the attachment apparatus as a result of excessive occlusal force.
- **First-degree occlusal trauma:** Injury resulting from excessive occlusal forces applied to a tooth or teeth with normal support.
- **Second-degree occlusal trauma:** Injury resulting from normal occlusal forces applied to a tooth or teeth with inadequate support.

According to Flezar et al, pocket reduction of clinically mobile teeth did not respond as well to various forms of periodontal surgery as firm teeth with comparable initial disease severity [47]. In another study, Trejo and Weltman were able to demonstrate that interproximal intraosseous defects of teeth with limited presurgical tooth mobility (i.e., Miller's class 1 and 2 mobility) will respond favorably to regenerative therapy [48].

Therefore, before any regenerative procedures, the clinician should consider immobilizing or splinting mobile teeth to remove this possible risk factor.

F. According to the literature, these are some of the complications that have been reported for GTR with allograft:
1. Membrane exposure
2. Inflammatory reaction
3. Infection
4. Incision line opening
5. Loss of graft or reduced graft
6. Potential of disease transfer from the cadaver
Management of these complications is as follows:
1. **Membrane exposure:** The literature supports the removal of exposed nonresorbable membranes but not before sufficient time has elapsed for bone formation. Often these problems can be managed with good oral hygiene and use of topical 0.12% Chlorhexidine rinse until time of removal.
2. **Inflammatory reaction:** With the use of resorbable membrane, a confined inflammatory

event does take place upon degradation of the graft. As mentioned earlier this does not seem to affect the result of the augmentation. Surgical trauma can also cause significant inflammation that may put overwhelming pressure on the tissues resulting in suture line opening. To avoid this event a careful atraumatic surgical technique is required, and the use of steroids such as prednisone may be helpful.

3. **Infection:** Careful aseptic surgical technique, including thorough postoperative rinsing of the surgical site with sterile saline, can reduce the chances of infection. Pre- and postoperative systemic antibiotics have shown to improve augmentation results. Antibiotics such as penicillin, amoxicillin, clindamycin, azithromycin, or metronidazole can be used. If the infection cannot be controlled with antibiotics, the removal of the bone graft may be necessary.

4. **Incision line opening:** As mentioned, a careful atraumatic surgical technique as well as the use of steroids may reduce the likelihood of this happening. More importantly, however, the surgeon must release the flap from the underlying periosteum to ensure tension-free closure.

5. **Loss of graft:** The clinical situation should be reevaluated. The option of performing a second GTR procedure can be discussed.

6. **Potential of disease transfer from the cadaver:** According to the literature, the use of DFDBA includes the possible, although remote, potential of disease transfer from the cadaver [12].

Other complications with performing GTR surgery include ankylosis between bone and tooth that may or may not result in root resorption. Recession of the gingival tissue as a result of bone/graft loss as well as recurrence of deep pockets may also be an issue [12].

Case 3

Treatment of Intrabony Defects Using Growth Factors

CASE STORY

The patient was a 30-year-old female who was referred to private practice/periodontology clinic for examination and consultation. Her chief concern related to the fractured maxillary right lateral incisor. She had been aware of a problem due to the root fragment protruding through the buccal gingival margin (Figure 1).

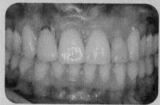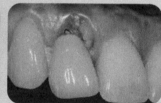

Figure 1: (A) Initial evaluation. (B) Tooth #7 presents with root fracture.

LEARNING GOALS AND OBJECTIVES

- To understand the use of recombinant human platelet-derived growth factor for implant site development
- To introduce the concepts of growth factor mediated wound healing for oral regeneration
- To observe the results of a clinical case using novel clinical application of tissue engineering principles

Medical History

The patient was in excellent medical health with a noncontributory medical history (no history of hospitalization, no daily medications, negative smoking history).

Dental History

The dental history provided a report of root canal therapy and crown restoration, approximately 10 years ago. The patient had noted a crack in the tooth (#7) about 14 months ago but had no dental pain and did not understand the need for timely treatment.

Examinations

Extra- and intraoral examinations were generally within normal limits (Figure 2). Mucogingival defects were noted for teeth #3–12,14, and 19–31. Probing depths ranged from 2 to 4mm for maxillary sites, 2–4mm with localized 9-mm probing depth buccal of tooth #7, and 5mm mesial of #7 for the buccal and palatal surfaces. Mandibular probing depths ranged from 2 to 4mm with localized 5-mm probing for the interproximal lingual of teeth #30/31. There was a generalized pattern of gingival recession ranging from 2 to 4mm. Mobility grade 3 was noted for the maxillary right lateral incisor.

Radiographic Examination

Periapical radiograph revealed 100% bone loss for the maxillary right lateral incisor. There was significant loss of lamina dura for the adjacent canine and central incisor. Vertical fracture was evident in the radiograph, which confirmed a hopeless prognosis for this tooth (Figure 3).

Treatment Options

Treatment options were presented to the patient, including replacement with a dental implant-supported crown restoration, a fixed partial denture, and a removable partial denture. The patient was highly motivated to have a fixed restoration and wanted an implant-supported crown.

This case presents challenges for obtaining a healthy foundation for a dental implant and an

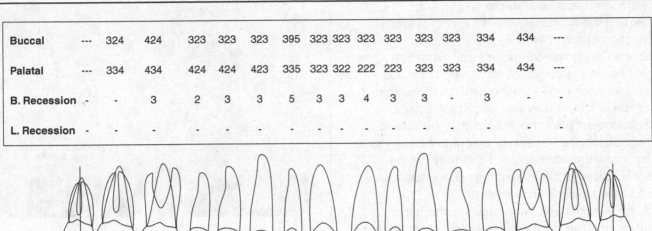

Buccal	---	324	424	323	323	323	395	323	323	323	323	323	323	334	434	---
Palatal	---	334	434	424	424	423	335	323	322	222	223	323	323	334	434	---
B. Recession	-	-	3	2	3	3	5	3	3	4	3	3	-	3	-	-
L. Recession	-	-	-	-	-	-	-	-	-	-	-	-	-	-	-	-

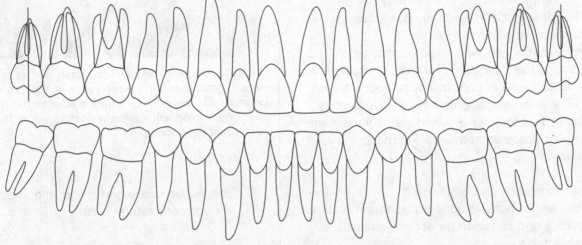

Buccal	434	434	423	323	333	333	222	222	222	223	323	323	332	434	434	434
Lingual	434	435	534	423	323	322	222	223	323	323	323	323	323	424	434	434
B. Recession	-		3	3	3	3	3	-	3	3	2	3	4	-	3	3
L. Recession	-	-	-	-	-	3	2	3	3	2	3	-				

Figure 2: Initial probing depths and periodontal measurements (mm).

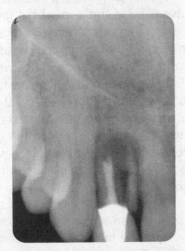

Figure 3: Periapical radiography reveal root fracture with bone loss.

aesthetic result for this patient, whose smile displays the free gingival margin of the papilla in the aesthetic zone:

- There is vertical and horizontal loss of alveolar bone including the complete buccal plate
- There is gingival recession and no attached gingiva, with approximately 1 mm keratinized tissue for the lateral incisor
- There is the need to regenerate the bone support for the adjacent teeth to improve their prognosis
- There is the challenge of providing ridge augmentation procedures and maintaining the gingival papillae
- Due to the gingival recession, the adjacent teeth would benefit from a root coverage procedure
-

The standard approach to dental implant replacement would include the following steps:

1. Extraction of tooth #7
   - Due to the advanced bone loss, extraction alone will cause resorption of remaining bone and shrinkage of papilla during healing. Once this tissue is lost, it may be difficult to recover;
   - Subsequent graft procedures may be able to reestablish the necessary amount of bone tissue for implant placement, but this may not be sufficient to achieve aesthetic goals due to increased clinical crown length.
   - Surgical extraction with ridge augmentation advancing the buccal flap for closure presents a challenge: there is poor quality of buccal tissue, which will be unpredictable to achieve primary closure. This technique would also decrease the vestibule space and advance the mucogingival junction

or

2. Flapless extraction and grafting:
   - Placement of passive bone replacement material in such a noncontained defect is generally unpredictable

or

3. Growth factor enhanced therapy:
   - The goal of the proposed therapy is to use a minimally invasive approach to stimulate bone regeneration through the use of a growth factor enhanced matrix, combining recombinant human platelet-derived growth factor BB (rhPDGF-BB) with mineralized freeze-dried bone allograft (FDBA). The growth factor upregulates the wound healing process to a clinically significant level, allowing for improved healing
   - The goal of the preservation procedure performed at the time of extraction is to recover the vertical bone height without flap surgery and with preservation of the aesthetic form of the gingival tissues and papillae. Therefore, even if there is the need for additional lateral ridge augmentation, the case can be converted to a less complex problem, which is more predictable to treat than a vertical defect
   - The patient is advised there may be multiple steps of bone augmentation and that the site will be evaluated with three-dimensional tomography to determine the bone available for implant placement. Soft tissue grafting is planned to be combined with dental implant placement, once it is determined to be adequate bone, with

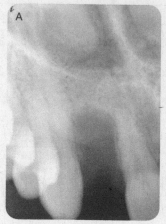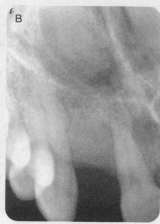

Figure 4: (A) Intraoperative radiograph reveals removal of all root fragments and the preservation of the fragile interproximal periodontium for the adjacent teeth. (B) Periapical radiograph 4 months postgrafting with evidence of significant bone formation.

connective tissue grafting for the implant site and the adjacent natural teeth

Treatment

Extraction and ridge preservation with growth factor enhanced matrix rhPDGF-BB and FDBA (Figures 4A and B):

- With local anesthesia the lateral incisor is extracted and the extraction socket debrided and degranulated. A periapical radiograph is exposed to confirm removal of all of the root fragments.
- 0.5 ml rhPDGF-BB (0.3 mg/ml) is combined with 0.5 g FDBA (growth factor enhanced matrix) and allowed to bind for approximately 10 minutes prior to being condensed incrementally into the socket.
- The site is overfilled to the level of the gingival margin and a collagen membrane (BioGide, Osteohealth) is placed over the coronal aspect of the graft and stabilized with medical adhesive (Peryacril, Glustitch). The patient is provided with an essex appliance for 2 weeks to allow healing; then a removable partial denture is delivered to provide the provisional tooth replacement during the remaining healing period. It is important that there is no pressure on the edentulous ridge during the early healing period (Figure 5).

The site is allowed to heal for 5 months and then a cone beam computerized tomography (CT) scan is obtained to evaluate the bone available for dental implant placement (Figure 6). The CT scan is taken with the patient wearing a barium stent to identify the

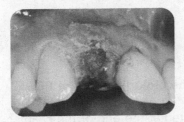

Figure 5: Immediate postoperative view of extraction socket grafted with growth factor-enhanced matrix combining rhPDGF-BB with FDBA protected by a collagen membrane and a medical adhesive.

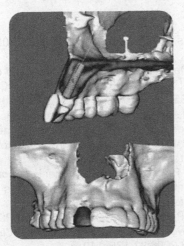

Figure 6: Cone beam CT scan 5 months postoperatively is used to determine if there is adequate bone for implant placement. The barium stent guides the surgical plan. (A) Sagittal view with projection of the planned implant at ideal placement position. (B) Anterior view with barium stent highlighted.

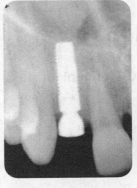
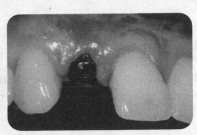

Figure 7: Implant after second-stage surgery. Note the tissue height preservation.

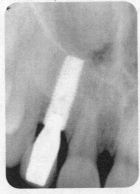
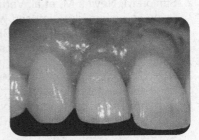

Figure 8: Definitive crown delivered to the patient. Note the improved gingival margin and the decreased gingival recession. Prosthodontist: Nancy S. Arbree, DDS, FACP, MS. Dental technician: Paul Chen.

tooth position of the future implant-supported crown. This allows for analysis as to whether the potential implant position is adequate to meet the restorative goals. The implant is planned using a viewing software (Simplant, Materialise Dental), and in the three-dimensional view it is readily visible that the implant can be placed in the proper position. It is interesting to note the lack of bone width throughout the patient's maxilla noted from the protuberance of the roots of the other anterior teeth.

A procedure is planned consisting of a dental implant placement combined with soft tissue grafting, a connective tissue graft, to provide root coverage for the adjacent teeth and to enhance the soft tissue profile of the dental implant site for function and aesthetics. Additional particulate bone grafting can also be used to provide contour grafting to the edentulous ridge if necessary during the same procedure. The

procedure is provided utilizing the barium stent as a guide to implant placement and a 4.0 × 13-mm implant is placed in a submerged fashion. A connective tissue graft harvested from the palate is placed to provide root coverage for the maxillary right canine extending mesially to the right central incisor and the buccal flap is advanced for closure over the grafted sites.

The implant is allowed to heal for 5 months before providing second-stage surgery with placement of a healing abutment with a modified punch technique. The tissues were allowed to heal for 4 weeks prior to beginning the restorative procedures (Figure 7).

The maintenance of tissue height and width provides an aesthetic framework for the design of an aesthetic implant-supported crown restoration. The final restoration meets the patient's functional and aesthetic needs (Figure 8).

Self-Study Questions

A. What are the benefits of Ð GF for implant site development?

B. What are the aesthetic challenges for predictable aesthetic outcomes?

C. What is the biologic effect of PDGF?

Answers located at the end of the chapter.

References

1. Simion M, Rocchietta I, et al. Vertical ridge augmentation by means of deproteinized bovine bone block and recombinant human platelet-derived growth factor-BB: a histologic study in a dog model. Int J Periodontics Restorative Dent 2006;26:415–423.
2. Simion M, Nevins M, et al. Vertical ridge augmentation using an equine block infused with recombinant human platelet-derived growth factor-BB: a histologic study in a canine model. Int J Periodontics Restorative Dent 2009;29:245–255.
3. Nevins ML, Camelo M, et al. Minimally invasive alveolar ridge augmentation procedure (tunneling technique) using rhPDGF-BB in combination with three matrices: a case series. Int J Periodontics Restorative Dent 2009;29:371–383.
4. Nevins ML, Camelo M, et al. Human histologic evaluation of mineralized collagen bone substitute and recombinant platelet-derived growth factor-BB to create bone for implant placement in extraction socket defects at 4 and 6 months: a case series. Int J Periodontics Restorative Dent 2009;29:129–139.
5. Hollinger JO, Hart CE, et al. Recombinant human platelet-derived growth factor: biology and clinical applications. J Bone Joint Surg Am 2008;90(suppl 1): 48–54.
6. Homsi J, Daud AI. Spectrum of activity and mechanism of action of VEGF/PDGF inhibitors. Cancer Control 2007;14:285–294.
7. Matsuda N, Lin WL, et al. Mitogenic, chemotactic, and synthetic responses of rat periodontal ligament fibroblastic cells to polypeptide growth factors in vitro. J Periodontol 1992;63:515–525.
8. Oates TW, Rouse CA, et al. Mitogenic effects of growth factors on human periodontal ligament cells in vitro. J Periodontol 1993;64:142–148.
9. Sarment DP, Cooke JW, et al. Effect of rhPDGF-BB on bone turnover during periodontal repair. J Clin Periodontol 2006;33:135–140.
10. Cooke JW, Sarment DP, et al. Effect of rhPDGF-BB delivery on mediators of periodontal wound repair. Tissue Eng 2006;12:1441–1450.
11. Nevins M, Giannobile VV, et al. Platelet-derived growth factor stimulates bone fill and rate of attachment level gain: results of a large multicenter randomized controlled trial. J Periodontol 2005;76:2205–2215.

TAKE-HOME POINTS

A. Preclinical studies and case reports provide proof of principle that rhPDGF-BB, when combined with other graft matrices, can support improved bone formation and wound healing in alveolar ridge reconstruction and implant therapy. Simion et al [1] reported a canine study that demonstrated the potential for a deproteinized cancellous bovine block, which when infused with rhPDGF-BB regenerated significant amounts of new bone in severe mandibular vertical ridge defects without placement of a barrier membrane. The xenogenic block grafts were infused with rhPDGF-BB and stabilized in alveolar defects using two dental implants with or without collagen membranes. The histologic findings revealed robust osteogenesis throughout the block graft, with significant graft resorption and replacement. In contrast, alveolar ridge defects treated with traditional GBR without the growth factor supported little or no bone formation.

Simion et al [2] reported similar findings using rhPDGF-BB in combination with a novel equine hydroxyapatite and collagen (eHAC) bone block in the canine model. Moreover, recent case reports demonstrate that FDBA and anorganic bovine bone can serve as effective scaffolds to deliver rhPDGF-BB for lateral ridge augmentation and reconstruction, following extraction for implant placement [3,4].

B. Extraction socket grafting presents the dilemma as to whether to raise a flap or proceed with a flapless approach. Often there is the need for flap elevation to be able to debride the defect thoroughly. Alternative techniques such as a submarginal incision may preserve the gingival form and allow access to a periapical defect with the limitation of secondary healing at the coronal aspect of the socket. For sockets with a complete loss of the buccal plate flap, advancement will provide primary closure and the best protection of the bone graft. However this requires surgical skill and experience, and the soft tissues must be managed to prevent a wound dehiscence that can

result in tissue volume shrinkage and loss of interdental papilla, which can be difficult to recover in the future. The use of procedures combining hard and soft tissue grafting can result in optimal preservation of ridge form. The soft tissues are often supported by the root prominence, and there is the need for additional volume of tissue beyond that easily regenerated with the bone graft procedure. These combined procedures are performed for optimal aesthetic preservation.

In the case of flapless socket preservation, additional soft tissue thickness can be provided to enhance the tissue biotype either at the time of extraction with tunneling techniques or at the time of implant placement using flap access. This will minimize the need for additional surgery after the implant has integrated by diagnosing and intercepting this, so that the tissue thickness is augmented in combination with the implant placement procedure.

C. PDGF exerts potent stimulatory effects as a chemoattractant and mitogen for mesenchymal cells (including osteogenic cells), as well as a promoter of angiogenesis, complementing the actions of vascular endothelial growth factor (VEGF) [5,6]. PDGF-BB has been shown to enhance the chemotactic and mitogenic activity of periodontal ligament cells at concentrations as low as $1\,ng/ml$ [7,8]. PDGF-BB triggers a cascade of biologic and cellular events at the surgical wound during the initial postoperative period that lasts for weeks as documented in human clinical trials [9]. These events are characterized by the recruitment and differentiation of mesenchymal cell populations, as well as new vessel formation, ultimately supporting wound healing and regeneration [5].

Cooke et al [10] examined the effects of PGDF-BB on levels of VEGF and bone turnover in periodontal wound fluid in 16 patients who were randomized to receive treatment of intrabony defects with either β-tricalcium phosphate (TCP) carrier alone, β-TCP plus $0.3\,mg/ml$ rhPDGF-BB, or β-TCP plus $1.0\,mg/ml$

rhPDGF-BB. These patients had participated in a large clinical trial evaluating the efficacy and safety of PDGF-BB in the treatment of intraosseous periodontal defects [11]. Pyridinoline cross-linked carboxyterminal telopeptide of type I collagen (ICTP) is an indicator of osseous metabolic activity and provided a marker of bone turnover. Low-dose rhPDGF-BB application was found to elicit increases in ICTP at 3–5 days in the wound healing process, with the 1.0 mg/ml rhPDGF-BB group showing the most pronounced difference in VEGF at 3 weeks. Thus a single dose of rhPDGF-BB exhibited demonstrable, sustained metabolic actions at the clinical site of application.

Case 4

Treatment of Intrabony Defects Using Alloplastic Materials

CASE STORY

A 54-year-old Caucasian female presented to the dental clinic with a chief complaint of: "I have a broken tooth." She reported that the tooth had fractured while eating nuts. She reported no pain or swelling. She was concerned with the appearance of the missing tooth and was having difficulty eating. Upon examination by the restorative dentist, tooth #13 had been found to be fractured below the gingival margin (Figure 1). After informing the patient that the tooth was not restorable, she had been told of her restorative options for replacing the tooth. The patient elected to pursue implant therapy to replace the tooth and was referred to the Periodontal Department for an evaluation.

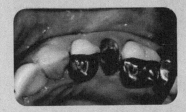

Figure 1: Preoperative presentation.

LEARNING GOALS AND OBJECTIVES

- To understand the events following wound healing
- To identify indications for grafting and understand what can be accomplished.
- To identify different materials that can be used for grafting

Medical History

The patient's medical history was reviewed with no significant findings. She was taking no medications other than a daily multivitamin. She had no known drug allergies.

Review of Systems

- Vital signs
  - Blood pressure:114/68 mm Hg
  - Heart rate: 62 beats/minute
  - Respiration: 12 breaths/minute

Social History

The patient did not use tobacco products. She drank alcohol socially and reported drinking one to three drinks per week. She was married with two children who were currently in college. She was an elementary school teacher.

Extraoral Examination

- No significant findings. The patient had no masses or swelling and the temporomandibular joint is within normal limits.

Intraoral Examination

- The soft tissues of the mouth including tongue appeared normal. Oral cancer screen was negative.
- A gingival examination revealed coral pink tissue with stippling and knife edge margins. Mild plaque accumulation was present on the buccal surfaces of the maxillary second molars with mild marginal inflammation.

Occlusion

There were no occlusal discrepancies or interferences.

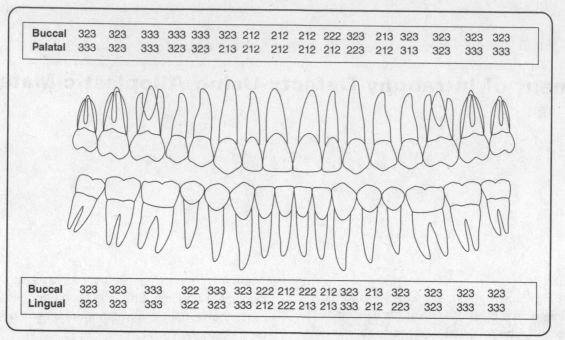

| | Buccal | 323 | 323 | 333 | 333 | 333 | 323 | 212 | 212 | 212 | 222 | 323 | 213 | 323 | 323 | 323 | 323 |
| | Palatal | 333 | 323 | 333 | 323 | 323 | 213 | 212 | 212 | 212 | 212 | 223 | 212 | 313 | 323 | 333 | 333 |

| | Buccal | 323 | 323 | 333 | 322 | 333 | 323 | 222 | 212 | 222 | 212 | 323 | 213 | 323 | 323 | 323 | 323 |
| | Lingual | 323 | 323 | 333 | 322 | 323 | 333 | 212 | 222 | 213 | 213 | 333 | 212 | 223 | 323 | 333 | 333 |

Figure 2: Probing pocket depth measurements.

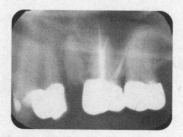

Figure 3: Periapical radiograph depicting the fractured root and the interproximal bone levels.

Radiographic Examination

A periapical radiograph was ordered (Figure 3).

Diagnosis

Tooth #13 was diagnosed as nonrestorable due to the amount of tooth structure lost.

Treatment Plan

The treatment plan for this patient is an atraumatic extraction of tooth #13 with immediate implant placement and simultaneous osteotome sinus augmentation.

Treatment

Prior to surgery, a surgical guide was fabricated (Figure 4A) and a periapical radiograph was taken (Figure 4B). Immediately prior to surgery, 20 ml of blood were

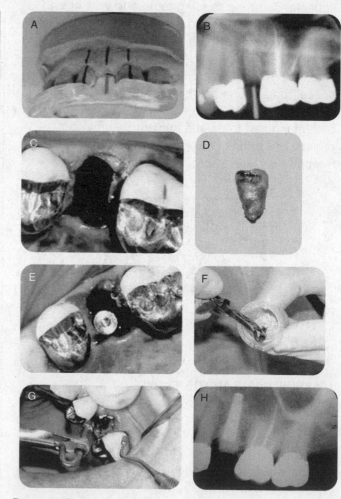

Figure 4: Surgical procedure.

withdrawn and processed for the preparation of 1 ml of platelet-rich plasma (PRP). After local infiltration with lidocaine 2% and epinephrine 1:50,000, the root was gently extracted using periotomes and forceps, minimizing trauma to the soft and hard tissues (Figures 4C and D). No flaps were elevated. After degranulation of the extraction socket, a 3-mm elevation of the sinus floor was achieved with osteotomes and the site was prepared for implant placement. Subsequently, one endosteal implant of 13 mm, 3.75 mm was placed (tapered Screw-Vent MP-1 HA Dual Transition Surface, Centerpulse Dental Inc). A preparation of calcium

sulfate and PRP (CS-PRP) was used to fill the residual gap between the socket wall and the implant body (Figures 4F and G). A barrier of pure calcium sulfate was used to cover the head of the implant and the grafted area. A Vicryl 5-0 suture was used to hold the barrier in place. No attempt was made to cover the calcium sulfate barrier with soft tissue. The immediate postoperative radiograph revealed the presence of grafted material both apical to and around the neck of the implant (Figure 4I). The patient was prescribed a 7-day course of amoxicillin 250 mg tid starting 1 day before the surgery.

Self-Study Questions

A. What is an alloplast?

B. What are some of the commonly used alloplast materials?

C. What are the indications for using an alloplast?

D. What is the difference between regeneration and repair?

E. Why would a practitioner choose an alloplast over an autograft, allograft, or xenograft?

F. What is the diagnosis of this case according to the American Academy of Periodontology (AAP classification system?

G. Describe the differences between at least two different prognosis systems.

H. To establish a correct prognosis, what information should be gathered?

I. What are the treatment options for this clinical case?

J. How would you perform socket preservation in this clinical case?

K. How do you measure treatment success for this clinical case?

L. What is the correct maintenance protocol for the presented clinical case?

Answers located at the end of the chapter.

References

1. Lindhe J., Lang N, et al. Clinical Periodontology and Implant Dentistry. Copenhagen, Denmark: Blackwell Munksgaard, 2006.
2. Nasr HF, Aichelmann-Reidy ME, et al. Bone and bone substitutes. Periodontology 2000 1999;19:74–86.
3. Carranza F, Newman M, et al. Clinical Periodontology. St. Louis, MO: Mosby, 2006. Chapter 67 p982.
4. Meffert RM, Thomas JR, et al. Hydroxylapatite as an alloplastic graft in treatment of human periodontal osseous defects. J Periodontol 1985;56:63.
5. Snyder AJ, Levin MP, et al. Alloplastic implants of tricalcium phosphate ceramic in human periodontal osseous defects. J Periodontol 1984;55:273.
6. Froum SJ, Weinberg MA, et al. Comparison of bioactive glass synthetic bone graft particles and open debridement in the treatment of human periodontal defects. A clinical study. J Periodontol 1998;69:698.
7. Froum SJ, Kusher L, et al. Human clinical and histologic responses to durapatite implants in intraosseous lesions. J Periondontol 1982;53:719.
8. Froum S, Stahl SS. Human intraosseous healing responses to the placement of tricalcium phosphate ceramic implants II. 13 to 18 months. J Periodontol 1987;58:103.
9. Annals of Periodontology 1996;1:621–670.
10. Darby I, Chen S, et al. Ridge preservation techniques for implant therapy. I J Oral Maxillofac Implants 2009;24:260–271.
11. Armitage GC. Development of a classification system for periodontal diseases and conditions. Ann Periodontol 1999;4:1–6.
12. Becker W, Berg L, et al. The long term evaluation of periodontal treatment and maintenance in 95 patients. Int J Periodontics Restorative Dent 1984;4:54–71.
13. McGuire MK, Nunn ME. Prognosis versus actual outcome. II. The effectiveness of clinical parameters in developing an accurate prognosis. J Periodontol 1996;67:658–665.
14. Kwok V, Caton JG. Prognosis revisited: A system for assigning periodontal prognosis. J Periodontol 2007;78:2063–2071.
15. Albrektsson T, Zarb G, et al. The long-term efficacy of currently used dental implants: a review and proposed criteria of success. Int J Oral Maxillofac Implants 1986;1:11–25.
16. Iacono VJ; Committee on Research, Science and Therapy, the American Academy of Periodontology. Dental implants in periodontal therapy [position paper]. J Periodontol 2000;71:1934–1942.

TAKE-HOME POINTS

A. Alloplastic materials are synthetic, inorganic, biocompatible, and/or bioactive bone graft substitutes that are claimed to promote bone healing through osteoconduction [1].

B. Hydroxyapatite (HA): Three forms are available for periodontal use. These include a solid particulate nonresorbable form, a porous nonresorbable form derived from the exoskeleton of coral, and a resorbable nonceramic HA.

ß-Tricalcium phosphate (ß-TCP): A porous form of calcium phosphate.

Polymers: Includes the polymer polyhydroxyethylmethacrylate (PHEMA), which is often referred to as HTR (hard tissue replacement).

Bioactive glasses (bio-glasses): Bio-glasses are composed of SiO_2, NaO_2, P_2O_5 and are resorbable or nonresorbable depending on the relative proportion of these components. When bio-glasses are exposed to tissue fluids, a double layer of silica gel and calcium phosphate is formed on the surface. The material promotes absorption and concentration of proteins through this layer allowing the osteoblasts to form extracellular bone matrix that theoretically may promote bone formation [2].

Calcium sulfate: Calcium sulfate (plaster of Paris) is biocompatible and porous, thereby allowing fluid exchange, which prevents flap necrosis. The material resorbs completely in 2–3 weeks [3].

C. Alloplasts can be used in place of autografts, allografts, or xenografts when performing bone grafts in the oral cavity. The periodontal literature is replete with studies that examine the clinical and histologic outcomes of alloplastic materials used to treat periodontal intrabony defects. When compared with open flap debridement, materials such as HA, β-TCP, and bioactive glass all showed significant gains in clinical attachment levels [4–6].

When results were examined histologically, the graft particles were often encapsulated in fibrous connective tissue with pocket closure primarily through long junctional epithelium [7,8]. The 1996 World Workshop in Periodontics concluded that "synthetic graft materials function primarily as defect fillers. If regeneration is the desired treatment outcome, other materials are recommended" [9]. Alloplastic materials can also be used successfully for ridge augmentation or sinus augmentation procedures. Histologic samples of bone grafting with different alloplastic materials show varying amounts of bone regeneration [10]. Particles of nonresorbable alloplasts usually become encapsulated by connective tissue, which may interfere with osseointegration of a dental implant if that is the desired goal of the grafting procedure. To avoid encapsulation of the alloplast by connective tissue, a completely resorbable alloplast is preferred to an nonresorbable one.

D. When the periodontium is damaged by inflammation or as a result of surgical treatment, the defect heals either through periodontal regeneration or repair. In periodontal regeneration, healing occurs through the reconstitution of an new periodontium, which involves the formation of alveolar bone, periodontal ligament (PDL), and new cementum in an area where the periodontium has been lost. Repair is healing by replacement with epithelium or connective tissue, or both, that matures into various nonfunctional types of scar tissue, termed *new attachment*. Histologically, patterns of repair included long junctional epithelium, new connective tissue adhesion, and/or ankylosis. Fully resorbable alloplast may favor regeneration, whereas nonresorbable alloplast tends to favor repair.

E. Several factors may influence a practitioner to choose an alloplast as a graft material. Alloplastic materials are synthetically derived so there is an unlimited supply with no risk of disease transmission or antigens that initiate cross-reactivity. Alloplastic materials are also a viable option for patients who have moral or religious objections to using human- or animal-derived graft materials.

F. On October 1999, the International Workshop for a Classification of Periodontal Diseases and Conditions was held and a new classification system for periodontal diseases was generated [11]. According to this classification, a root fracture is classified within the "Developmental or Acquired Deformities and Conditions" group and defined as a "Localized tooth-related factor that modifies or predisposes to plaque-induced gingival diseases/periodontitis."

G. Becker et al in 1984 [12] proposed a classification with three categories: good, questionable, and hopeless. In their studies, this system predicted correctly most of the prognoses in well-maintained patients. However, it was unable to predict outcomes in poorly maintained patients.

McGuire and Nunn [13] subsequently developed a more detailed prognostication system with five different categories: good, fair, poor, questionable, and hopeless. A tooth with a fair prognosis presents with approximately 25% attachment loss; a tooth with a poor prognosis presents with a 50% attachment loss; a tooth with a questionable prognosis presents with an attachment loss >50%; and a tooth with hopeless prognosis presents with inadequate attachment to maintain the tooth in health, comfort, and function.

More recently, Kwok and Caton [14], arguing that tooth loss is influenced by natural and iatrogenic reasons, proposed a prognostication system based on the probability of disease progression. Four categories are proposed: favorable, when future loss of periodontal supporting tissue is unlikely; questionable, when future periodontal breakdown may occur if the periodontium is not stabilized with comprehensive periodontal care; unfavorable, when periodontal breakdown is likely to occur even with comprehensive periodontal care; and hopeless, when the tooth must be extracted.

H. Practitioners use several factors when assessing the prognosis of individual teeth and the overall case. McGuire evaluates prognosis based on the amount of periodontal support or clinical attachment loss of each tooth. Additional factors considered include the elimination or control of the disease etiology, patient compliance and ability to maintain the tooth, crown-to-root ratio and root form, furcation involvement, and mobility. To restore the tooth in consideration, a root canal, post and core, and a crown would be necessary. Crown lengthening would be required to achieve adequate biologic width and ferrule. The amount of ostectomy required to achieve the treatment goals would result in a greater compromise of support of the fractured tooth as well as the adjacent teeth. See Chapter 3 for a detailed discussion on crown lengthening. Based on these criteria the tooth is given a hopeless prognosis.

I. Whenever a tooth has been given a hopeless diagnosis, the patient should be presented with all viable treatment options. This includes leaving the space unrestored. If the patient prefers this option, he or she must be informed of the sequela involved with a missing tooth such as supereruption of mandibular teeth. The patient can have a fixed or removable partial denture. Or the patient can have an implant placed. If the patient elects to pursue implant therapy, a delayed or immediate placement option can be discussed with the patient. In this particular case, due to proximity to the maxillary sinus, a sinus elevation procedure will likely be needed to accommodate a dental implant.

J. After atraumatic extraction of the tooth, the extraction site should be thoroughly debrided, ensuring the removal of all granulomatous tissue and irrigated with sterile saline. To preserve the ridge width, a bone graft material should be placed into the site. The practitioner has the option of a variety of grafting materials with different properties. These options include autograft harvested from another site, allograft, xenograft, or alloplast. Factors that influence the decision on what material to use include the desire to have a material that is osteoinductive, osteoconductive, or osteogenic. For additional information on socket preservation see Chapter 7, Case 3.

K. The established criteria for successful implant treatment include the following:
1. The absence of persistent signs or symptoms such as pain, infection, neuropathies, paresthesias, and violation of vital structures
2. Implant immobility
3. No continuous peri-implant radiolucency
4. Negligible progressive bone loss (<0.2 mm annually after physiologic remodeling during the first year of function)
5. Patient/dentist satisfaction with the implant-supported restoration [15]

L. Patients should be on a regular recall schedule to monitor the maintenance, including plaque control, of the implant-supported prosthesis. Maintenance programs should be designed individually because there is a lack of data detailing precise recall intervals, methods of plaque and calculus removal, and appropriate antimicrobial agents for maintenance around implants [16].

Case 5

Guided Bone Regeneration

CASE STORY

The patient was a 35-year-old female who had been referred to the Department of Periodontology for a consultation regarding prosthetic rehabilitation of the edentulous spaces in the maxillary right and left quadrant. The existing fixed bridges were failing, and she wanted to have fixed implant restorations to replace these missing teeth. Her existing bridges had been removed and the abutment teeth had been reprepared and then temporarily recemented (Figure 1).

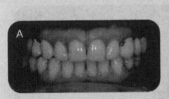 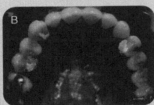

Figure 1: (A) Intraoral photo of both maxillary and mandibular teeth in occlusion and (B) occlusal view of maxillary arch.

LEARNING GOALS AND OBJECTIVES

■ To identify the indications for guided bone regeneration (GBR)
■ To understand the variety of GBR techniques that are available and determine the optimal one for a particular site
■ To be introduced to surgical techniques and biomaterials used to perform GBR

Medical History

There were no significant medical problems and the patient had no known allergies. She had been previously diagnosed with depression but was no longer on any medication for this condition. The only medications she was currently taking were oral contraceptives.

Review of Systems

- Vital signs
  - Blood pressure: 128/79 mm Hg
  - Pulse rate: 68 beats/minute (regular)

Social History

The patient was of Hispanic descent and married with three children. She did not drink alcohol, smoke, or use recreational drugs.

Extraoral Examination

No significant findings were noted. The patient had no masses or swelling, and the temporomandibular joints are within normal limits (Figure 2).

Intraoral Examination

- The oral cancer screen was negative.
- The gingival examination revealed generalized mild marginal erythema.
- A hard tissue examination was completed.
- The edentulous ridges in the maxillary right and left quadrant are deformed in the buccolingual and apico-coronal directions (Seibert class 3) (Figure 1).
- The tongue was serrated laterally.
- Saliva was of normal flow and consistency.
- Amalgam tattoo was present on ridge in #18 region.
- Slightly inflamed palatal tonsils were noted.

Occlusion

- Supereruption #14, distoversion #19 leading to left posterior bite collapse.
- No significant mobility or traumatic occlusion was noted (Figure 3).

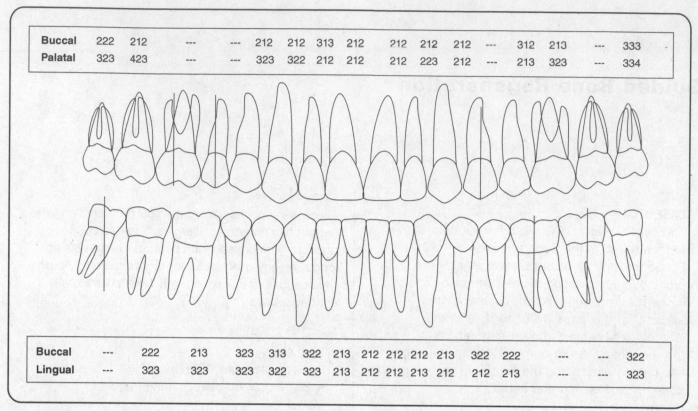

| Buccal | 222 | 212 | --- | --- | 212 | 212 | 313 | 212 | 212 | 212 | 212 | --- | 312 | 213 | --- | 333 |
| Palatal | 323 | 423 | --- | --- | 323 | 322 | 212 | 212 | 212 | 223 | 212 | --- | 213 | 323 | --- | 334 |

| Buccal | --- | 222 | 213 | 323 | 313 | 322 | 213 | 212 | 212 | 212 | 213 | 322 | 222 | --- | --- | 322 |
| Lingual | --- | 323 | 323 | 323 | 322 | 323 | 213 | 212 | 212 | 213 | 212 | 213 | --- | --- | 323 |

Figure 2: Probing pocket depth measurements (following phase 1 therapy).

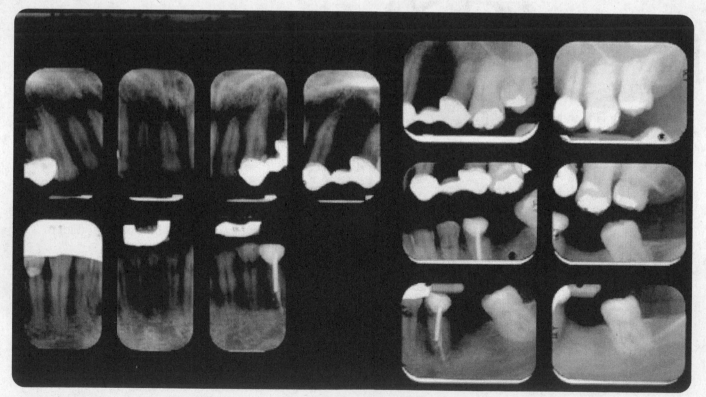

Figure 3: Radiographic evaluation (periapicals of the maxillary left posterior teeth).

Treatment Plan

Prosthodontic, endodontic, and orthodontic consultations were required to establish a comprehensive treatment plan. A cone beam computerized tomography (CT) scan was ordered for the maxillary arch to understand the anatomy, the condition of the deficient ridges, and the proximity of the maxillary sinus (Figure 4).

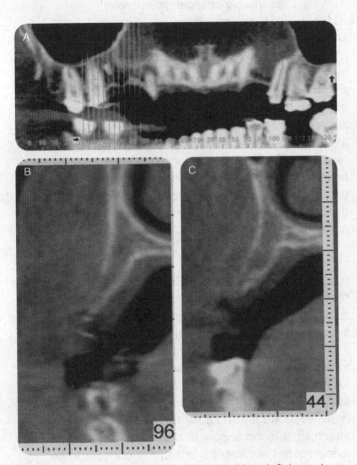

Figure 4: CT scans displaying horizontal ridge deficiency in #12 region.

The CT clearly indicates sufficient bone in the vertical dimension. However, to accommodate the appropriate implant for this site, 6–7 mm of width is required.

The final treatment plan for this region included GBR, prosthetic and occlusal rehabilitation including an implant supported fixed partial denture #4-x-6 (Figure 5).

Treatment

The patient received oral hygiene instructions and a prophylaxis 8 weeks prior to surgery.

Preoperative Consultation

The medical history was assessed. The consent form addressing benefits and risks associated with the procedure was reviewed with the patient. The patient was apprehensive about the procedure. Following a full disclosure of the treatment procedure, the patient became more comfortable. Accessibility to the surgical site was acceptable. The CT scan demonstrated that <3 mm of bone was present horizontally at edentulous site #12. No major anatomic obstacles were present. The site was significantly deficient in osseous width so a GBR technique involving tenting screws and a rigid resorbable membrane was selected. The following prescriptions were delivered to the patient: amoxicillin 500 mg (tid for 10 days starting 24 hours before the procedure), ibuprofen 600 mg (every 4–6 hours as needed), Vicodin ES (every 6 hours), and Peridex 0.12% (bid).

Guided Bone Regeneration Procedure

A posterior superior alveolar, middle superior alveolar, greater palatine nerve block, and local infiltrations were achieved with lidocaine 2% (epinephrine 1/100,000). A full-thickness flap was elevated in the maxilla right quadrant to expose the cortical bone (Figure 6A–C).

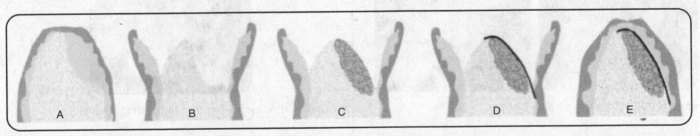

Figure 5: (A) Horizontal defect evident with soft tissue fill. (B) crestal incision is made and the tissue is reflected to expose the osseous defect. (C) defect filled with allograft bone. (D) Membrane placed over grafts and endogenous bone. (E) Primary soft tissue closure is obtained and then sutured.

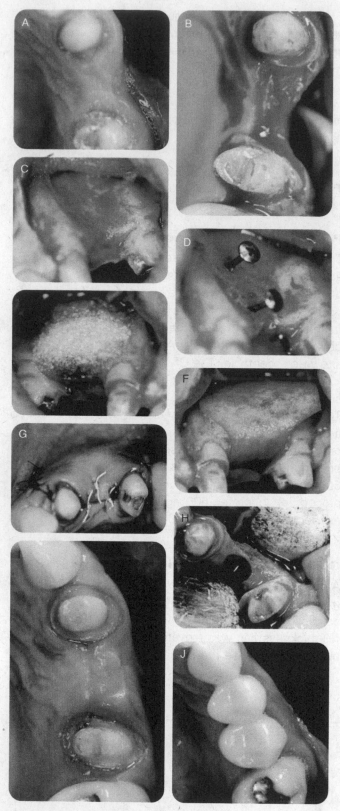

Figure 6 (A–J): Intraoral surgical photos.

Two vertical relaxing incisions were made to improve visibility and reduce the possibility of tissue tearing. Following surgical access to the region, the buccal aspects of the deficient ridge were decorticated with a round diamond bur to enhance osseous bleeding. Two 10-mm tenting screws were placed and deemed immobile (Figure 6D). Rehydrated mineralized freeze-dried bone allograft (FDBA) was then placed in excess onto this site (Figure 6E).

A rigid resorbable collagen membrane (Osseoguard-Collagen Matrix, Inc, Franklin Lakes, NJ, USA) was placed over the bone allograft (Figure 6F), and the flap was repositioned and sutured back to its initial position (Figure 6G). Healing was uneventful. Six months following GBR the site was anesthetized and exposed. A 4.1-mm osteotomy was performed allowing for sufficient buccal and lingual bone to assure long-term stability of tissues and prevent recession (Figure 6H). Photographs taken prior to finalization with permanent fixed implant crowns demonstrate significant improvement in ridge width (Figure 6I and J). Figure 7 shows the radiograph taken on the day of the procedure.

Discussion

Guided bone regeneration (GBR) is a predictable procedure for regenerating bone in a deficient maxillary or mandibular ridge, provided the determinants of success and the potential risk factors are identified. The degree of postoperative bone loss determines the technique the clinician chooses. There are certain tenets of tissue engineering that must be enforced for successful predictable augmentation. A scaffold is required (bone particles) for the patient's bone cells to attach to, a blood supply to the site is required (decorticate the patient's bone), the graft must be

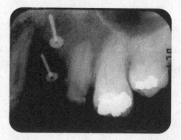

Figure 7: Radiograph on the day of the procedure.

separated from the soft tissue to prevent fibroblast and squamous cell infiltration (membrane), and the graft must be stabilized. Larger defects can be treated with the technique described or with a titanium reinforced nonresorbable membrane to stabilize the graft. Autogenous bone may also be added to the

bone mixture in such a situation to provide more of the patient's own bone-producing cells.

The healing for this procedure was uneventful. The tenting screws were removed and the permanent dental implant placed 5 months following the GBR procedure.

Self-Study Questions

A. Define the Siebert classification system for edentulous ridge osseous defects.

B. What is the rationale for performing GBR?

C. When is GBR indicated? When is it contraindicated?

D. Which biomaterials can be used in a GBR? Is there histologic evidence of bone formation?

E. What are the techniques used for GBR therapy?

F. Are implants placed in GBR site as successful as implants placed in pristine bone? Does the surgical technique have an influence on the implant survival rate in the long term?

G. What are the complications associated with GBR? How do you manage these complications?

Answers located at the end of the chapter.

References

1. Chiapasco M, Zaniboni M. Clinical outcomes of GBR procedures to correct peri-implant dehiscences and fenestrations: a systematic review.Clin Oral Implants Res 2009;20(Suppl 4):113–123.
2. Shanaman RH. The use of guided tissue regeneration to facilitate ideal prosthetic placement of implants. Int J Periodont Restor Dent 1992;2:257.
3. Wachtel HC, Langford A, et al. Guided bone regeneration next to osseointegrated implants in humans. Int J Oral Maxillofac Implants 1991;6:127–135.
4. Seibert J, Nyman S. Localized ridge augmentation in dogs: a pilot study using membranes and hydroxyapatite. J Periodontol 1990;61:157–165.
5. Seibert JS. Reconstruction of deformed, partially edentulous ridges, using full thickness onlay grafts. Part I. Technique and wound healing. Compend Contin Educ Dent 1983;4:437–453.
6. Fiorellini JP, Nevins ML. Localized ridge augmentation/preservation. A systematic review. Ann Periodontol 2003;8:321–327.
7. Li J, Wang HL. Common implant-related advanced bone grafting complications: classification, etiology, and management. Implant Dent 2008;17:389–401.
8. Lindhe J, Karring T, et al. Clinical Periodontology and Implant Dentistry. 4th ed. Hoboken, NJ: Wiley-Blackwell, 2003.
9. Newman MG, Takei H, et al. Carranza's Clinical Periodontology. 3rd ed. Maryland Heights, MO, Elsevier/Saunders, 1995.
10. Zellin G, Gritli-Linde A, et al: Healing of mandibular defects with different biodegradable and non-biodegradable membranes: an experimental study in rats. Biomaterials 1995;16:601.
11. Friedmann A, Strietzel FP, et al. Histological assessment of augmented jaw bone utilizing a new collagen barrier membrane compared to a standard barrier membrane to protect a granular bone substitute material, Clin Oral Implant Res 2002;13:587.
12. Sandberg E, Dahlin C, et al. Bone regeneration by the osteopromotive technique using bioabsorbable membranes: an experimental study in rats. Int J Oral Maxillofac Surg 1993;51:1106.
13. Hollinger JO, Brekke J, et al. Role of bone substitutes. Clin Orthop 1996;324:55–65.
14. Tolman DE. Reconstructive procedures with endosseous implants in grafted bone: a review of the literature. Int J Oral Maxillofac Implants 1995;10:275–294.
15. Mowlem R. Cancellous chip bone grafts: Report on 75 cases. Lancet 1944;2:746–748.
16. Mellonig JT. Autogenous and allogeneic bone grafts in periodontal therapy. Crit Rev Oral Biol Med 1992;3:333–352.

17. Mulliken JB, Glowacki J. Induced osteogenesis for repair and construction in the craniofacial region. Plast Reconstr Surg 1980;65:553–560.

18. Cammack GV II, Nevins M, Clem DS III, et al. Histologic evaluation of mineralized and demineralized freeze-dried bone allograft for ridge and sinus augmentations. Int J Periodontics Restorative Dent 2005;25:231–237.

19. Simion M, Trisi P, Piattelli A. Vertical ridge augmentation using a membrane technique associated with osseointegrated implants. Int J Periodontics Restorative Dent 1994;14:496–511.

20. Cochran DL, Douglas HB. Augmentation of osseous tissue around nonsubmerged endosseous dental implants. Int J Periodontics Restorative Dent 1993;13:506–519.

21. Mellonig JT, Nevins M. Guided bone regeneration of bone defects associated with implants: An evidence-based outcome assessment. Int J Periodontics Restorative Dent 1995;15:168–185.

22. Proussaefs P, Lozada J, et al. The use of titanium mesh in conjunction with autogenous bone graft and inorganic bovine bone mineral (Bio-Oss) for localized alveolar ridge augmentation: a human study. Int J Periodontics Restorative Dent 2003;23:185–195.

23. Becker W, Becker BE, et al. A comparison of demineralized freeze-dried bone and autologous bone to induce bone formation in human extraction sockets. J Periodontol 1994;65:1128.

24. Becker W, Schenk R, et al. Variations in bone regeneration adjacent to implants augmented with barrier membranes alone or with demineralized freeze-dried bone or autologous grafts: a study in dogs, Int J Oral Maxillofac Implants 1995;10:143.

25. Becker W, Urist MR, et al. Human demineralized freeze-dried bone: inadequate induced bone formation in athymic mice-a preliminary report. J Periodontol 1995;66:822.

26. Landsberg C, Grosskopf A, et al. Clinical and biological observations of demineralized freeze-dried bone allografts in augmentation procedures around dental implants. Int J Oral Maxillofac Implants 1994;9:586.

27. Carranza FA Sr. A technic for reattachment. J Periodontol 1954;25:272.

28. Moskow BS, Tannenbaum P. Enhanced repair and regeneration of periodontal lesions in tetracycline-treated patients: case reports, J Periodontol 1991;62:341.

29. Esposito M, Grusovin MG, et al. Interventions for replacing missing teeth: horizontal and vertical bone augmentation techniques for dental implant treatment. Cochrane Database Syst Rev 2009:CD003607.

30. Simion M, Trisi P, et al. Vertical ridge augmentation using a membrane technique associated with osseointegrated implants. Int J Periodontics Restorative Dent 1994;14:496–511.

31. Meijndert L, Meijer HJ, et al. Evaluation of aesthetics of implant-supported single-tooth replacements using different bone augmentation procedures: a prospective randomized clinical study. Clin Oral Implants Res 2007;18:715–719.

32. Donos N, Mardas N, et al. Clinical outcomes of implants following lateral bone augmentation: systematic assessment of available options (barrier membranes, bone grafts, split osteotomy). J Clin Periodontol 2008;35(8 Suppl):173–202.

33. Chiapasco M, Abati S, et al. Clinical outcome of autogenous bone blocks or guided bone regeneration with e-PTFE membranes for the reconstruction of narrow edentulous ridges. Clin Oral Implants Res 1999;10:278–288.

34. Fiorellini JP, Nevins ML. Localized ridge augmentation/preservation: a systematic review. Ann Periodontol 2003;8:321.

35. Rominger JW, Triplett RG. The use of guided tissue regeneration to improve implant osseointegration [see comments]. J Oral Maxillofac Surg 1994;52:106.

TAKE-HOME POINTS

A. The Siebert classification was developed to facilitate communication between clinicians as to the severity of ridge deformities as well as indicate the potential outcome of regenerative procedures based on their value within the classification system [4,5].
- Class I: Bucco-lingual loss of tissue with normal apico-coronal ridge height
- Class II: Apico-coronal loss of tissue with normal buccolingual ridge width
- Class III: Combination of bucco-lingual and apico-coronal loss of tissue, resulting in loss of normal height and width of the ridge.

Typically, the higher the Siebert class, the more difficult it is to regenerate the ridge to its original form. There is a caveat to this rule, however. Not always do we require vertical and/or horizontal augmentation to place implants. If the remaining ridge displays sufficient bone for implant placement, no regenerative procedure may be necessary. Furthermore, when placing an implant in an aesthetic area such as the maxillary anterior region, augmentation may be necessary for aesthetic reasons only.

B. According to Chiapasco and Zaniboni, in a systematic review in 2009, GBR is a procedure that allows spaces maintained by a barrier membrane to be filled with bone [1]. Bone loss can be a result of several factors: tooth loss, traumatic extractions, periodontal disease, infection, and so on. Thus the rationale for GBR procedures is to recreate the osseous ridge for either aesthetic or functional reasons. Primarily, this procedure is used to rebuild the ridge for eventual implant placement. Most importantly, the implant should be placed so the eventual restoration is placed in the original tooth position and provides a natural emergence of the tooth from the soft tissues (prosthetically driven) [2].

The term *GBR* was initially coined by Wachtel et al to describe the principles of guided tissue regeneration (GTR) applied to bone structures [3]. Other authors contributed greatly to the early understanding of GBR [4].

C. According to the 2003 Periodontal World Workshop, GBR is indicated for patients who had previous bone loss/destruction such that insufficient bone remained for implant placement [6].

There is no absolute contraindication for GBR, but the following conditions may present more risk of complications [7]:
- Elderly patients: Commonly present systemic conditions that may compromise healing.
- Bisphosphonates: Intravenous – great risk of osteonecrosis of the jaws; oral – low risk of osteonecrosis.
- Diabetes: Uncontrolled diabetes is associated with delayed healing, failure of bone grafts, and further bone loss.
- Radiation: Risk of osteoradionecrosis but is apparently low. Probably more risk after the first year postexposure.
- Alcoholism: Risk of more adverse results.
- Severe bone loss, especially in the vertical dimension: Limited and unpredictable results. In the anterior region this condition can lead to multiple surgeries that may negatively affect aesthetics.
- Active infectious oral disease, especially periodontal disease: May promote infection, including patients with poor oral hygiene and poor compliance.
- All other conditions that would be a contraindication for any oral surgery, such as uncontrolled high blood pressure, cancer, or blood dyscrasias.

D. The GBR procedure is based on the use of a membrane to prevent epithelial and connective tissue growth into the regenerating site and a bone filler that primarily provides a scaffold where cells can attach. Membranes can be classified as resorbable or nonresorbable.

Resorbable membranes: Can be a tissue, such as a connective tissue graft or allogeneic dermal matrix, but usually refers to membranes made of collagen (BioGuide) and Poly-Lactic (e.g., Atrisorb) or polylactic acid [9,10] (e.g., Guidor). Polyglycolic acid, polyorthoesther, polyurethane, and polyhydroxybutyrate are also synthetic membranes used for GBR.

The advantages of a resorbable membrane are the elimination of surgical reentry for membrane removal as well as reduced complications if membrane becomes exposed. Disadvantages of using resorbable membranes include the possibility of early degradation prior to completion of bone formation as well as the presence of inflammation brought on by this degradation process [10]. More recently, new developments including cross-linking of collagen to increase resistance to biodegradation have been developed [11]. Fortunately, the mild inflammatory reaction caused by bioresorbable membranes does not seem to interfere with osteogenesis [9]. In addition to these attributes, resorbable membranes are also user friendly. However, their lack of resiliency results in a collapse of the membrane into the defect area [12]. Resorbable membranes are best reserved for clinical indications that allow the graft material or hardware (tenting screws, plates) to maintain the space required [9].

Nonresorbable membranes: Usually made of polytetrafluoroethylene (PTFE) or expanded PTFE (ePTFE), and can be reinforced by titanium structure to give more stability. Titanium mesh and titanium foil are also occasionally used. Typically, nonresorbable membranes are removed after 6–12 months [8].

The primary advantage of a nonresorbable membranes is stabilization of the graft. The disadvantages relate to its difficulty in handling and the possibility of its exposure during the healing process. Exposed membranes become contaminated with oral bacteria, which may lead to infection of the site and result in bone loss [9]. It is important to remove these membranes at a designated time period during the healing process. If the membrane is removed too early, bone loss can also occur [9].

The available sources of bone materials include the following [13]:
1. Autograft: patient's own bone
2. Allograft: processed cadaver bone from another human (FDBA and DFDBA [demineralized freeze dried bone allograft])
3. Alloplast: synthetic bone substitutes such as tricalcium phosphate
4. Xenograft: cadaver bone from an animal such as bovine or porcine

These products are provided in a particulate form of various sizes as well as in block form. Particulate grafts from the preceding list may also be combined [13].

The particulate autograft is still considered the gold standard for most ridge augmentation procedures primarily due to its inherent osteogenic behavior [14,15]. Blood vessels are able to penetrate the spaces between the particles compared with a block graft and thus provide for more rapid in growth of blood vessels. A larger osteoconduction surface area, more exposure of osteoinductive growth factors, and easier biologic remodeling are also advantages of the particulate graft [9].

However, autografts have limitations that include donor site morbidity, increased cost, potential resorption, size mismatch, and an inadequate volume of graft material [16,17]. Bone allografts overcome many of the shortfalls of autogenous grafts but are considered primarily osteoconductive and to some degree osteoinductive (DFDBA) in nature. The literature suggests that DFDBA may have greater osteoinductive potential because of the availability of morphogenic proteins. However, a histologic study comparing FDBA with DFDBA for ridge augmentation demonstrated regeneration of 42% new bone area with no statistical difference between the two materials [18].

Bone allograft is bone collected from a human cadaver that is commercially available from tissue banks. It is obtained from cortical or cancellous bone within 12 hours of death of the donor, defatted, cut in pieces, washed in absolute alcohol, and deep frozen. The material may then proceed to the next steps (mineralized, FDBA) or be demineralized (DFDBA). Both products then are ground and sieved to a particle size of 250–750 μm and freeze-dried. They are then vacuum-sealed in glass vials [9].

The use of particulate allograft bone replacement substitute has been reported for numerous applications, including ridge augmentation [19,20].

Successful horizontal ridge augmentation has been described with the use of a variety of different techniques and materials including allograft bone [14,21]. Vertical ridge augmentation with bone allograft has proven to be more difficult primarily due to the problem of osteogenic cells and blood vessels to gain access to the far reaches of the graft. Success was demonstrated using titanium mesh with autogenous particulate grafts [22].

From a histologic standpoint, biopsies of some studies using bone allografts indicate viable bone cells and visible osteocytes in lacunae, and a 9-month specimen showed no remaining allograft material [9]. However, there are some contradictory results using DFDBA and membrane combinations [23–25].

To enhance the quality and quantity of regenerated bone, there is a growing interest in growth factors. Products now clinically available include recombinant platelet-derived growth factor (rhPDGF) (Gem 21; Osteohealth Inc, Shirley, NY, USA), the recombinant human bone morphogen protein 2 (rhBMP-2; Infuse Medtronics Inc, Minneapolis, MN, USA). Platelet-rich growth factors derived from the patient's own blood are compounds rich in different growth factors.

E. GBR encompasses a variety of different applications including socket preservation, sinus elevation, peri-implant GBR, and ridge augmentation. Our focus is on ridge augmentation.

Typically the surgery begins with a crestal incision within the keratinized tissue. A full-thickness buccal and lingual flap is elevated to completely expose the osseous defect (Figure 5A and B). The exposed cortical bone is then perforated (decorticated) to allow for the osteogenic potential of the autogenous bone including blood supply, osteoblasts, and growth factors to enter into the graft (Figure 5B). Bone allograft is then placed with slight overfill to compensate for some bone resorption during the healing phase (Figure 5C). The membrane is then placed confirming that it overlaps the existing ridge.(Figure 5D). To achieve primary closure, a periosteal releasing incision is necessary (Figure 5E) to achieve tension-free closure [26]. Most reports suggest removing sutures approximately 10–14 days after surgery. It is also suggested that no prosthesis be inserted for 2–3 weeks after surgery, to avoid

pressure over the wound during the early healing period.

Additional concepts for flap management associated with ridge augmentation include the following [9]: It is desirable to make incisions remote relative to the placement of barrier membranes (e.g., vertical releasing incisions at least one tooth away from the site to be grafted). In the anterior maxilla, keeping vertical incisions remote is also an aesthetic advantage [9].

Systemic antibiotics are generally used after regenerative periodontal therapy, even though studies to support their use are minimal. There have been some case reports that have demonstrated rebuilding of periodontal lesions after scaling, root planing, and curettage, with systemic and local treatment using penicillin or tetracycline, in combination with other forms of therapy. [27,28].

F. Conclusions from a recent meta-analysis of randomized controlled clinical trials looking at different bone grafting studies for ridge augmentation suggest there are too few studies, and most have insufficient numbers of subjects [29]. Even though various techniques are effective in augmenting bone horizontally and vertically, it is unclear which are the most efficient [29].

According to the literature, vertical ridge augmentation using bone allograft did not demonstrate predictable results and is often associated with more complications, including implant failure [8]. Lindhe et al suggested that "short implants appear to be a better alternative to vertical bone grafting of resorbed mandibles" [8]. According to Simion et al, vertical bone augmentation was limited to approximately 4mm with autogenous particulate bone [30].

Meijndert and colleagues provided the best evidence for the success of horizontal ridge augmentation. This group demonstrated implant success when they were placed in augmented ridges with block grafts and particulate grafts (Bio-Oss) [31]. This finding is consistent with a systematic review by Donos et al. They also concluded that the stability of these grafts and implants placed in them appears to be similar to pristine bone [32]. In terms of the membranes, the results of this study also indicated that both resorbable and nonresorbable demonstrated good results.

The review by Donos concluded that "The implant survival at the augmented sites irrespective of the procedure used varied from 91.7% to 100% and from 93.2% to 100% at the control sites for a period between 12 and 59.1 months." This results include implants placed at the same time of augmentation [32]. "Significant increase of the ridge dimensions (87%–95%) can be expected for this procedure and block grafts appear to be slightly better" [31,33,34].

Further evidence to support these conclusions is illustrated in a systematic review of survival rates of dental implants after ridge augmentation therapy by Fiorellini and Nevins [34]. They reported that the survival rates for implants placed in augmented bone with using several GBR procedures were similar to implants placed in native bone.

G. A systematic review by Li and Wang reported that the complications most reported for particulate GBR are as follows [7]:
1. Membrane exposure
2. Inflammatory reaction
3. Flap sloughing (associated with use of nonabsorbable membrane)
4. Infection
5. Incision line opening
6. Loss of graft or reduced graft
7. Sublingual edema

Management of these complications is as follows:
1. *Membrane exposure:* In a study where implants were placed in conjunction with nonresorbable barrier membranes and FDBA, a success rate of 96.8% was achieved with complete bone fill. This study reported an exposure rate of 29% of the membranes, but little effect on the bone regeneration was noted [9,34,35]. The literature supports the removal of the exposed nonresorbable membranes but not before sufficient time has elapsed for bone formation. Often these problems can be managed with good oral hygiene and use of topical 0.12% chlorhexidine rinses until that time.
2. *Inflammatory reaction:* With the use of resorbable membrane a confined inflammatory event does take place upon degradation of the graft. As mentioned earlier this does not seem to affect the result of the augmentation. Surgical trauma can also cause significant inflammation that may put overwhelming pressure on the tissues, resulting in suture line opening. To avoid this event, a careful atraumatic surgical technique is required and the use of steroids such as prednisone may be helpful.
3. *Flap sloughing:* Because there is no blood supply below the flap when using nonresorbable membranes, a compromised environment exists. It is essential to maintain an appropriate thickness of the flap as well as a good base blood supply to minimize this possibility.
4. *Infection:* Careful aseptic surgical technique, including thorough postoperative rinsing of the surgical site with sterile saline, can reduce the chances of infection. Pre- and postoperative systemic antibiotics have shown to improve augmentation results. Antibiotics such as penicillin, amoxicillin, clindamycin, azythromycin, or metronidazole can be used. If the infection cannot be controlled with antibiotics, the removal of the bone graft may be necessary.
5. *Incision line opening:* As mentioned, a careful atraumatic surgical technique as well as the use of steroids may reduce the likelihood of this happening. More importantly, however, the surgeon must release the flap from the underlying periosteum for tension-free closure.
6. *Loss of graft or reduced graft:* The clinical situation should be reevaluated. The options of placing shorter implants or performing a complementary GBR can be discussed.
7. *Sublingual edema/Bleeding:* Some drawbacks of GBR are that the augmentation procedures, especially in the vertical dimension, can result in more serious complications (including a life-threatening sublingual edema and bleeding), major discomfort, and pain. Pressure can be applied on the bleeding point with a gauze until hemostasis is observed (tamponade). Vessel ligature and electrocautery have also been reported, although they need to be used with caution.

5

Mucogingival Therapy

Clinical Cases in Periodontics, First Edition. Nadeem Karimbux.
© 2012 John Wiley & Sons, Inc. Published 2012 by John Wiley & Sons, Inc.

Case 1

Pedicle Flaps

CASE STORY

A 32-year-old Caucasian female presented with a chief complaint of: "my lower front teeth are sensitive." She reported experiencing sensitivity of her lower teeth when drinking hot and cold liquids. She also expressed concern about the appearance of her lower gums. Her general dentist had referred her for periodontal treatment of her gingival recession (Figure 1).

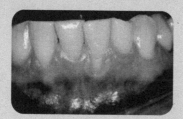

Figure 1: Preoperative picture. Courtesy of David S. Greenfield, DMD.

LEARNING GOALS AND OBJECTIVES

■ To be able to diagnose mucogingival defects and deformities
■ To identify the possible etiology for gingival recession
■ To understand which surgical techniques should be applied to correct gingival recession defects

Medical History

There were no significant findings in reviewing the patient's medical history. She did not report taking any medications or supplements. The patient reported having no known drug allergies. She had had an annual physical with her primary care physician.

Review of Systems

- Vital signs
  - Blood pressure 121/70 mm Hg
  - Pulse rate: 70 beats/minute (regular)
  - Respiration: 15 breaths/minute

Dental History

The patient reported that she saw her general dentist twice yearly for a cleaning and checkup. She had received orthodontic treatment as a teenager to correct crowding of her maxillary and mandibular arches. She reported brushing twice daily with a medium-bristle toothbrush. The patient tried to floss daily but sometimes she forgot.

Social History

The patient had been born and raised in Massachusetts. She currently resided in Boston with her husband and 4-year-old daughter. The patient was a high school English teacher. She reported drinking alcohol socially and had between one and three drinks per week and denied the use of tobacco products.

Extraoral Examination

The patient had no detectable lesions, masses, or swelling, and the temporomandibular joint was within normal limits.

Intraoral Examination

There were no detectible masses or lesions of the tongue, floor of the mouth, hard/soft palate, or buccal mucosa. Oral cancer screening was negative.

Hard Tissue Examination

The patient had no carious lesions. The restorations were intact on radiographic and clinical examination.

Periodontal Examination

- The full-mouth charting revealed probing depths of 1–3 mm with some bleeding on probing in the posterior quadrants.
- Mild gingival inflammation was present in the posterior quadrants adjacent to the second molars.
- An isolated recession defect was present on tooth #24 measuring 3 mm from the cementoenamel junction (CEJ).
- There was a minimal amount of attached keratinized tissue adjacent to the recession defect with mild localized marginal inflammation.

Occlusion

There were no occlusal discrepancies or interferences.

Radiographic Examination

- A recent full-mouth series revealed no carious lesions or pathologic findings.
- The bone levels appeared to be within normal limits with intact crestal lamina dura.

Diagnosis

According to the American Academy of Periodontology the patient's gingival condition is classified under developmental or acquired deformities and conditions [1]. It is further grouped into mucogingival deformities and conditions around teeth with gingival/soft tissue recession and a lack of keratinized gingiva.

The recession defect can be classified according to the Miller Classification System of gingival recession defects [2]. This defect is a Miller class 1 because it does not extend beyond the mucogingival junction and there is no interproximal bone loss. For a more in-depth discussion of classification of gingival recession, refer to Chapter 5, Case 3.

Treatment Plan

The proposed treatment plan for this patient is a dental prophylaxis including oral hygiene instructions. After establishing proper home care, the recession will be treated with a pedicle graft to repair the isolated gingival defect.

Discussion

Prior to treatment of gingival recession it is important to identify the possible etiology of the defect. The patient received orthodontic treatment, which can result in gingival recession if the teeth are moved labially beyond their bony housing. The patient also has a thin biotype, which is characterized by a thin scalloped gingiva and buccal plate that make the patient more prone to recession [3]. Improper toothbrushing technique such as overzealous brushing with a medium or hard-bristle toothbrush, can also lead to gingival recession. Once a dental prophylaxis was completed and the patient demonstrated the ability to maintain proper oral hygiene, the treatment of the recession defect could proceed.

In this case the desired treatment outcome was to achieve root coverage and increase the width of attached tissue around tooth #24. After considering the possible treatment options, the decision to use a laterally positioned pedicle graft was made. (Refer to question D to review indications for laterally positioned pedicel graft.)

The lateral pedicle graft was performed under local anesthesia with no complications. (See question C for a step-by-step guide to the procedure.) The patient was seen for postoperative appointments at 2, 4, and 6 weeks. At 6 weeks there is almost full root coverage with an increase in the amount of attached keratinized tissue around #24. The patient also reported a decrease in sensitivity in her lower front teeth (Figure 2).

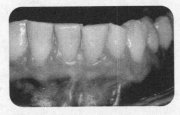

Figure 2: Six-week postoperative picture. Courtesy of David S. Greenfield, DMD.

Self-Study Questions

A. What is a pedicle graft?

B. What are the surgical techniques that use pedicle grafts for root coverage?

C. How is a laterally positioned pedicle flap performed?

D. What are the indications/contraindications for using these techniques?

E. What are the benefits/limitations of using pedicle flaps compared with free autogenous grafts?

F. How else can pedicle flaps be used in the oral cavity?

Answers located at the end of the chapter.

References

1. Armitage GC. Development of a classification system for periodontal diseases and conditions. Ann Periodontol 1999;4:1–6.
2. Miller PD Jr. Root coverage using the free soft tissue autograft citric acid application. III. Int J Periodontal Rest Dent 1985;2:6,15.
3. Ochenbein C, Ross S. A reevaluation of osseous surgery. Dent Clin North Am 1969;13:87–102.
4. Grupe HE, Warren RF Jr. Repair of gingival defects by a sliding flap operation. J Periodontol 1956;27:92.
5. Cohen DW, Ross SE. The double papillae repositioned flap in periodontics. J Periodontol 1968;39:65–70.
6. Harris R. The connective tissue and partial thickness double pedicle graft: a predictable method of obtaining root coverage. J Periodontol 1992;63:447–486.
7. Mariotti A. Efficacy of chemical root surface modifiers in the treatment of periodontal disease. A systematic review. Ann Periodontal 2003;8:205.
8. Rose LF, Mealy BL, et al. Periodontics Medicine, Surgery and Implants. Philadelphia, PA: Mosby, 2004. Chapter 21 p432.
9. Rose LF, Mealy BL, et al. Periodontics Medicine, Surgery and Implants. Philadelphia, PA: Mosby, 2004. Chapter 21 pp432–434.
10. Wennstrom JL. Mucogingival therapy. Ann Periodontol 1996;1:671–701.
11. Fugazzotto PA. Maintenance of soft issue closure following guided bone regeneration: technical considerations and report of 723 cases. J Periodontol 1999;70:1085–1097.
12. Nemcovsky CE, Zvi A, et al. Healing of dehiscence defects at delayed-immediate implant sites primarily closed by a rotating palatal flap following extraction. Int J Oral Maxillofac Implants 2000;15:4.

TAKE-HOME POINTS

A. A pedicle graft (also called pedicle flap) is a full- or split-thickness flap designed in such a way that it remains connected at its base. The flap can then be rotated or positioned at an adjacent location while still maintaining its own blood supply through its connection. The blood supply nourishes the graft and facilitates the vascular union with the recipient site. This differs from a free autogenous tissue graft that is completely severed from its blood supply but can be attached to another part of the oral cavity.

B.
1. **Laterally positioned flap:** This technique, first described by Grupe and Warren in 1956, uses donor gingiva from a healthy tooth to cover the exposed root of an adjacent tooth [4].
2. **Double papilla flap:** This technique, described by Cohen and Ross in 1968, is used to cover defects where there is an inadequate amount of gingival on the adjacent area for a laterally positioned flap [5]. In this method, the papillae from each side of the problem tooth are reflected and rotated over the midfacial aspect of the recipient tooth and sutured. Harris described a modification of this technique by placing a subepithelial connective tissue graft under the double pedicle flaps [6].
3. **Coronally positioned flap:** This technique can be used when there is an adequate amount of keratinized tissue and thickness of gingiva adjacent to the recession defect. The gingiva is released and advanced coronally to cover the recession defect. The procedure can be performed with or without vertical releasing incisions and it is often used in combination with other mucogingival techniques.

C. Before beginning the procedure, the bone level on the facial of the donor site should be evaluated with bone sounding. If the distance from the bone to the CEJ is >2 mm, there is a risk of recession on the donor tooth. Leaving a collar of tissue at the donor site can reduce this risk. The root surface where coverage will be attempted should be thoroughly planed and smoothed to remove surface irregularities or defects. Some practitioners might use chemicals such as EDTA, citric acid, or tetracycline to condition the root surface. However, there is no definitive evidence in humans that chemically treated roots are more biologically acceptable than mechanically prepared surfaces for soft tissue grafting [7].

The first incisions are made to prepare the recipient site for the donor tissue. An incision starting in the papilla between the donor and recipient site is made from the level of the CEJ continuing at an oblique angle beyond the base of the defect. A small horizontal incision at the level of the expected root coverage is made on the opposite side of the recipient site and then extended apically to meet the first incision. The epithelium between these incisions is removed in preparation to receive the pedicle graft.

The next incision is made from the line angle of the tooth adjacent to the donor site and extended parallel to the first incision. The following incision extends across the donor site connecting the first and third incision. This incision can be sulcular, or if there is a concern of recession, this incision can be made so a collar of tissue remains. The tissue collar should have at least 0.5 mm of attached tissue (Figure 3).

The flap is reflected with a split-thickness dissection. Full-thickness dissection may be necessary in some portions to maintain adequate flap thickness and prevent perforations. The flap

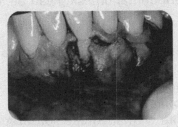

Figure 3: Incision design for lateral pedicle flap. Courtesy of David S. Greenfield, DMD.

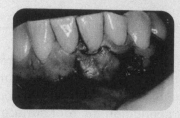

Figure 4: Rotation of pedicle flap. Courtesy of David S. Greenfield, DMD.

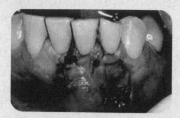

Figure 5: Flap sutured to recipient site. Courtesy of David S. Greenfield, DMD.

can now be mobilized and rotated to the recipient site. If there is tension on the flap at the recipient site, additional release of the tissue may be done (Figure 4).

Once the pedicle flap is in the correct position and tension free, it is sutured in place using 5-0 or 6-0 simple interrupted sutures. The leading edge of the flap is secured first with sutures in the papilla and mucosa. The trailing edge is secured with a suture in the papilla. If there is periosteum left intact from the split-thickness dissection, additional sutures can be placed to stabilize the flap (Figure 5).

The graft should be stable and immobile, which can be confirmed by movement of the lip. If desired, a periodontal dressing can be applied to the area [8].

D. Indications for the use of pedicle grafts for root coverage include the following [9]:
1. An isolated area of recession with no bone loss on the proximal surface.
2. A donor site with adequate soft tissue width and thickness, sufficient vestibular depth, and adequate bone thickness with no dehiscence.

Contraindications for the procedure include the following:
1. A donor site with thin tissue is not recommended because it is prone to future recession.
2. If the distance from the crest of bone to the CEJ on the facial surface of the donor tooth is >2 mm, there is a risk of recession after the tissue is rotated.

E.
1. There is only one surgical site with a pedicle graft (palatal donor site not needed), which limits the risk of postoperative morbidity.
2. The pedicle maintains its own blood supply, which increases the chance for graft survival and root coverage.
3. There is a harmonious blend of tissue color and contour after healing compared with free autogenous tissue grafts that can have less aesthetic results.
4. It is more difficult to treat multiple teeth using pedicle grafting techniques compared with free autogenous grafts, which can be harvested according to the size needed.
5. There is less risk of recession from the donor site of free autogenous grafts compared with pedicle flaps.
6. Root coverage is less predictable using pedicle grafting techniques with a mean root coverage of 62.5% for laterally positioned or double papilla flaps. The mean root coverage for connective tissue grafts in combination with various flap techniques is 89.3% [10].

F. A variety of surgical techniques using pedicle grafts are described in the dental literature. Fugazzotto reported a technique using a rotated palatal pedicle graft to help obtain primary closure in guided bone regeneration procedures [11]. After palatal reflection, a layer of connective tissue is dissected away from the base (apical) of the flap while maintaining its connection at the coronal portion. This method helps achieve tension-free primary closure over the grafted site. Nemcovsky et al have demonstrated a technique that uses rotated palatal tissue to achieve primary tissue closure over extraction sites [12]. They reported the use of full- and partial-thickness rotated palatal flaps to cover extraction sites as well as coverage of immediate implants placed in the maxilla. In the technique demonstrated here, a subepithelial connective tissue graft is harvested adjacent to and one tooth distal to the extraction site. This graft is rotated to cover the grafted extraction site while maintaining its attachment adjacent to the area. This technique helps achieve primary closure to aid in the formation of adequate bone and soft tissue formation (Figures 6–8).

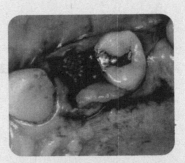

Figure 7: Allograft placed in extraction socket and connective tissue rotated under sulcular tissue on palate. Courtesy of Kasumi Barouch, DDS.

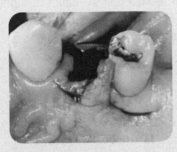

Figure 6: Connective tissue harvested from palate. Courtesy of Kasumi Barouch, DDS.

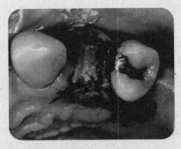

Figure 8: Connective tissue sutured in place while maintaining connection at base of graft. Courtesy of Kasumi Barouch, DDS.

Case 2

Connective Tissue Grafts

CASE STORY
This patient was a 36-year-old male whose general dentist had noticed the recession on teeth #3, 4, and 5 was progressing and had referred him to a periodontist. The dentist had also been concerned with the cervical abrasion/erosion, lack of keratinized tissue, and associated frenum close to the gingival margin on tooth #5 (Figure 1).

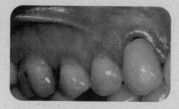

Figure 1: Preoperative clinical presentation.

LEARNING GOALS AND OBJECTIVES
- To identify the indications and rationales for soft tissue grafting
- To understand the surgical technique for subepithelial connective tissue grafting including:
  - Zucchelli incision designs and technique for multiple recession sites.
  - Root preparation
  - Harvesting of donor tissue
  - Suturing of graft and flap
- To understand the rationale for root preparation
- To understand the presurgical and postsurgical considerations

Medical History
The patient's medical history was not significant. The patient was not taking any medications and denied having any allergies.

Review of Systems
- Vital signs
  - Blood pressure: 128/76 mm Hg
  - Pulse rate: 68 beats/minute
  - Respiration: 14 breaths/minute

Social History
The patient admitted to smoking cigarettes as a young adult but had not smoked for at least 10 years. He denied using chewing tobacco. He was a social drinker and admitted to drinking one or two alcoholic beverages three to four times a week.

Dental History
The patient had received fairly regular dental care throughout most of his childhood and adult years, with periodic cleanings and examinations approximately every 6 months. He had had orthodontic care as a teenager; treatment lasted approximately 2 years.

Oral Hygiene Status
The patient brushed his teeth three to four times a day, using a medium or soft brush, and admitted to brushing somewhat "aggressively." He flossed three to four times a week.

Family History
One of his parents had been treated for recession, but both parents had all or most of their own teeth.

Extraoral Examination
No significant findings were present.

Intraoral Examination

- Oral cancer screening was negative. Soft tissues including buccal mucosa, hard and soft palate, floor of the mouth, and tongue all appeared normal.
- There was generally an adequate amount of attached keratinized gingiva present on all remaining teeth (Table 1).
- The patient had excellent oral hygiene with a minimal amount of plaque accumulation and gingival inflammation.
- See Figure 2 for periodontal charting.
- There was some mild clinical attachment loss with no probing depths >3 mm, no tooth mobility, and no furcation invasion.
- Tissue color, contour, and consistency: Generalized pink color with normal contour except for recession as noted below. Consistency was firm with normal stippling.
- Bleeding on probing was localized and very slight.

Table 1: Keratinized/Attached Gingiva

Tooth #	1	2	3	4	5	6	7	8
Recession	X	2	3	2	4	0	0	0
Width of keratinized tissue	X	4	3	4	1	4	4	4
Width of attached gingiva	X	2	1	2	0	2	2	2

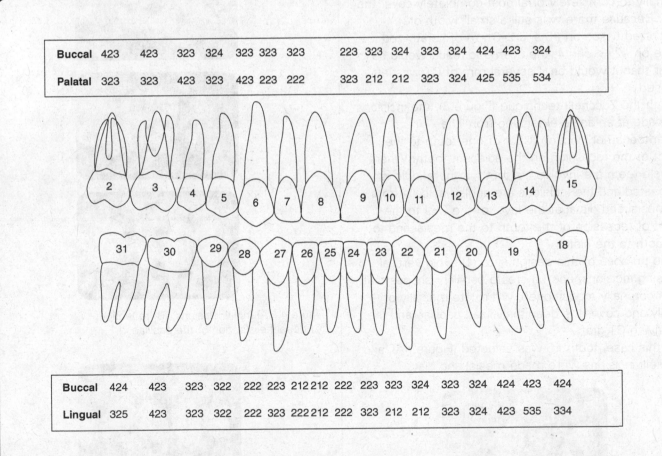

Figure 2: Probing pocket depth/recession measurements during initial visit.

Radiographic Examination

There was no bone loss evident on radiographic examination.

Diagnosis

• Recession with inadequate attached gingiva, localized #3 and 5.
• Cervical abrasion/erosion, #3–5.

Treatment Plan

• Oral hygiene instructions to modify traumatic brushing technique
• Subepithelial connective tissue graft, #3, 4, and 5.

Treatment

After evaluation of the thickness and anatomy of the palate by "sounding," administration of local anesthetic, and evaluation of the amount of keratinized tissue present on the facial of teeth #3–5, treatment of #3–5 with a SCTG using the right palate as a donor site was recommended.

A decision was made to reposition the overlying flap coronally to completely or almost completely cover the graft. Because there was still a small width of keratinized tissue on #5 and 2–3 mm of keratinized tissue on #2, 3, and 4, the cosmetic result would be better than it would be if several mm of CT was left exposed.

With the Zucchelli technique (Figure 3), the incisions are made at an angle extending from the cementoenamel junction (CEJ) of one tooth to the height of the recession on the adjacent tooth. Where multiple teeth are involved, a tooth in the middle is designated and the incisions are angled apically from the mesial and distal at the level of the CEJ to the height of recession of the tooth to the mesial and to the tooth to the distal.

The purpose of this design is to (1) avoid vertical releasing incisions, and (2) create papillary shapes that, when coronally repositioned, will rotate mesially or distally and cover the deepithelialized papillae and the underlying CT graft.

In this case, tooth #5 was selected (Figure 4A), and Zucchelli incisions were made mesial and distal

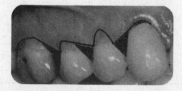

Figure 3: Zucchelli technique.

starting at the CEJ. Additional incisions were made starting at the distal CEJ of #4, angling to the apical extent of the recession of #3. Another similar incision was made starting at the distal cervical of tooth #3.

A partial-thickness flap was reflected (Figure 4B), freeing the flap apically to allow the flap to easily be coronally repositioned. To avoid perforating the flap with sharp dissection, it may be necessary to elevate carefully over any exostoses.

The papillae are carefully deepithelialized (Figure 4C) using a 12b scalpel blade. The amount of tissue removed is approximately ≤1 mm, leaving as much of the underlying connective tissue papilla as possible.

Root Preparation

Root plane to smooth the roots and remove or round out" any grooves, at times creating a saddle shape (Figure 5). It may be necessary to use a high-speed

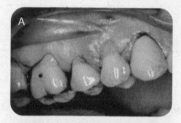
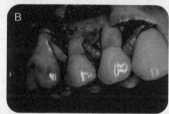
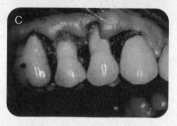

Figure 4: (A) Initial incisions; (B) reflection; (C) deepithelialization of the papillae.

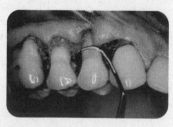

Figure 5: Root planing.

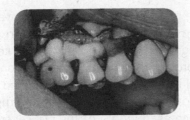

Figure 6: Application of EDTA solution.

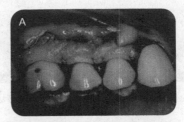

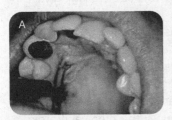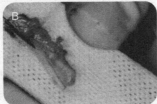

Figure 7: (A) Harvesting of the graft; (B) trimming of the graft.

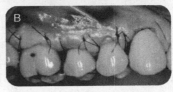

Figure 8: (A) Suturing of the connective tissue graft; (B) suturing of flap.

handpiece lightly and carefully with football-shaped finishing burs, medium, fine, and extrafine diamonds if the grooving on the root is severe or if an existing restoration needs to be removed.

Chemically treat the root with EDTA solution 17% (Pulpdent) for 2 minutes by applying saturated cotton pellets or burnishing with a saturated cotton pellet for 45 seconds (Figure 6).

After measuring the length of graft needed to cover the roots, mark the approximate positions at the beginning and end of the graft on the palate with the point of the probe.

Make the first incision 4 mm from the gingival margin. Make the second incision 1–2 mm closer to the tooth and parallel to the first incision (Figure 7A).

The depth of the incisions can safely extend 7 mm from the CEJ on a shallow palate, 12 mm on an average palate, and 17 mm on a high palate [1].

If the palate is thin, it may be necessary to elevate the graft form the palatal bone instead of making a second incision.

At the apical extent of the incision, angle the scalpel toward the palate to free the graft. Do the same at the mesial and distal borders of the graft.

Remove the epithelium by trimming it with a sharp scalpel (Figure 7B).

Suturing

Suture the graft with individual sling sutures using 5-0 chromic gut suture. Tie on the lingual, if possible, to allow for better flap to graft contact (Figure 8A). Suture the flap with 6-0 monofilament nylon or Gore CV-6 suture. Use one sling suture per tooth (Figure 8B).

Enter the flap from the facial about 3 mm from the gingival margin, approximately at the mesial line angle of the tooth. Proceed interproximally, not engaging the interproximal connective tissue papilla but going coronal to it, wrapping around the lingual, passing through the distal embrasure to the facial, again keeping the suture coronal to the papilla. Pass the suture needle through the facial flap 3 mm apical to the gingival margin at the distal line angle, pass through the distal embrasure coronal to the papilla, wrap around the lingual to the mesial embrasure, pass through it, and tie the suture on the facial. Repeat for each tooth. Also place a sling suture to secure the gingival flap one tooth mesial and one tooth distal to the graft.

Postoperative Instructions

- Ice the area for 24–48 hours, 20 minutes on and 20 minutes off
- Sleep on back with head slightly elevated
- Rinse with chlorhexidine 0.12% rinse bid
- Avoid brushing or flossing for 2–4 weeks
- Eat a soft diet and try to avoid eating on the side of the surgery
- After 2 weeks can use an ultra-soft brush to gently remove debris with roll technique

Prescriptions

- Motrin 800 mg: 1 tablet tid starting 1 hour before procedure
- Vicodin 5/500: 1–2 tablets every 4–6 hours as needed for pain

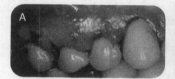
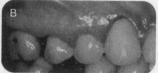

Figure 9: (A) Suture removal at 2 weeks; (B) 8 weeks postsurgery.

- Doxycycline: 100 mg. 1 tablet bid day of surgery, then 1 tab every day for 10 days
- Chlorhexidine rinse 0.12%: rinse for 30–60 seconds bid

Postoperative Follow-up

Patients should be seen 7–14 days after the surgery to remove dressing/sutures (Figure 9A). Additional follow-up to observe patient home care and healing should be planned accordingly (Figure 9B).

Discussion

Indications

The need for an adequate band of attached gingiva has been a topic in the periodontal literature for at least 50 years. It has been argued that without an adequate band of attached gingiva, the stability of the gingival margin would be at risk with the potential for further attachment loss, recession, pocket formation, and inflammation.

The amount of attached gingiva needed to prevent further recession and attachment loss has also been debated and is unclear. Early papers suggested that 5–6 mm of keratinized tissue with a probing depth of 2–3 mm would result in a functional band of attached gingiva of 2–3 mm that was necessary to obtain stability of the marginal gingiva. Lang and Loe [2] stated that 80% areas ≥2 mm keratinized gingiva (KG) and 1 mm attached gingiva (AG) remained healthy while inflammation persisted in areas with <2 mm KG and 1 AG even with good oral hygiene. Several other studies found that areas with minimal width of KG were no more prone to inflammatory changes.

The 1989 World Workshop [3] concluded there were several parameters that should be considered when determining if an adequate zone of attached gingiva is present and the minimum amount of attached gingiva that is acceptable.

The American Academy of Periodontology Consensus Statement on Mucogingival Conditions [4] defines an inadequate amount of keratinized tissue as <2 mm of width, of which <1 mm is attached gingiva. It states that a minimal amount or absence of attached

gingiva alone is not a justification for gingival augmentation. The presence of "recession, loss of supporting bone, absence or reduction of keratinized tissue, and probing depths extending beyond the mucogingival junction" must be considered as well as resulting "root sensitivity, loss of tooth structure (abrasion), increased length of the clinical crown, and inflammation and bleeding of the marginal tissue." Ultimately, the clinician's best judgment must be used to determine whether or not to treat mucogingival conditions [4].

With those considerations, gingival grafting to increase the width of attached gingiva may be indicated if there is <2 mm width of keratinized tissue in which <1 mm is attached gingiva, the recession is progressive, the gingival margin would be stressed by a restorative margin at or below the gingival margin, a removable partial denture would stress the gingival margin, orthodontic treatment is planned (and the teeth are to be moved labially), in progress or completed, or an inability to maintain the gingival margin free of inflammation, bleeding, and/or plaque accumulation [3]. Grafting for root coverage should also be considered when recession has resulted in root abrasion, root sensitivity, and/or compromised aesthetics.

There are several reasons for performing connective tissue grafts. These include areas where there is inadequate attached gingiva (Figures 10A and B), to improve aesthetics, decrease root sensitivity, improve cleansibility, and reduce the exposure of furcations (Figures 11A and B), stop progressive recession (Figures 12A and B), treat root wear/erosion/cervical abrasion (Figures 13A and B) cover exposed crown margins (Figures 14A and B), cover an exposed implant collar (Figures 15A and B), covering lingual recession (Figures 16A and B), and root coverage and ridge augmentation prior to a fixed bridge (Figures 17A and B).

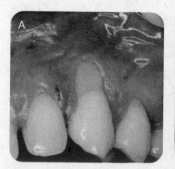
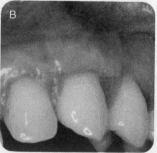

Figure 10: (A,B) Inadequate attached gingiva with recession.

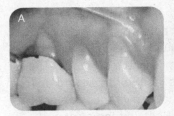
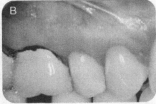

Figure 11: (A,B) Treatment with subepithelial connective tissue graft.

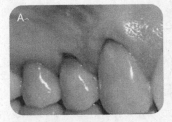
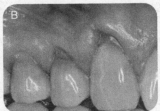

Figure 12: (A,B) Progressive recession.

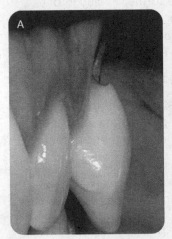
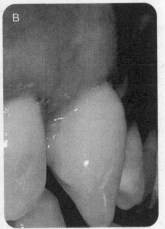

Figure 13: (A,B) Root wear/erosion/cervical abrasion.

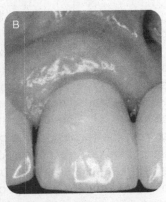
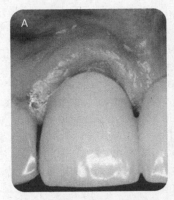

Figure 14: (A,B) Covering exposed crown margins.

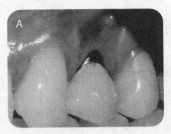
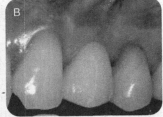

Figure 15: (A,B) Covering an exposed implant collar.

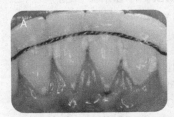
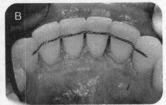

Figure 16: (A,B) Covering lingual recession.

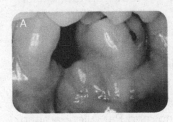
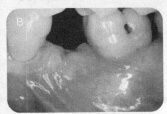

Figure 17: (A,B) Root coverage and ridge augmentation prior to a fixed bridge.

Treatment with subepithelial connective tissue graft can accomplish the following (see Figures 3 and 4):

- Improve aesthetics
- Decrease root sensitivity
- Improve cleansability
- Reduce exposure of furcations (improving long-term prognosis)

Techniques

The early procedures developed to augment the zone of attached gingiva included denudation of the bone, denudation of the periosteum, apically repositioned flap, and free gingival grafts. The bone denudation procedure produced a beautiful result but also caused attachment loss and significant morbidity, taking

months to heal with the need to wear periodontal packing for most of the time. Leaving exposed periosteum decreased the bone loss, but the morbidly and healing period were still significant. Free gingival grafts, using the stratified squamous epithelium and the underlying connective tissue from the palate as donor material, decreased morbidity at the recipient site, but morbidity at the palatal donor site gave free gingival grafts an unpleasant reputation among patients.

All of these procedures were quite successful in creating adequate zones of attached gingiva and eliminating or minimizing the risk of further recession. However, these procedures were not indicated for root coverage, and there was little that could be done to correct the recession that often resulted in unsatisfactory aesthetics, root sensitivity, chemical erosion, mechanical abrasion, and caries. Pedicle flap procedures were developed and used successfully to obtain root coverage, but an adequate adjacent donor site was needed and not always available limiting the use of this procedure.

Root coverage with a free gingival graft was described by Holbrook and Ochsenbein [5] in 1983. The procedure required taking a rather large graft from the surface of the palate, often measuring 12–15 mm in the vertical dimension, and suturing the graft in place with a complex pattern of mattress sutures to closely adapt the graft to the root and periosteum apical and lateral to the root. Root coverage was fairly predictable with this procedure, but an acrylic appliance was needed to cover the donor area because of the large palatal wound. However, even with the best attempts at wound coverage, postoperative morbidity was prolonged.

The subepithelial connective tissue graft was developed by Langer and Langer [6] to create an increased zone of attached gingiva and to partially or completely cover roots, improving aesthetic outcomes, decreasing root sensitivity, covering areas of erosion and abrasion, and protecting the root from additional root wear.

The subepithelial connective tissue graft has become the standard of care for treatment of recession. The techniques used for subepithelial connective tissue grafts are varied, and well-publicized modifications of the Langer technique were developed by P. D. Miller [7], John Bruno, and Pat Allen, among others.

Conclusion

As the demand for aesthetics in dentistry has increased, subepithelial connective tissue grafts have increasingly become an integral component of periodontal therapy. Although the purest indication for soft tissue grafting is a lack of attached gingiva, indications for subepithelial connective tissue grafts have grown to include root coverage, either partial or complete, for many reasons including improving aesthetics, root sensitivity, cervical abrasion, and covering a crown margin or an exposed implant collar.

All of the various techniques, although similar, have subtle differences in outcomes and indications. The technique presented here is ideal for achieving uniform aesthetic tissue contours and rarely requires a second procedure of gingivoplasty. Because the existing keratinized tissue is coronally repositioned over the CT graft to the level of the CEJ, the sometimes unsightly line, demarcating where the flap and connective tissue joined, is absent.

Langer's technique can result in horizontal suture lines at the base of the papillae that require a soft tissue plasty. Bruno's technique requires a second procedure to reposition the mucosa apically that was coronally advanced to completely cover the CT graft. This second procedure exposes the connective tissue that then matures into a beautiful band of keratinized attached gingiva.

In the future, we will see further evolution of materials and techniques for increasing zones of attached gingiva, covering roots and implants, and reconstructing lost papillae. Periodontal plastic surgery continues to be a challenging and exciting area of the specialty of periodontology. Together with restorative procedures, periodontal plastic surgery helps us get closer to achieving our goal of restoring our patients' dentition to its most natural and aesthetic potential.

References

1. Reiser G, et al. The subepithelial connective tissue graft palatal donor site: Anatomic considerations for surgeons. Int J Peridontics Restorative Dent 1996;16:131–137.
2. Lang NP, Loe H. The relationship between the width of attached gingiva and gingival health. J Periodontol 1972;43:623.
3. Nevins M, Becker N, et al., eds; American Academy of Periodontology. World Workshop in Clinical Periodontics. Chicago, IL: AAP, 1989/ pp7–10.
4. American Academy of Periodontology Consensus Statement on Mucogingival Conditions, May 2009. Available at: http://www.perio.org/members/tpi/policy/policy18.html.
5. Holbrook T, Ochsenbein C. Complete coverage of the denuded root surface with a one-stage gingival graft. Int J Periodontics Restorative Dent 1983;3:8–27.
6. Langer B, Langer L. Subepithelial connective tissue graft technique for root coverage. J Periodontology 1985;56:715–720.
7. Miller PD Jr. A classification of marginal tissue recession. Int J Periodontics Restorative Dent 1985;5:8–13.
8. Zucchelli G, De Sanctis M. Treatment of multiple recession-type defects in patients with esthetic demands. J Periodontology 2000;71:1506–1514.

Case 3

Free Gingival Grafts

CASE STORY

A 65-year-old Caucasian female presented for consultation regarding soft tissue grafting about the mandibular anterior teeth (Figure 1) as recommended by her periodontist. The patient had been diagnosed and treated for periodontitis 16 years ago and continued with periodontal maintenance every 3 months. The patient reported recent difficulty with adequate plaque control, food impaction, and sensitivity in this mandibular anterior region.

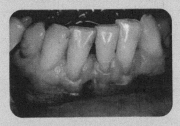

Figure 1: Initial presentation: mandibular anterior area.

LEARNING GOALS AND OBJECTIVES

- ■ To be able to recognize a mucogingival defect and identify areas of insufficient attached gingiva
- ■ To understand the treatment goals achievable with a free gingival graft (autologous epithelialized connective tissue graft) and to make appropriate treatment choices
- ■ To appreciate the surgical steps in performing a free gingival graft (FGG):
  - Root preparation
  - Surgical preparation of recipient bed
  - Graft harvesting from donor site
  - Adaptation of graft and suturing technique for graft immobilization and vascularization

Medical History

The patient reported a history of hyperthyroidism that had been treated with one course of radiation 30 years ago, and she was currently on Levothroid for subsequent hypothyroidism. There were no other significant medical problems, and the patient had no known allergies.

Dental History

The patient reported a history of nonsurgical periodontal treatment and periodontal surgery in the maxillary right quadrant 16 years ago and subsequent 3-month recalls. The patient had a history of multiple restorations and extraction of some of her molars along with extraction of tooth #25 when she had been in her teenage years, possibly due to crowding, but no orthodontic treatment was rendered.

Social History

The patient did not drink alcohol and she was a former cigarette smoker. The patient smoked 12 pack-years and stopped smoking 25 years ago.

Oral Hygiene

The patient reported tooth brushing at least once a day using an electric soft toothbrush that was replaced every 6–8 weeks. She said she flossed two times a day.

Extraoral and Intraoral Examinations

- • There were no significant findings. The patient had no extraoral or intraoral masses or swelling, and the temporomandibular joint was within normal limits.
- • A periodontal examination revealed localized mild marginal gingival erythema, with rolled margins, edematous papillae, and bleeding on probing in area #23–24, 26, and 27. There was gingival recession present on the buccal aspect of teeth #4–6, 10, 11, 19, 21–24, 26, 28, 30, and 31, with probing depths ranging from 1 to 3mm throughout, no mobility

Probing Buccal	-	-	222	222	323	312	212	223	323	313	213	323	323	333	223	-
Recession	-	-	1	1	2	3	-	1	-	3	3	2	2	3	3	-
Keratinized gingiva	-	-	4	4	3	1	2	3	3	1	1	2	2	3	3	-
Probing Palatal	-	-	323	323	323	323	211	222	212	222	222	322	222	323	323	-

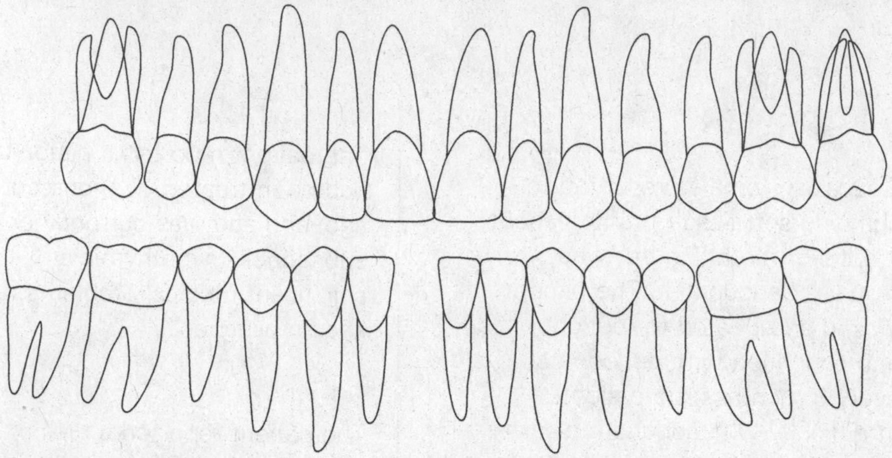

Probing Buccal	-	323	323	323	323	323	322	-	222	222	222	222	223	323	323	-
Recession	-	2	3	-	2	-	2	-	2	3	1	3	-	3	-	-
Keratinized gingiva	-	2	2	2	2	2	1	-	2	1	1	1	1	1	1	-
Probing Lingual	-	323	323	323	323	323	222	-	222	222	222	323	323	333	333	-

Figure 2: Probing pocket depth, keratinized gingiva, and recession measurements.

present, keratinized gingiva ranging from 1 to 4 mm with generalized lack of attached gingiva (Figures 1 and 2). Aberrant inferior labial frenum was found.
- Edentulous sites #1, 2, 16, 17, 25, and 32: there were numerous restoration and discolored anterior composites present.
- The remaining soft tissues of the mouth appeared within normal limits.

Occlusion

Angle class I occlusion on left side and angle class III occlusion on right side.

Radiographic Examination

Periapical radiographs of the mandibular incisor area are presented in Figure 3 depicting mild horizontal bone loss localized to the anterior mandibular teeth.

Diagnosis

After reviewing the history and the clinical and radiographic examinations, the patient was diagnosed with gingivitis on a reduced periodontium and mucogingival defects: gingival recession, decreased vestibular depth, and aberrant frenum attachment.

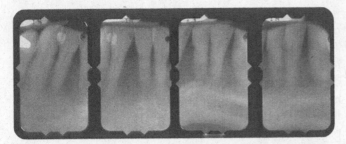

Figure 3: Periapical radiographs depicting the interproximal bone levels.

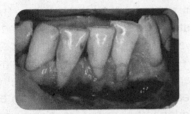

Figure 4: Preparation of the recipient site.

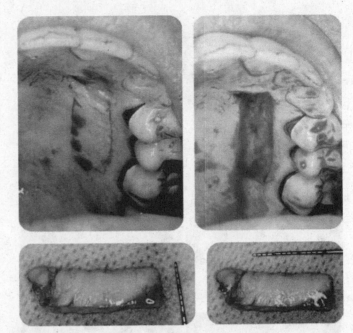

Figure 5: Harvesting of epithelio-connective tissue graft from the donor site.

Treatment Plan

The treatment plan included surgical treatment for correction of the mucogingival defects, followed by periodontal maintenance every 3 months.

Treatment

Surgical treatment for this patient included a FGG area #23–24-x-26, vestibuloplasty, and a labial frenectomy. Topical anesthetic was applied, and 5.4 ml of 0.5% Marcaine plus 1:200,000 epinephrine were locally infiltrated in the buccal and lingual area #22–27, and 1.8 ml of 2% lidocaine plus 1:100,000 epinephrine was given via left greater palatine and nasopalatine blocks.

Preparation of recipient site included the following steps:

- Scaling and root planing of teeth #22–24, 26 using hand and rotary instruments was completed.
- Horizontal incisions were made just coronal to the mucogingival junction from the mesial of #22 to the distal of #26 (Figure 4).
- Vertical incisions were made at the mesial and distal aspects of the horizontal incision short of the mesial line angles of #22 and #27 and 3 mm apical to the mucogingival junction.
- A split-thickness flap was dissected providing for deepening of the vestibule, a labial frenectomy, and the appropriate size of the recipient graft bed, followed by deepithelization of keratinized tissue coronal to the horizontal incision.

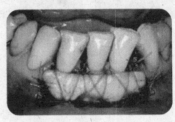

Figure 6: Epithelio-connective tissue graft sutured to the recipient bed.

- The residual flap was excised and loose connective tissue removed to provide a uniform firm bed.
  Harvesting of palatal epithelial-connective tissue graft (Figure 5):
- Using a #15 blade a 22 mm × 8 mm × 1.5 mm graft was harvested from donor area: palatal from D of #10 to middle of #14 starting approximately 3 mm apical to cementoenamel junction (CEJ) of teeth
- The donor site was sutured with 4-0 chromic gut
- Gelfoam and Coe-Pak were used.
  Graft stabilization (Figure 6):
- Single interrupted 5-0 chromic gut sutures (P-3 needle) were used to stabilize the flap apically to the periosteum
- The graft was positioned coronally to partially cover the recession on the mandibular incisors
- Single interrupted sutures engaged the lateral border of the graft to stabilize it to the adjacent mucosa

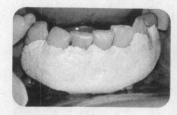
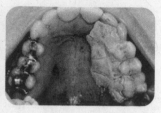

Figure 7: Recipient and donor sites were protected with periodontal dressing.

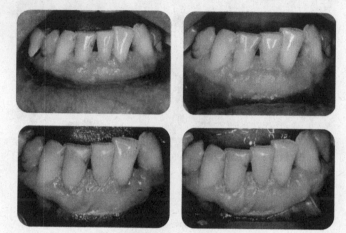

Figure 8: Postoperative follow-up.

- Continuous compressing cross-mattress sutures were placed over the graft, without engaging the graft, to immobilize the graft and compress it against the underlying vascular bed and root surfaces
- Moist gauze was used to compress the graft to ensure intimate adaption to the bed and development of a minimal clot
- Periodontal dressing (Coe-Pak) was placed over the recipient site, covering the sutured graft (Figure 7).
- The patient tolerated the procedure well.
- Postoperative instructions (oral and written), ice packs, and prescriptions were given for Tylenol #3 (#15) and Peridex.

The patient was followed postoperatively to monitor healing at 2 weeks (Figure 8, top left), 1 month (top right), 4 months (bottom left) and 1 year (bottom right).

Discussion

The FGG belongs to a broader category of gingival reconstructive surgery termed mucogingival surgery or periodontal plastic surgery (A). FGG for gingival augmentation has been used for >40 years [1]. These procedures are designed to correct, prevent, or ameliorate mucogingival defects defined as "deviations

from the normal anatomic relationship between the gingival margin and the mucogingival junction (C) [2]. The most common mucogingival deformity is gingival recession, although the rationale for its treatment continues to evolve and be debated. When recession is associated with the absence or lack of keratinized tissue, this defect is considered more vulnerable to progressive attachment loss. Although with adequate plaque control and professional follow-up these defects may be able to be maintained, evidence has demonstrated that without regular dental care, untreated mucogingival defects are more likely to progress than treated ones [3]. Having <1 mm of attached keratinized tissue is generally recognized as a mucogingival defect [2,4]. This finding, coupled with progressive recession, a need for cervical margin restorative care, or inadequate plaque control, indicates a need for treatment (C). Aberrant frenum attachment, planned orthodontic treatment, root abrasion, and sensitivity in conjunction with inadequate keratinized tissue can also be considered indications for treatment (E). The absence of keratinized tissue around dental implants has been shown to be associated with both recession and bone loss (D). It is evident from recent data that both the maintenance of marginal tissue and the preservation of alveolar bone about implants are aided by the presence of marginal keratinized tissue. Gingival augmentation is routinely used to enhance aesthetics through root coverage, correction of ridge deformities, and socket preservation.

In this case, to correct or minimize the soft tissue defects found in the mandibular anterior area, including multiple areas of recession, aberrant labial frenum, and reduced vestibular depth, an autogenous free gingival tissue graft was chosen to optimally treat this area (E). The choice of a FGG will provide the opportunity of simultaneously increasing the zone of attached gingival, deepening of the vestibule, frenectomy, and establishing improved contours for plaque control. The recession found on teeth #23, 24, 26 correspond to Miller class III recession defects; therefore only partial root coverage can be expected [5]. In the case of class I or II recession defects, complete root coverage can be obtained with a one-stage free gingival graft procedure. Bernimoulin et al [6] demonstrated a second surgical procedure to provide complete root coverage by coronally positioning a mature free gingival graft with a pedicle flap. A later study by Laney et al [7] compared the relative success of soft tissue coverage of denuded roots (class I or II according to Miller's classification) using two surgical procedures—autogenous FGG and a second stage coronally positioned flap (CPF)—could not demonstrate a significant difference in success between FGG and CPF at 3 months. Livingston [8] reported successful coverage of multiple and adjacent denuded root surfaces with a free gingival autograft. The surgical case presented in this chapter successfully achieved the multiple goals outlined here. Careful attention to each step in the surgical protocol can provide superior outcomes. By harvesting a thick palatal graft, the following are expected: significant enhancement in the predictability of root coverage (K) [9], augmentation in gingival dimensions with resultant increased resistance to further recession, and increase in vestibular depth

as well as greater primary contraction but less secondary contraction compared with thin grafts [1]. Furthermore, using a thick palatal graft can likely lead to creeping attachment (I) [10] between 1 month to 1 year after the surgery, with no significant difference between 1 and 5 years, as reported later by Matter [11]. The periodontal dressing placed on both the donor and recipient sites provided comfort to the patient the first few days after the surgery (K).

To summarize, the conducted treatment significantly improved the patient's oral health, hygiene, function, and aesthetics. Continued periodontal recall and maintenance along with proper plaque control has to be followed to maintain the obtained results.

Self-Study Questions

A. What is a mucogingival defect?

B. What is the etiology of a gingival recession?

C. What is the rationale for the treatment of mucogingival defects?

D. Do we need keratinized tissue about dental implants?

E. What are the indications and contraindications for using a FGG?

F. What are the advantages and disadvantages of using a FGG?

G. What is Miller's classification of recessions, and how can they aid in predicting the potential for root coverage?

H. What are the critical anatomic considerations in donor tissue harvesting? What is the anticipated result in case of free gingival grafts of different thicknesses?

I. What healing is expected after a FGG?

J. Is chemical root treatment necessary for successful root coverage with a FGG?

K. What are the possible complications after the surgery, and how can we prevent them? How can smoking affect the treatment result?

L. What other surgical techniques can be used in place of free soft tissue grafting?

Answers located at the end of the chapter.

References

1. Sullivan HC, Atkins JH. Free autogenous gingival grafts.1. Principles of successful grafting. Periodontics 1968;6:5–13.
2. American Academy of Periodontology consensus statement on mucogingival conditions. May 2009.
3. Kennedy JE, Bird WC, et al. A longitudinal evaluation of varying widths of attached gingiva. J Clin Periodontol 1985;12:667–675.
4. Lang NP, Löe H. The relationship between the width of keratinized gingiva and gingival health. J Periodontol 1972;43:623–627.
5. Miller PD Jr. A classification of marginal tissue recession. Int J Periodontics Restorative Dent 1985;5: 8–13.
6. Bernimoulin JP, Lüscher B, et al. Coronally repositioned periodontal flap. Clinical evaluation after one year. J Clin Periodontol 1975;2:1–13.

7. Laney JB, Saunders VG, et al. A comparison of two techniques for attaining root coverage. J Periodontol 1992;63:19–23.

8. Livingston HL Total coverage of multiple and adjacent denuded root surfaces with a free gingival autograft. A case report. J Periodontol 1975;46:209–216.

9. Miller PD Jr. Root coverage using a free soft tissue autograft following citric acid application. Part 1: Technique. Int J Periodontics Restorative Dent 1982;2:65–70.

10. Matter J, Cimasoni G. Creeping attachment after free gingival grafts. J Periodontol 1976;7:574–579.

11. Matter J. Creeping attachment of free gingival grafts. A five-year follow-up study. J Periodontol 1980;51:682–685.

12. Miller PD Jr. Regenerative and reconstructive periodontal plastic surgery. Mucogingival surgery. Dent Clin North Am 1988;32:287–306.

13. Consensus report. Mucogingival therapy. Ann Periodontol 1996;1:702–706.

14. Camargo PM, Melnick PR, et al. The use of free gingival grafts for aesthetic purposes. Periodontol 2000 2001;27:72–96.

15. Levin L, Samorodnitzky-Naveh GR, et al. The association of orthodontic treatment and fixed retainers with gingival health. J Periodontol 2008;79:2087–2092.

16. Maynard JG Jr, Wilson RD. Physiologic dimensions of the periodontium significant to the restorative dentist. J Periodontol 1979;50:170–174.

17. Ericsson I, Lindhe J. Recession in sites with inadequate width of the keratinized gingiva. An experimental study in the dog. J Clin Periodontol 1984;11:95–103.

18. Zigdon H, Machtei EE. The dimensions of keratinized mucosa (KM) around implants affect clinical and immunological parameters. Clin Oral Implant Res 2008;19:387–392.

19. Schrott AR, Jimenez M, et al. Five-year evaluation of the influence of keratinized mucosa on peri-implant soft-tissue health and stability around implants supporting full-arch mandibular fixed prostheses. Clin Oral Implants Res 2009;20:1170–1177.

20. Karring T, Lang NP, et al. The role of gingival connective tissue in determining epithelial differentiation. J Periodontal Res 1975;10:1–11.

21. Agudio G, Nieri M, et al. Free gingival grafts to increase keratinized tissue: a retrospective long-term evaluation (10 to 25 years) of outcomes. J Periodontol 2008;79:587–594.

22. Paolantonio M, di Murro C, et al. Subpedicle connective tissue graft versus free gingival graft in the coverage of exposed root surfaces. A 5-year clinical study. J Clin Periodontol 1997;24:51–56.

23. Reiser GM, Bruno JF, et al. The subepithelial connective tissue graft palatal donor site: anatomic considerations for surgeons. Int J Periodontics Restorative Dent 1996;16:130–137.

24. Mörmann W, Schaer F, et al. The relationship between success of free gingival grafts and transplant thickness. Revascularization and shrinkage–a one year clinical study. J Periodontol 1981;52:74–80.

25. Orsini M, Orsini G, et al. Esthetic and dimensional evaluation of free connective tissue grafts in prosthetically treated patients: a 1-year clinical study. J Periodontol 2004;75:470–477.

26. Oral reconstructive and corrective considerations in periodontal therapy. Greenwell H, Fiorellini J, et al; Research, Science and Therapy Committee. J Periodontol 2005;76:1588–1600.

27. Oliver RC, Löe H, et al. Microscopic evaluation of the healing and revascularization of free gingival grafts. J Periodontal Res 1968;3:84–95.

28. Pasquinelli KL. The histology of new attachment utilizing a thick autogenous soft tissue graft in an area of deep recession: a case report. Int J Periodontics Restorative Dent 1995;15:248–257.

29. Miller PD Jr. Root coverage with the free gingival graft. Factors associated with incomplete coverage. J Periodontol 1987;58:674–681.

30. Ruggeri A Jr, Prati C, et al. Effects of citric acid and EDTA conditioning on exposed root dentin: An immunohistochemical analysis of collagen and proteoglycans. Arch Oral Biol 2007;52:1–8.

31. Vanheusden AJ, Goffinet G, et al. 1999 In vitro stimulation of human gingival epithelial cell attachment to dentin by surface conditioning. J Periodontol 1999;70:594–603.

32. Baker DL, Stanley Pavlow SA, et al. Fibrin clot adhesion to dentin conditioned with protein constructs: an in vitro proof-of-principle study. J Clin Periodontol 2005;32:561–566.

33. Kassab MM, Cohen RE, et al. The effect of EDTA in attachment gain and root coverage. Compend Contin Educ Dent 2006;27:353–360.

34. Ibbott CG, et al. Effects of citric acid treatment on autogenous free graft coverage of localized recession. J Periodontol 1985;56:662–665.

35. Brasher W, Rees T, et al. Complications of free grafts of masticatory mucosa. J Periodontol 1975;46:133.

36. Griffin TJ, Cheung WS, et al. Postoperative complications following gingival augmentation procedures. J Periodontol 2006;77:2070–2079.

37. Rossmann JA, Rees TD. A comparative evaluation of hemostatic agents in the management of soft tissue graft donor site bleeding. J Periodontol 1999;70:1369–1375.

TAKE-HOME POINTS

A. A mucogingival defect is generally defined as any significant deviation from the normal anatomic relationship between the gingival margin and the mucogingival junction [2]. The most common defects present as gingival recession, minimal keratinized marginal tissue (gingiva), a shallow vestibule, and aberrant frenum attachment. Most associate the term *mucogingival defect* with an absence of an adequate zone of attached keratinized tissue (<1mm of attached gingiva). The amount of attached gingiva is determined by measuring from the free gingival margin to the mucogingival junction and then subtracting the sulcular probing depth from it.

Periodontal plastic surgery [12] is defined as a means of treatment for mucogingival problems with the intent to prevent or correct anatomic, developmental, and traumatic or plaque disease–induced defects of the gingival, alveolar mucosa, or bone. The goal is the creation of form and appearance that are acceptable and pleasing to the patient and the therapist [13]. The final results following mucogingival surgical therapy should be an increase of the apico-coronal and bucco-lingual dimensions of the gingival tissues and in the establishment of proper vestibular depth where necessary. When performed for root coverage, mucogingival procedures should additionally result in coverage of the previously denuded root surface to the level of the CEJ and also include biologic attachment between the grafted tissue and the root surface, resulting in a shallow sulcus [14].

B. The most common reason for gingival recession is generally attributed to mechanical trauma/ aggressive brushing in an anatomically susceptible site. The anatomic position of the tooth in relation to the bony envelope of the jaw is an important factor in the patient's susceptibility to recession. Teeth with prominent roots extending outside the envelope of the alveolar process and teeth in buccal version generally demonstrate recession.

Progressive periodontal disease can also lead to recession, some evidence indicates that orthodontic therapy can promote recession if the arches are expanded or plaque control is poor [15]. Restorative dentistry that is significantly subgingival, overcontoured, or with poor marginal integrity can contribute to recession [16]. Occlusal trauma such as bruxism can sometimes be associated with recession.

C. The rationale for the treatment of mucogingival defects can be divided into two categories: (1) treatment for aesthetic criteria and (2) treatment to prevent progressive attachment loss. Although the FGG can be used to cover roots and correct ridge deformities, other procedures such as the subepithelial connective tissue graft (SECTG) have supplanted its use due to superior aesthetics. When <1mm of attached keratinized tissue is noted in conjunction with recession, treatment for gingival augmentation should be strongly considered. The study by Kennedy et al [3] demonstrated that it is possible to maintain periodontal health and attachment for a period of 6 years through rigorous control of gingival inflammation via scaling, root planing, oral hygiene, and maintenance at 3- to 6-month intervals despite the absence of attached gingiva. In patients who had discontinued participation in this study for a period of 5 years, reestablishment of gingival inflammation associated with additional recession was revealed. In the same study, in the experimental sites, where FGG was performed in areas with recession and inadequate or no attached gingiva, the dimension of keratinized and attached gingiva increased. A reduction in recession and gain in clinical attachment was also exhibited and was stable >6 years. In these patients who were treated by a FGG and discontinued participation in the study, no gingival inflammation and additional recession were observed in areas treated by a free graft as compared with the untreated sites [3].

Other parameters also influence the need for treatment such as the level of plaque control and the patient's maintenance schedule. The need for restorative treatment or orthodontics in conjunction with a mucogingival defect can indicate treatment. Maynard and Wilson [16] suggested that

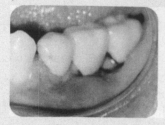
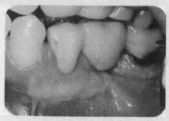

Figure 9: FGG prior to a restoration and bone grafting/implant placement procedures: preoperative and 7-month post-FGG photographs.

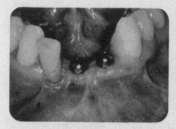
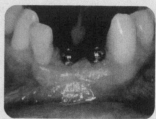

Figure 10: FGG prior to implant restorations to recreate lost attached gingiva and deepen the vestibule: preoperative and 2-month postoperative FGG photographs.

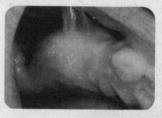
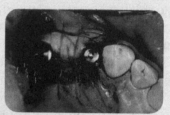

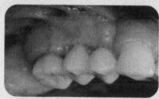

Figure 11: Epithelio-connective tissue palatal pedicle graft performed during second stage implant: preoperative, immediate, and 5-month postoperative photographs.

if intracrevicular margins, defined as those placed into and confined within the gingival crevice, are planned for a restorative procedure, keratinized tissue is necessary (as shown in Figure 9). Additionally, Ericsson and Lindhe [17] demonstrated that submarginal metal stripes caused increase gingival recession in areas with minimal keratinized tissue in beagle dogs. The patient's age, susceptibility to periodontitis, and medical health are other important factors to consider.

D. Having marginal keratinized mucosa (KM) about implants appears to impart significant benefits. Zigdon and Machtei [18] found in their retrospective study that KM around dental implants affects both the clinical and the immunologic parameters at these sites:

- Negative correlation between mucosal thickness and MR (mucosal margin to the implant-abutment interface) as well as between KM width and MR, periodontal attachment level, and prostaglandin E_2 levels
- Similarly, a thick mucosa (>1 mm) associated with lesser recession compared with a thin (<1 mm) mucosa

In patients exercising good oral hygiene and receiving regular implant maintenance therapy, implants with a reduced width <2 mm of peri-implant keratinized mucosa were more prone to lingual plaque accumulation and bleeding as well as buccal soft tissue recession over a period of 5 years (Schrott et al [19]).

Additionally, more soreness to plaque control measures and to food impaction is reported by patients with an absence of keratinized tissue

adjacent to implants. Figure 10 is an example of use of FGG to recreate lost attached gingiva and deepening of the vestibule around previously placed implants. An epithelio-connective tissue palatal pedicle graft can also be performed during a second stage implant to recreate keratinized tissue around implants soon to be restored (Figure 11).

E. Since the advent of the subepithelial connective tissue graft, the indications for use of the FGG have greatly diminished. However there remain multiple important indications for its use. In regions where a very shallow vestibule exists and coronal manipulation of the gingival flap would exacerbate this situation and possibly hinder future plaque control, a free gingival graft should be considered. Presence of a coronally positioned frenum may also compromise the use of a SECTG, and a FGG can be considered. These situations occur most frequently in the mandibular anterior region. Because these sites are also less aesthetically critical, a FGG may become a superior choice.

In addition to the superior esthetics of the SECTG, the postoperative healing of the donor site heals with significantly less discomfort and time. This factor can be taken advantage of by combining a portion of both techniques (Figure 12). A traditional FGG recipient site bed can be made, but the harvesting of the graft can be done with a SECTG technique. This will allow one to take advantage of the superior healing of the palate. The SECTG will produce a keratinized graft as the epithelial coverage is dictated by the underlying CT [20]. The main disadvantage using just CT is that

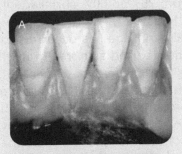
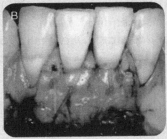
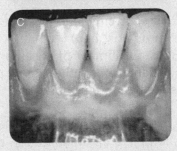

Figure 12: Connective tissue used as a free graft. (A) Recession associated with mucogingival involvement on the buccal of #24 and 25. (B) Connective tissue harvested from palate and used as a free graft. (C) Healing with keratinization and significant root coverage. Note the approximately 40% shrinkage of the vertical height of the graft but minimal horizontal shrinkage.

the shrinkage of the graft is extensive. The way to avoid this and also increase the handling properties of the graft is to harvest a "composite" graft containing a portion of only CT graft and a portion of epithelial and connective tissue, comprising a wide band of keratinized tissue. A 3-mm band of keratinized tissue with the rest being connective tissue is generally adequate. Importantly, partial closure of the palatal site can be obtained and the discomfort associated with this technique is no different than with the classical harvest of a SECTG.

Free gingival grafts have few contraindications mostly related to systemic and/or anatomic constraints such as the following:

- Bleeding/coagulation disorders or medications (i.e., use of acetylsalicylic-based medication) that can produce uncontrolled bleeding
- Impingement on critical anatomy such as the mental foramen
- Improper access to donor (i.e., reduced mouth opening) or recipient sites

F. These are the advantages of using a FGG:
- Predictable procedure to provide an adequate band of keratinized tissue and stable up to 25 years of follow-up [21]
- Technically less demanding and the procedure is shorter compared with SECTG
- Will not compromise vestibular depth and also provides an increase in vestibular depth
- Can be used in conjunction with frenectomy
- Can be used for root coverage [9].
  These are the disadvantages of using a FGG:
- Percentage of root coverage is less than with the SECTG [22]
- Can be perceived as less aesthetic than the SECTG
- Increased soreness from donor site than SECTG, pedicle, and acellular dermal graft
- Limitation in quantity and quality of donor tissue
- Limitations for reconstruction of interdental papilla

As mentioned earlier, better aesthetics can be achieved with the SECTG. FGG generally appear significantly paler than adjacent tissue. In most cases this has to do with the contrast of the adjacent mucosa and not the adjacent keratinized tissue.

In general, the best area to harvest keratinized tissue for grafting is the hard palate. Due to anatomic constraints, this tissue could be limited (H). To date, reconstruction of a lost interdental papilla could not be achieved with a FGG.

G. In 1985, Miller published a classification of marginal tissue recession [5]:

- Class 1: Recession does not extend to MGJ, no interdental bone or soft tissue loss; 100% coverage expected
- Class 2: Recession to or beyond MGJ but no interdental bone or soft tissue loss; 100% coverage anticipated
- Class 3: Recession extends to or beyond MGJ; loss of interdental bone or soft tissue, apical to the CEJ but coronal to the level of the recession defect; partial root coverage anticipated (Figure 13)
- Class 4: Recession extends to or beyond MGJ with loss of interdental bone or soft tissue apical to the level of the recession defect; no root coverage can be anticipated

H. The surgeon must be completely familiar with the anatomy of the palatal donor as well as recipient sites for appropriate surgical treatment. Reiser et al [23] found variations in the size and shape of the hard palate and identified the average location of the neurovascular bundle from the CEJ of the maxillary premolars and molars to vary with the palatal height:

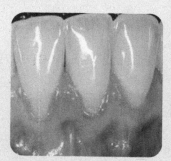 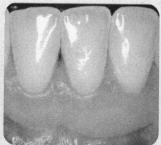

Figure 13: Root coverage with a FGG. Recession and mucogingival involvement #24 and 25 (left); site healed at 8 weeks with root coverage, elimination of mucogingival defect (right).

- High palatal vault to 17mm
- Average palatal vault to 12mm
- Shallow palatal vault to 7mm

Additionally, the same authors using cadaver dissection demonstrated that the surgeon can gain substantial donor tissue thickness in the area from the mesial line angle of the palatal root of the first molar to the distal line angle of the canine. Palatal exostosis can be encountered over the molar palatal area, thus limiting the thickness of the graft. By extending the harvesting area anteriorly from the distal line angle of the canine, palatal rugae can be encountered with subsequent less aesthetic results (Figure 5).

The thickness of the graft has a direct effect on its healing behavior. Gingival grafts demonstrated anywhere from 25% to 50% shrinkage in vertical height over 1 year [24]. The thinner the graft, the more vertical shrinkage has occurred [24]. Connective tissue used as a free graft showed >43% vertical shrinkage over 1 year [25]. Thinner gingival grafts (approximately 1mm) worked predictably when placed over the vascular bed but achieved very poor results with root coverage [26]. Thick grafts (1.5–2mm) proved to be the better choice for substantial root coverage [9]. These thicker grafts also required a larger vascular bed for predictable root coverage. Generally 75–80% of the graft needed to be in close apposition to the vascular bed.

I. Sullivan and Atkins [1] described initial stages of graft maturation after a free autogenous gingival graft:

- Days 0–2: Plasmatic circulation (direct diffusion of nutrients from its host bed)
- Days 2–8: Reestablishment of vascularization
- Days 4–10: Organic connective tissue union (fibrous tissue attachment) between the graft and its bed

At histologic evaluation following FGGs, Oliver et al [27] found complete epithelialization by 14 days and keratinization by 28 days. In a case report histologic study in humans, Pasquinelli [28] reported on new attachment and new bone growth, with minimal sulcus depth of 1mm, after 10.5 months following treatment of a deep buccal recession with a thick (1.5 mm) free autogenous gingival graft.

Creeping attachment following a FGG was described by Matter and Cimasoni [10] and Matter [11] as a postoperative coronal migration of gingival marginal tissue resulting in partial or total coverage of a previously denuded root, with firm tissue attached to root surface and probing that does not show any sulcular depth. Creeping attachment occurred between 1 month and 1 year after surgery, and none was observed after 1 year. In addition, he listed various factors that seem to significantly influence creeping attachment, including the width of the recession, position and thickness of the graft, bone resorption, position of the tooth, and hygiene of the patient [10].

J. Root conditioning for enhancing root coverage continues to be controversial. Many agents have been advocated to condition roots before gingival grafting including citric acid, tetracycline-HCl, and EDTA. Miller [9,29] advocated this from an anecdotal clinical standpoint. Citric acid and EDTA have been shown to expose collagen fibrils and sound dentin while preserving the structural and biochemical properties of the dentin matrix [30]. Enhanced cell attachment was observed after chemical root conditioning in an in vitro study by Vanheusden et al [31]. Citric acid removes the smear layer that may aid in healing [32]. Using EDTA has more recently been shown to enhance root coverage [33]. However, a study by Ibbott et al [34] showed there is no significant improvement in root coverage with citric acid pretreatment. Due to the limitations of any definitive studies, root conditioning continues to be debated.

K. Although complications are generally limited after FGG surgery, the most common ones are excessive hemorrhage at donor site, swelling, and discomfort [35,36]. To avoid postoperative bleeding, several measures have been described: use of compressing suture (placed proximal to the bleeding site [23]), hemostatic agents [37], periodontal dressing (suggested to cover the donor site for 2 weeks [36]) and use of a palatal stent or denture, or a combination of them. By using a periodontal dressing or palatal stent, the bleeding is prevented by the mechanical pressure as well as by protecting the area from direct trauma to the open wound left behind for healing by secondary intention, thus having less sensitivity associated with direct trauma. In addition, in patients who have coagulation disorders or use acetylsalicylic-based medication before or during the initial healing process, the likelihood of bleeding is increased [35]. Duration of the procedure was positively associated with postoperative pain and swelling after FGG [36].

The study by Miller [5] showed that smoking interfered with complete root coverage after FGG surgery. Heavy smoking, in excess of 10 cigarettes per day, correlated 100% with failure to obtain root coverage; patients who were "light" or "occasional" smokers (five cigarettes or fewer per day) responded as favorably as the nonsmokers to root coverage using FGGs. A successful protocol was followed consisting of patients refraining from smoking during the initial 2 weeks of healing after the surgery subsequently resulting in root coverage comparable with nonsmokers. Furthermore, patients who were smokers were found to have three times more postoperative swelling as reported by Griffin and colleagues [36].

L. In addition to FGG, various techniques can be used to treat mucogingival problems and recession: subepithelial connective tissue graft, lateral pedicle graft, coronally advanced pedicle flap, guided tissue regeneration, and acellular dermal allograft.

Case 4

Treatment of Mucogingival Deformities Using Alloplastic Materials

CASE STORY

A 45-year-old Caucasian female presented with a chief compliant of: "I don't like the recession on my upper teeth" (Figures 1–3).The patient noticed this recession had become worse over time and was associated with occasional sensitivity to cold.

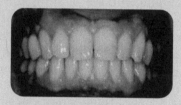

Figure 1: Preoperative presentation.

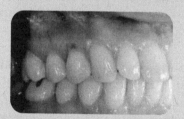

Figure 2: Pre-op presentation (right side).

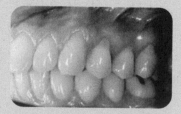

Figure 3: Pre-op presentation (left side).

LEARNING GOALS AND OBJECTIVES

- To be able to diagnose recession and inadequate attached gingiva
- To identify the possible treatments and prediction of outcomes for situations where a patient presents with soft tissue recession and root sensitivity
- To understand the importance of oral preventive treatment in such cases

Medical History

There were no significant medical problems at this time. The patient previously had undergone genetic testing and was found to have a variation of the *BRCA* gene, putting her at an increased risk for development of breast and ovarian cancer. As a result, she had a mastectomy and reconstruction in 2006, as well as an oophorectomy in 2007. At the time of presentation, the patient reported that she took Celexa 20 mg once daily, as well as a multivitamin, fish oil, and flax oil daily. She also reported an allergy to cats, dogs, pollen, and gluten.

Review of Systems

- Vital signs
  - Blood pressure: 105/78 mm Hg
  - Pulse rate: 72 beats/minute (regular)
  - Respiration: 16 breaths/minute

Social History

The patient drank alcohol socially (one to two glasses of wine per week) and had no history of smoking.

Extraoral Examination

No significant findings were noted. The patient had no masses or swelling, and the temporomandibular joint was within normal limits.

Oral Hygiene

The patient reported brushing twice per day using an electric toothbrush and flossing once per day. On clinical examination, the patient's hygiene was found to be excellent (Figure 4).

Intraoral Examination

- The soft tissues of the mouth (except gingiva) including the tongue appeared normal.
- A gingival examination revealed generalized pyramidal papillae with knife-edged margins and gingival recession on the maxillary posterior teeth bilaterally.

Occlusion

There were no occlusal discrepancies or interferences.

Radiographic Examination

Bite-wing radiographs were taken (Figure 5). No abnormal findings were detected radiographically.

Diagnosis and Treatment Plan

After reviewing the patient's history and clinical examination, it was concluded that the patient's gingival recession was likely secondary to a history of aggressive oral hygiene habits. The treatment plan includes an initial phase of scaling and polishing with oral hygiene instruction and modification of brushing and flossing techniques.

Overall, the patient's extensive areas of recession could be classified as a combination of Miller classification I and II. The papillae were broad and noted to completely fill the embrasure space. Given these clinical findings, and due to the patient's request of not using autogenous tissue for grafting, a decision was made to use an acellular dermal matrix for root coverage of the maxillary right and left quadrants.

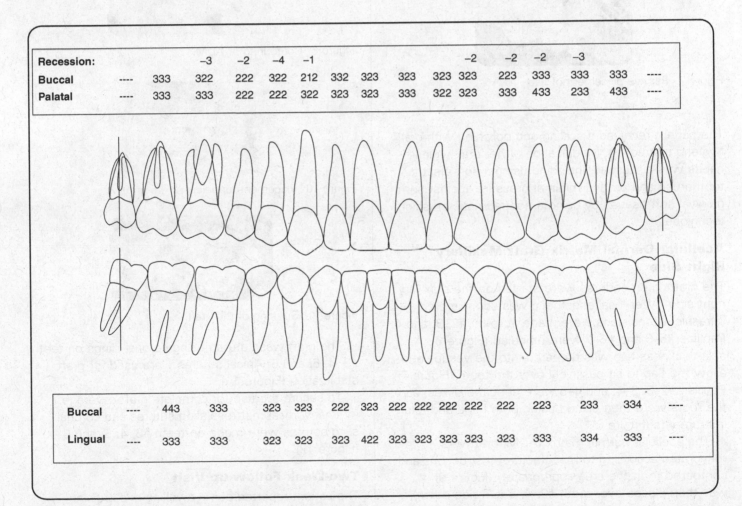

Recession:			−3	−2	−4	−1				−2	−2	−2	−3	
Buccal	----	333	322	222	322	212	332	323	323	323 323	223	333	333 333	----
Palatal	----	333	333	222	222	322	323	323	333	322 323	333	433	233 433	----

Buccal	----	443	333		323	323	222	323	222 222 222 222	222	223		233	334	----
Lingual	----	333	333		323	323	323	422	323 323 323 323	323	333		334	333	----

Figure 4: Probing pocket depth and recession measurements.

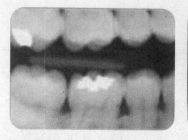
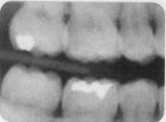
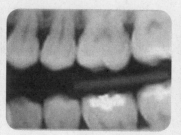
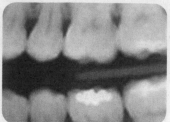

Figure 5: Bite-wing radiographs.

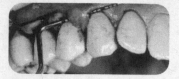

Figure 6: Tunnel procedure.

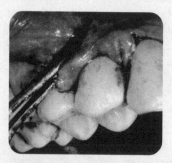

Figure 7: Passive placement of flap.

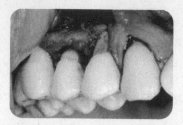

Figure 8: Root planing.

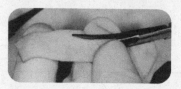

Figure 9: Contouring of ADM.

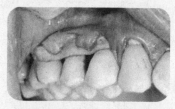

Figure 10: Placement/tunneling of the graft.

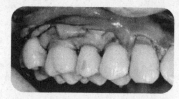

Figure 11: Suturing of the graft.

Treatment

The patient received a scaling and polishing with oral hygiene instruction. Modification of her oral hygiene habits was discussed, including using a soft electric toothbrush and putting minimal pressure against her gingival soft tissues by using a nontraumatic brushing technique.

Acellular Dermal Matrix Graft Maxillary Right Side

The grafting procedures were started on the maxillary right side. After local anesthetic was administered, intrasulcular incisions were made at teeth #2, 3, and 4. Papillae #5–6 and #6–7 were tunneled (Figure 6). A split-thickness flap was prepared into the vestibule to allow the flap to sit passively over the teeth (Figure 7). Papillae #2–3, 3–4, and 4–5 were deepithelialized, and the roots were then planed using both hand and rotary instruments (Figure 8).

The acellular dermal matrix (ADM) graft was rehydrated according to manufacturer instructions and contoured to fit the area appropriately (Figure 9). It was then placed over teeth #3, 4, 5 (CT side down), and tunneled under papillae #5–6 and 6–7 (Figure 10).

The graft was sutured using coronal slings on teeth #3, 4, 5, and 6. Apical sutures were used for graft stabilization (Figure 11).

To secure the flap for complete graft coverage, internal vertical mattress sling sutures and coronal sling sutures were made on teeth #3, 4, 5, and 6 (Figure 12).

Two-Week Follow-up Visit

The patient reported some swelling and bruising externally for 3–5 days postoperatively, with minimal

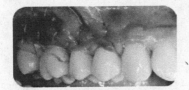

Figure 12: Flap positioned to cover graft.

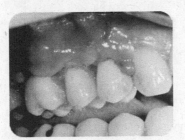

Figure 13: Two-week postoperative view.

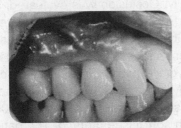

Figure 14: Eight-week follow-up visit.

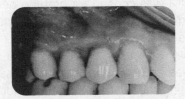

Figure 15: Twelve-week follow-up visit.

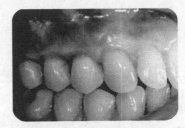

Figure 16: Seventeen-week follow-up visit.

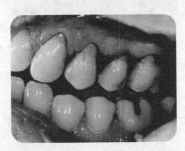

Figure 17: Initial incisions.

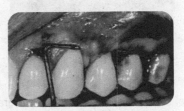

Figure 18: Tunneling near teeth #11/12.

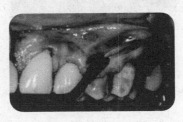

Figure 19: Release of flap for final positioning.

postoperative pain. Healing was within normal limits, with some erythema, particularly in the area of #5–6 (Figure 13).

Eight-Week Follow-up Visit

The maxillary right side is healing well. The erythema has subsided, and the patient has begun to brush gently using the modified Stillman method of brushing (Figure 14).

Figures 15 and 16 show the 12-week and 17-week follow-up visits, respectively.

ADM Graft Maxillary Left Side

After local anesthetic was administered, papillae #10–11, #11–12, were tunneled, with intrasulcular

incisions #12, 13, 14, and 15, recreating interproximal papillae #12–13, 13–14, 14–15 (Figures 17 and 18). A split-thickness flap was created for appropriate release (Figure 19).

The ADM was hydrated according to the manufacturer's instructions and contoured to fit the recipient bed (Figure 20). It was then tunneled beneath papillae #10–12 and placed under flap #12–14 (Figure 21).

To stabilize the graft, apical sutures and coronal sling sutures were completed. A combination of internal vertical mattress and coronal slings were used to achieve complete coverage of the graft (Figure 22).

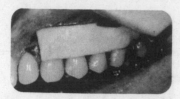

Figure 20: Contoured ADM try-in

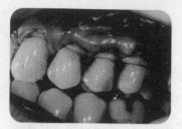

Figure 21: Placement and tunneling of the graft.

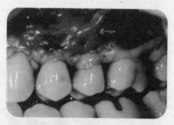

Figure 22: Final suturing of flap to cover the graft.

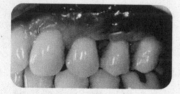

Figure 23: Three-week follow-up visit.

Three-Week Follow-up Visit

The maxillary left side was healing well, with some slight erythema still present (Figure 23).

Figures 24 and 25 show the 5- and 10-week follow-up visits, respectively.

Discussion

This patient presented with a chief complaint of extensive recession on the maxillary arch. On examination, her oral hygiene was observed to be excellent, probing depths were normal, and there was

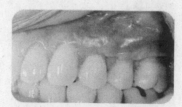

Figure 24: Five-week follow-up visit.

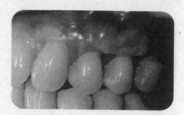

Figure 25: Ten-week follow-up visit.

no significant interproximal bone loss detected radiographically. Occlusion was evaluated, and there were no interferences on protrusion or lateral excursions. Given these findings, it was established that the patient's recession was likely secondary to her aggressive hygiene habits. The recession could be classified as Miller's classification I or II; hence it would be reasonable to anticipate up to 100% root coverage with soft tissue grafting. The patient was presented with soft tissue grafting options, which included connective tissue autografts, or ADM matrix allografts. ADM was chosen for grafting because the patient preferred to not have her palatal tissue used as the donor site for such extensive grafting.

After review of appropriate oral hygiene practices, the patient was prepared for her grafting surgeries. When evaluating the tissues in planning for her allograft procedure, some important elements were examined. The papillae in this case were thick and full with at least 3-mm width to allow for sufficient blood supply to the graft. In addition, there was adequate vestibular depth and no significant muscle attachments, which could potentially make coronal repositioning and stabilization of the flap quite difficult.

For any patient with recession, it is imperative to identify the cause of such lesions and attempt necessary functional and/or behavioral adjustments before any surgical intervention. If not addressed, such factors could lead to long-term recurrence of recession, even subsequent to surgical grafting procedures.

Self-Study Questions

A. What is acellular dermal matrix (ADM), and how is it processed?

B. How does ADM work?

C. What types of procedures can acellular dermal matrix allograft be used for?

D. What are the advantages/disadvantages of using acellular dermal matrix versus a connective tissue graft?

E. What are the long-term results of grafting using a ADM allograft?

Answers located at the end of the chapter.

References

1. Gapski R, Parks CH, et al. Acellular dermal matrix for mucogingival surgery: a meta-analysis. J Peridontol 2005;76:1814–1822.
2. Mahajan A, Dixxit J, et al. A patient-centered evaluation of acellular dermal matrix graft in the treatment of gingival recession defects. J Periodontol 2007;12:2348–2355.
3. Santos A, Goumenos G, et al. Management of gingival recession by the use of an acellullar dermal graft material: a 12-case series. J Periodontol 2005;76:1982–1990.
4. Luczyszyn SM, Papalexiou V, et al. Acellular dermal matrix and hydroxyapatite in prevention of ridge deformities after tooth extraction. Implant Dent 2005;14:176–184.
5. Cummings LC, Kaldahl WB, et al. Histologic evaluation of autogenous connective tissue and acellular dermal matrix grafts in humans. J Periodontol 2005;76:178–186.
6. Harris RJ. A comparative study of root coverage obtained with an acellular dermal matrix versus a connective tissue graft. J Periodontol 2000;20:51–59.
7. Langer G, Langer L. Subepithelial connective tissue graft technique for root coverage. J Periodontol 1985;56:715–720.
8. Harris RJ. A short-term and long-term comparison of root coverage with an acellular dermal matrix and a subepithelial graft. J Periodontol 2004;75:734–743.
9. Tal H, Moses Ofer, et al. Root coverage of advanced gingival recession: a comparative study between acellular dermal matrix allograft and subepithelial connective tissue grafts. J Periodontol 2002;73:1405–1411.
10. Hirsch A, Goldstein M, et al. A 2-year follow-up of root coverage using subpedicle acellular dermal matrix allografts and subepithelial connective tissue autografts. J Periodontol 2005;76:1323–1328.

TAKE-HOME POINTS

A. Acellular dermal matrix (ADM) is derived from prescreened donated human tissue that undergoes multiple steps of processing before its use in the mouth. First, the donated tissue is treated with a buffered salt solution to separate and eliminate the epidermis. It then undergoes a series of washes with a mild detergent to eliminate all remaining cells. The processed tissue is then freeze dried until it is ready to be used clinically.

B. Once the ADM is prepared, any cells that might lead to tissue rejection by the patient are removed. The remaining regenerative matrix consists only of collagens, elastin, vascular channels, and proteins that remain biologically active and are therefore recognized as human tissue. These remaining elements provide scaffolding so the patient's blood can infiltrate, bringing host cells into the area. These cells subsequently adhere to the proteins still found in the ADM and support repopulation and revascularization of the area, ultimately remodeling the ADM into the patient's own tissue.

C. ADM was first introduced into medicine in 1995 for use on burn patients. Since that time, its use has grown exponentially, encompassing many fields including urology, orthopedics, and dentistry. Given that ADM is still a relatively novel material for use by dental specialists (since 1997), there have been limited randomized controlled clinical trials available for comprehensive meta-analysis of ADM procedures versus commonly used mucogingival surgical procedures [1]. Clinical trends, however, have revealed that ADM can be successfully used in mucogingival procedures for root coverage [2,3], soft tissue augmentation, as well as acting as a barrier membrane for extraction socket grafting and guided bone regeneration [4]. One human histologic study found that, when compared with CTG, ADM has only a slightly different histologic presentation but was able to successfully cover roots with similar attachments to that of CTGs [5].

D. The advantages and disadvantages of using ADM versus connective tissue grafting include:

Advantages
- Ability to treat multiple sites in a single surgery
- Good handling properties (easy to use)
- Can be obtained in varying thicknesses (currently available in 0.3–1.8 mm) and sizes
- Ability to treat patients who have inadequate harvestable tissue
- Eliminates the need for a second surgical site (donor site)
- Avoids postoperative morbidity associated with harvesting palatal connective tissue
- Aesthetic results are comparable with those with connective tissue grafting [6]

Disadvantages
- Technique sensitive: The consensus clinical practice/opinion is to attempt complete coverage of ADM. Connective tissue grafts, in contrast, can be left slightly exposed [7].
- Some literature has shown that root coverage with subepithelial grafts had better stability over time versus coverage with an ADM (these results are not universal) [8].
- Some studies have demonstrated that autogenous grafting can result in greater gain of keratinized gingival when compared with ADM [9].

E. Given that acellular dermal matrix has only been used for dental purposes since the mid-1990s, long-term results for treatment are limited. Most available literature has shown that when compared with connective tissue grafting for root coverage, procedures using ADM are predictable and stable postoperatively [10].

Case 5

Frenectomy and Vestibuloplasty

CASE STORY

A 20-year-old African-American male presented with a chief complaint of: "I was told that I need to have some tissues removed between my two upper front teeth before orthodontic treatment." The patient had been referred from his orthodontist, who requested a periodontal consultation regarding the removal of maxillary labial frenum before orthodontic closure of the patient's midline diastema (Figure 1).

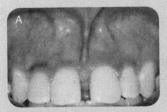 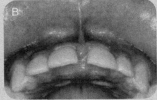

Figure 1: Preoperative presentation. (A) Buccal view; (B) occlusal view.

LEARNING GOALS AND OBJECTIVES
■ To be able to identify the clinical appearance of abnormal frenal attachments and shallow vestibules
■ To understand the potential complications associated with abnormal frenal attachments and shallow vestibules
■ To have a basic understanding of the surgical approaches of frenectomy and vestibuloplasty

Medical History

The patient denied any medical conditions and reported good general health. He was not taking any medications and had no allergies to any drug.

Review of Systems
- Vital signs
  - Blood pressure: 136/82 mm Hg
  - Pulse rate: 77 beats/minute
  - Respiration: 15 breaths/minute

Social History

The patient had never smoked but occasionally drank beer. He denied using recreational drugs.

Extraoral Examination

No abnormal swellings and masses were detected. Examination of temporomandibular joint and muscles of mastication appeared normal.

Intraoral Examination
- Soft tissue including buccal mucosa, tongue, floor of the mouth, and hard/soft palate all appeared within normal limits.
- A high maxillary labial frenal attachment between teeth #8 and #9 was observed; the frenum attached to the papilla between the two central incisors.
- Gingiva in general was healthy with stippling present, and there was adequate amount of attached keratinized gingiva. The papilla between #8 and #9 was blunt.
- Periodontal charting showed no probing pocket depth >3 mm. No tooth mobility, furcal involvement, gingival recession, or mucogingival defects were detected (Figure 2).

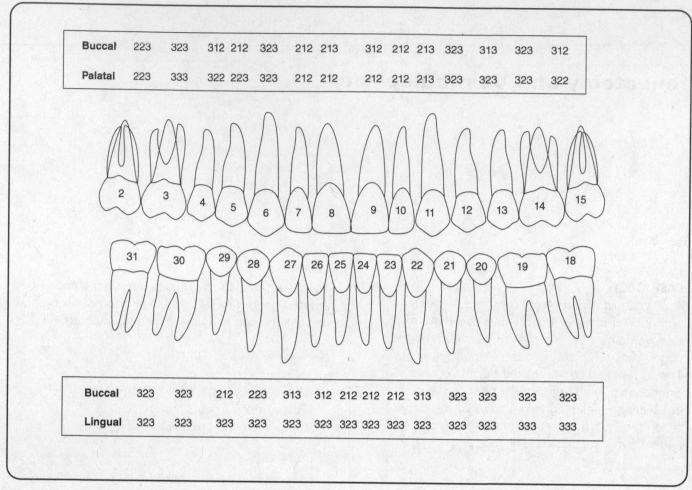

	Buccal	223	323	312 212	323	212 213	312 212 213	323	313	323	312
	Palatal	223	333	322 223	323	212 212	212 212 213	323	323	323	322

	Buccal	323	323	212	223	313	312 212 212 212	313	323	323	323	323
	Lingual	323	323	323	323	323	323 323 323 323 323	323	323	323	333	333

Figure 2: Probing pocket depth measurements during initial visit.

Occlusion

There was no occlusal disharmony detected.

Radiographic Examination

A panoramic and full-mouth radiographic series were taken. No abnormal findings were detected radiographically.

Diagnosis and Prognosis

Based on the clinical and radiographic examinations, the patient has an American Dental Association (ADA) overall diagnosis of type I gingivitis and an American Academy of Periodontology (AAP) diagnosis of dental plaque–induced gingivitis. In addition, the patient is diagnosed with an aberrant maxillary labial frenal attachment between teeth #8 and #9.

Treatment Plan

The following treatment plan and treatment sequence were discussed with the patient.

- Diagnostic phase: comprehensive periodontal examination, radiographic examination, study casts
- Disease control phase: oral hygiene instruction, adult prophylaxis
- Surgical phase: maxillary labial frenectomy
- Reevaluation phase: follow-up on healing of frenectomy
- Orthodontic treatment phase: closure of diastema

Treatment

After the disease control phase has been completed and the patient's oral hygiene has been optimized, a maxillary frenectomy was performed (Figure 3 provides detailed description of frenectomy). Once local anesthesia was obtained, a single interrupted suture was made at the base of the frenum in the vestibule. A horizontal incision to bone was then made just coronal to the suturing line to detach the frenum from the vestibule. Using a sharp 15C blade, the frenum and all of its underlying muscle fibers were then

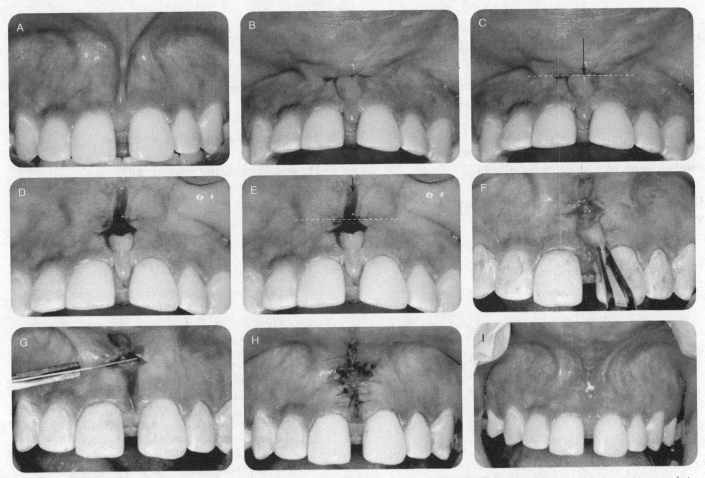

Figure 3: Maxillary labial frenectomy. (A) Preoperative presentation. (B) A single interrupted suture was made at the base of the frenum in the vestibule. (C) Note the positions of the two arrow tips (white dotted line represents single interrupted suture). (D) A horizontal incision to bone was made just coronal to the suturing line (i.e., white dotted line). (E) This incision frees the buccal mucosa, which is pulled away from the frenum (note the new position that the black arrow tip is pointing to) while the position of the frenal base remains unchanged. (F) Frenum and all of its underlying muscle fibers were removed. (G) An incision was made at the base of frenum to ensure total detachment of muscle fibers from the frenum. (H) Multiple single interrupted sutures were used to suture alveolar mucosa to the underlying periosteum. (I) Three-week postoperative presentation showed disappearance of maxillary labial frenum. Courtesy of Dr. Daniel Ho.

removed. Multiple single interrupted sutures were then used to suture the alveolar mucosa to the underlying periosteum to prevent recurrence of high frenal attachment. Hemostasis was achieved. Postoperative instructions were given. Chlorhexidine mouthwash and analgesics were prescribed. The patient presented 3-week postoperatively for a follow-up. Clinically, soft tissues healed well with evidence of epithelization, and maxillary labial frenum had completely disappeared.

Discussion

The presence of abnormal maxillary labial frenal attachments often hinders the orthodontist from

closing midline diastema for the patients. Even if diastema can be closed in these situations, patients often observe a relapse after orthodontic treatment [1]. Not only does frenectomy done prior to diastema closure allows orthodontists to easily close the gap, frenectomy helps prevent orthodontic relapse. Depending on the size of diastema and the extent of the frenal attachment, frenectomy can be done either at the start of the comprehensive orthodontic treatment or in the later phase of the treatment just prior to the need for closure. A period of 2–3 weeks is required for the soft tissue to heal after frenectomy before the orthodontist can start moving teeth again.

Self-Study Questions

A. What is a frenum and what are the complications associated with abnormal frenal attachment?

B. What is the vestibule and what are the clinical implications of a shallow vestibule?

C. What is meant by frenectomy, fiberotomy, and vestibuloplasty?

D. What other tools can be used to perform frenectomy?

E. How is vestibuloplasty performed?

F. How is fiberotomy performed?

Answers located at the end of the chapter.

ACKNOWLEDGMENTS
We would like to thank Dr. Maria Dona for providing Figure 5.

References

1. Edwards JG. The diastema, the frenum, the frenectomy: a clinical study. Am J Orthod 1977;71:489–508.
2. Fletcher SG, Meldrum JR. Lingual function and relative length of the lingual frenulum. J Speech Hear Res 1968;11:382–390.
3. Ballard JL, Auer CE, et al. Ankyloglossia: assessment, incidence, and effect of frenuloplasty on the breastfeeding dyad. Pediatrics 2002;110:63–69.
4. Mason C, Hopper C The use of CO_2 laser in the treatment of gingival fibromatosis: a case report. Int J Paediatr Dent 1994;4:105–109.
5. Morosolli AR, Veeck EB, et al. Healing process after surgical treatment with scalpel, electrocautery and laser radiation: histomorphologic and histomorphometric analysis. Lasers Med Sci 2010;25:93–100.
6. Haytac MC, Ozcelik O. Evaluation of patient perceptions after frenectomy operations: a comparison of carbon dioxide laser and scalpel techniques. J Periodontol 2006;77:1815–1819.
7. Shetty K, Trajtenberg C, et al. Maxillary frenectomy using a carbon dioxide laser in a pediatric patient: a case report. Gen Dent 2008;56:60–63.
8. Kalkwarf KL, Krejci RF, et al. Histologic evaluation of gingival response to an electrosurgical blade. J Oral Maxillofac Surg 1987;45:671–674.
9. Krejci RF, Kalkwarf KL, et al. Electrosurgery–a biological approach. J Clin Periodontol 1987;14:557–563.
10. Flocken JE. Electrosurgical management of soft tissues and restorative dentistry. Dent Clin North Am 1980;24:247–269.
11. Wade AB. Vestibular deepening by the technique of Edlan and Mejchar. J Periodontal Res 1969;4:300–313.
12. Bohannan HM. Studies in the alteration of vestibular depth. III Vestibular incision. J Periodontol 1963;34:209–215.
13. Edwards JG. A Long term prospective evaluation of the circumferential supracrestal fiberotomy in alleviating orthodontic relapse. Am J Orthod 1988;93:380–387.

TAKE-HOME POINTS

A. The frenum is a fold of tissue that consists predominantly of muscle fibers and is covered externally by oral mucosa. High frenal attachments are implicated in midline diastema formation and gingival recession due to frenal pull (especially in a thin biotype gingival apparatus). A high frenal attachment also acts as a barrier for thorough toothbrushing and other oral hygiene measures, leading to accumulation of plaque followed by gingival inflammation. Moreover, high frenal attachments in edentulous patients may affect denture stability, and hence frenum removal is required to improve the stability and retention of dentures.

In addition, a short lingual frenum may result in ankyloglossia, a congenital tongue anomaly associated with decreased tongue mobility and potential speech disturbance resulting in poor articulation [2]. Patients with ankyloglossia resulting from a short lingual frenum may also have poor feeding ability as well as unfavorable mechanical (e.g., playing wind instruments) and social well-being [3].

All the conditions just mentioned associated with abnormal frenal attachments are indications for frenectomy (Figure 4).

B. The oral cavity is divided anatomically into the oral cavity proper and the vestibule. The narrow area surrounded by the lips on one side and the dentition on the other side is called the vestibule. The area bounded by teeth with palate above and the floor of the mouth and tongue below is called the oral cavity proper.

Adequate vestibular depth aids in proper toothbrushing and allows one to effectively perform various other oral hygiene measures such as the use of interdental brushes. A shallow vestibule prevents proper positioning of toothbrushes. In addition, a shallow vestibule is an important factor that has to be taken into account when procedures affecting the final vestibular depth are planned. In procedures such as coronally positioned flap for root coverage as well as guided bone regeneration procedure where the buccal flap is overstretched, patients with a shallow vestibule may end up losing the whole vestibule after the procedures.

Apart from its implications in oral hygiene and periodontal surgery, shallow vestibules are not prosthetically favorable, especially in edentulous patients receiving complete or partial dentures. The flanges of the denture will not seat properly leading to poor retention of the prosthesis. All these conditions require vestibuloplasty.

C. Frenectomy is the complete surgical removal of abnormal frenal attachment including its band of tissues attaching to the bone. This procedure often involves incisions extending to the palate (in the maxillary anterior region). One of the serious drawbacks of this procedure is the potential loss of papillary height leading to compromised aesthetics in the maxillary anterior region.

Fiberotomy or supracrestal fiberotomy is a minor surgical procedure performed in teeth that have undergone orthodontic rotational movement. Orthodontically, rotated teeth are more prone for relapse, and this procedure if done appropriately will prevent relapse.

Vestibuloplasty is a procedure performed to restore the relative height of the alveolar ridge by apically positioning the muscle/fiber attachments into the vestibule (as opposed to restoring the absolute height of the alveolar ridge in a guided bone regeneration ridge augmentation technique).

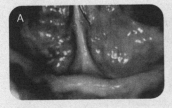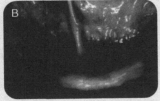

Figure 4: Mandibular lingual frenectomy. (A) Preoperative presentation; (B) 4-week postoperative presentation.

D. Laser surgery and electrosurgery are other tools that can be used to perform frenectomy apart from using scalpel blades. The major advantages of using laser surgery for intraoral soft tissue procedure are hemostasis, improved visibility of the surgical field, less severe scarring, and less postoperative pain and swelling [4,5]. Some recent studies have reported that frenectomies done with laser are usually more acceptable to patients, especially in the pediatric population [6,7]. The lasers are shown to seal the blood vessels, and with precise control of the depth it is an ideal surgical tool for soft tissue procedures. The major disadvantage associated with laser surgery is the delayed healing. It was shown that wounds created by lasers tend to heal 1–2 weeks later than healing of wounds following conventional techniques [4] (Figure 5).

Electrosurgery uses electric current delivered via a metal instrument to sever the tissues. The heat generated by the electric current allows electrosurgical instruments to denature the tissue cells and to create a thin layer of coagulated tissue [8,9]. The main advantages of using electrosurgery over conventional surgical techniques are hemostatic control with better visibility of the surgical field, minimized bacterial infection at incision site, less postoperative discomfort, less scar formation, reduction of chair time, and increased operative efficiency [10]. However, electrosurgery produces an unpleasant odor and is contraindicated in patients having some types of cardiac pacemaker [10].

E. Vestibuloplasty can be performed using a variety of different techniques [11]. One way is simply to reposition the buccal flap apically by making a partial-thickness horizontal incision either at or slightly coronal to the mucogingival junction. Once the buccal flap is moved to a more apical position, the flap is then secured to this new position by sutures, leaving the underlying tissue coronal to it exposed. A period of 2 weeks is allowed for the tissue to heal. The patient should be informed of discomfort expected after the surgery because some soft tissues are left exposed in oral cavity.

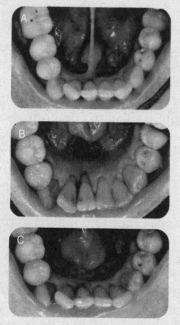

Figure 5: Mandibular lingual frenectomy using carbon dioxide laser surgery. (A) preoperative presentation; (B) during surgery; (C) 2 weeks postoperatively. Courtesy of Dr. Maria Dona.

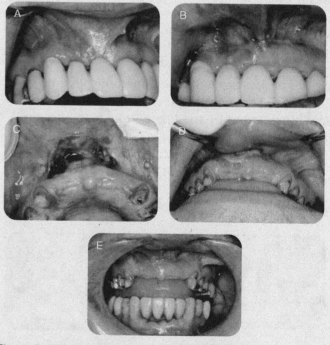

Figure 6: Vestibuloplasty clinical photos taken (A) preoperatively; (B) during surgery; (C) 1-week postoperatively;(D) 2-week postoperatively; and (E) 4-week postoperatively.

The soft tissue healing occurs via secondary intention (Figure 6).

Another way to perform vestibuloplasty is to deepen the vestibule by using gingival grafts. Typically harvested from the palate, the gingival graft is placed in the area where vestibule is to be deepened. Bohannan showed that vestibuloplasty done using gingival grafts has a more predictable long-term result when compared with those done without [12]. An apically repositioned flap in vestibuloplasty done without gingival grafts has the tendency to migrate coronally over time resulting in shallower vestibule.

F. Fiberotomy is performed using a scalpel blade that will be inserted into the sulcus of the teeth, severing the epithelial and connective tissue attachments including gingivodental fibers and transseptal fibers. Fiberotomy is not recommended during active orthodontic tooth movement as well as in the presence of gingival inflammation. Fiberotomy has been shown to be more effective in treating teeth in the maxillary anterior region than teeth in other sextants of the mouth [13]. Fiberotomy is highly successful in mitigating rotational relapses rather than labiolingual relapses [13].

6

Interdisciplinary Treatment

Clinical Cases in Periodontics, First Edition. Nadeem Karimbux.
© 2012 John Wiley & Sons, Inc. Published 2012 by John Wiley & Sons, Inc.

Case 1

Periodontics–Endodontics

CASE STORY

In June 1972, a general dentist referred a 50-year-old Caucasian female to a periodontist because she had periodontal disease. She reported having discomfort and pressure when chewing on her mandibular left molar about 1 month previously, which had lasted for several days. At the time that she presented to the periodontal clinic, the pain and pressure had disappeared (Figures 1 and 2).

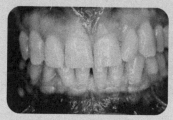

Figure 1: Intraoral picture of maxillary and mandibular teeth in occlusion.

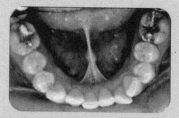

Figure 2: Intraoral occlusal picture of the mandibular teeth.

LEARNING GOALS AND OBJECTIVES

■ To be able to differentiate between a periodontal and endodontic lesion and to generate a differential diagnosis
■ To identify the possible etiology or etiologies for the problem and to perform therapy appropriately.
■ To understand the multifactorial processes of periodontal disease and endodontic disease and their treatment.

Medical History

The patient had some significant medical problems, which included gastric ulcer, minor depression, arthritis, mild functional heart murmur, and history of breast cancer 4 years previously. She had been hospitalized for a mastectomy, a hysterectomy, and a hip fracture. Allergies to Percocet and morphine were reported by the patient.

Medications

- Evista (raloxifene; for osteoporosis prevention)
- Tamoxifen (selective estrogen receptor modulator; for adjunctive therapy of breast cancer)
- Premarin (estrogen; for osteoporosis prevention, postmenopausal symptoms)
- Nexium (esomeprazole; for gastric ulcer risk reduction)

Dental History

About 1 month ago, the patient noticed that one tooth felt "high on the left side when biting my teeth together" and it was painful to masticate. She thought it was due to "my grinding my teeth." The patient said that she brushed her teeth twice a day and used dental floss once a day.

Past Dental History

The patient had maintenance hygiene therapy with her general dentist every 6 months and had a few amalgam restorations placed over the past 45 years.

Social History

The patient had a glass of wine occasionally and did not use tobacco or recreational drugs.

Review of Systems

- **Vital signs**
  - Blood pressure: 104/60 mm Hg
  - Pulse rate: 72 beats/minute (regular)
  - Respiration: 15 breaths/minute
  - Temperature: 37°C

Extraoral Examination

There were no significant findings. The patient had no masses or swelling, and the temporomandibular joint appears to be normal on palpation.

Intraoral Examination

- The patient demonstrated adequate intrasulcular brushing and flossing techniques.
- The soft tissues; lips, buccal mucosa, hard/soft palate, floor of the mouth, and tongue appeared normal in color, shape, texture, and consistency.
- Caries were not found during the clinical evaluation. Some restorations had marginal discrepancies.
- The gingiva displayed very slight marginal redness primarily associated with the lingual of the mandibular posterior teeth with slight bleeding on probing (Figures 1 and 2).
- Slight supra- and no subgingival calculus was seen because the patient had recently had her teeth cleaned 1 month ago. There was slight cervical and interproximal plaque. No gingival recession was found, although there was a slight loss of papillary height between teeth #24 and 25. Probing depths are seen on the chart (Figure 3) and were normal with the exception of a 10-mm facial pocket with bleeding and purulence in the furcation of tooth #19 (Figure 4).
- There was a high frenum attachment between teeth #8 and 9. There were slight exostoses on the facial alveolar ridge of the mandibular anterior teeth. There

was attrition and crowding of the lower anterior teeth, including a pronounced facial-distal rotation of tooth #23 (Figures 1 and 2).
- A pulp test of tooth #19 revealed no response to thermal stimulation and no response to an electrical test.
- The patient was asked to occlude on a bite stick (Tooth Sleuth). No pain was elicited.

Occlusion

Primary occlusal trauma was seen on tooth #19. There was a centric relation prematurity on teeth #14/19 with a 1-mm anterolateral slide to the right. There was a nonworking side contact on teeth 14/19 in the right lateral excursion. There was moderate attrition with the history of bruxism. Fremitus was not present (Figure 1 and 2).

Radiographic Examination

A complete mouth series of parallel technique periapical radiographs (Figures 5, 6, and 7) revealed:
- No evidence of interproximal bone loss
- Restorations with some marginal discrepancies
- Tooth #19 with about 20% bone loss in the furcation and a greater radiolucency than other teeth with furcations
- Periapical radiolucencies associated with tooth #19 on both the mesial and distal roots
- Impacted third molars
- No evidence of caries

Diagnosis

After reviewing the clinical history and performing the clinical-radiographic examination, the diagnoses of this patient were:

Differential Diagnosis for Tooth #19

1. Primary endodontic lesion with periapical radiolucencies
2. Primary periodontal lesion
3. Combined periodontal–endodontic lesion
4. Fractured tooth
5. Periapical cyst or granuloma
6. Buccal bifurcation cyst
7. Metastatic breast carcinoma

Definitive Diagnoses

1. Generalized slight marginal gingivitis
2. Primary endodontic lesion
   a. Necrotic pulp
   b. Presently asymptomatic apical periodontitis #19

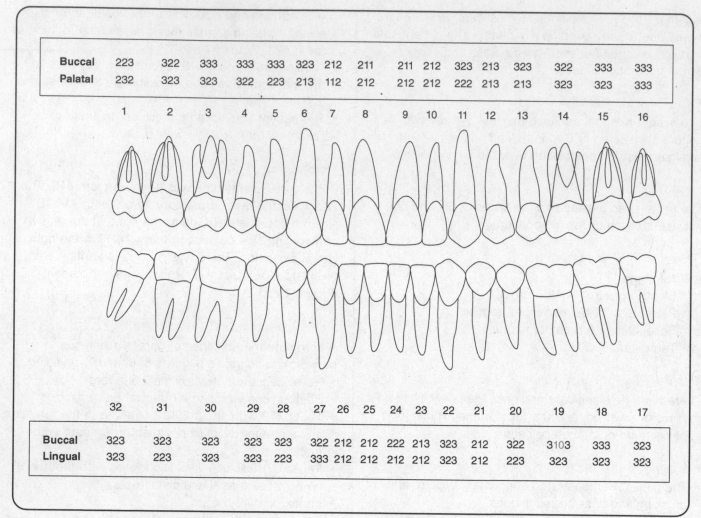

	1	2	3	4	5	6	7	8	9	10	11	12	13	14	15	16
Buccal	223	322	333	333	333	323	212	211	211	212	323	213	323	322	333	333
Palatal	232	323	323	322	223	213	112	212	212	212	222	213	213	323	323	333

	32	31	30	29	28	27	26	25	24	23	22	21	20	19	18	17
Buccal	323	323	323	323	323	322	212	212	222	213	323	212	322	3103	333	323
Lingual	323	223	323	323	223	333	212	212	212	212	323	212	223	323	323	323

Figure 3: Periodontal chart illustrating the full-mouth probing depth measurements.

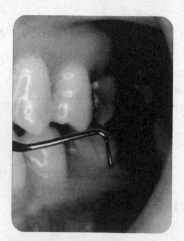

Figure 4: Intraoral picture of maxillary and mandibular posterior left molars in occlusion showing the 10-mm pocket in the furcation of tooth #19.

3. Primary occlusal trauma
4. Defective restorations
5. Impacted third molars

Treatment Plan

Phase 1

- Endodontic evaluation of tooth #19 and treatment as indicated.
- Oral hygiene technique reviewed, scaling (OHI/SCL)
- Oral surgery consultation for extraction of the impacted third molars. Due to the concern of sinus exposure, the patient's age, and the absence of symptoms related with the impacted teeth, the extractions were not performed.
- Occlusal guard maxilla
- Reevaluation of phase 1 therapy.

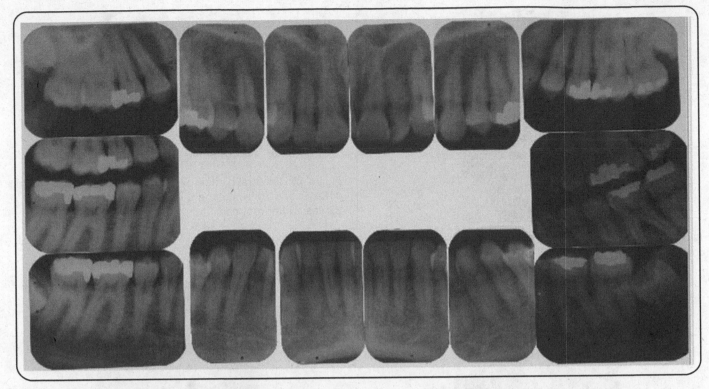

Figure 5: Complete mouth series of radiographs.

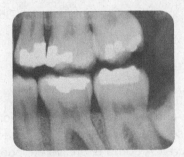

Figure 6: Bite-wing radiographs of the right-side molar region depicting the interproximal bone levels.

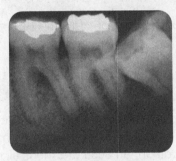

Figure 7: Periapical radiolucency on tooth # 19 with furcation involvement.

Phase 2

- Periodontal surgical therapy for tooth #19 if persistence of facial pocketing
  - Scaling, root planing, and gingival curettage
  - Guided tissue regeneration (if needed)

Phase 3

- Restorative:
  - Contour margins of defective restorations
  - Full crown or onlay #19

Phase 4

- Maintenance therapy (3/4 months of reevaluation)
  - OHI instruction

- Scaling and root planning (if needed)
- Evaluation of endodontic treatment and periodontal conditions

Treatment

The patient received root canal therapy for tooth #19. Three canals were filled with the warm gutta percha technique, and the access cavity was filled with Durelon. Following the root canal treatment, a final cast gold onlay was placed and maintenance hygiene therapy was then performed. The patient was followed for 35 years. A chronologic sequence of the case is presented in Figures 7, 8, 9, 10, and 11.

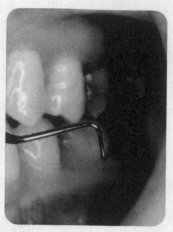

Figure 8: Tooth #19 with a 10 mm pocket in the facial furcation.

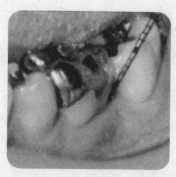

Figure 10: Intraoral picture of the mandibular posterior teeth #18, 19, and 20 illustrating the 2-mm pocket on tooth #19, 32 years after root canal therapy was performed.

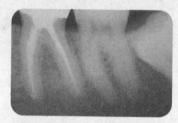

Figure 9: Periapical radiograph of tooth #19 (1-year follow-up).

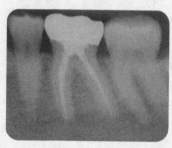

Figure 11: Periapical radiograph of tooth #19 (35-year follow-up).

Discussion

To arrive at a correct diagnosis, the patient's chief complaint and assessment of symptoms must be obtained. In addition, an accurate medical, dental, and social history is necessary. Following that, a comprehensive periodontal and endodontic evaluation needs to be completed. The examinations include an extraoral evaluation to assess the patient's general appearance that may involve the observation of localized skin redness, facial asymmetry, swelling, a sinus tract, tender or enlarged lymph nodes, or tenderness or discomfort upon palpation or movement of the temporomandibular joint. The intraoral examination consists of a visual and digital assessment of the teeth, gingiva, and other oral mucosa to detect areas of discoloration of the soft tissues, inflammation, ulcerations, swelling, and sinus tract formation. The dental examination includes an assessment for color changes, fractures, abrasion, erosion, caries, large restorations or other abnormalities, and clinical tests with the objective to discover the affected tooth or teeth. These clinical tests are periradicular tests (percussion and palpation) and pulp vitality tests (cold, heat, electric, and test cavity) [1]. In addition the Tooth Sleuth was used to help rule out a cracked tooth (vertical fracture). A comprehensive periodontal examination encompasses observing the patient's home care techniques, measurements of probing depth, bleeding, clinical attachment levels, plaque, calculus, gingival recession, furcation involvement, tooth mobility, and mucogingival deformities. Finally, the teeth are inspected for occlusal relationships and restorative needs [2]. In addition to these measurements, radiographs are a necessary adjunct to a thorough periodontal and endodontic examination [1,2].

Four main types of noxious stimuli are common causes of pulpal inflammation (Figures 12–16):
1. Mechanical damage due to dental procedures, attrition (parafunctional habits), abrasion, and barometric changes
2. Thermal injury due to large uninsulated metallic restoration, cavity preparation, polishing, and chemical reaction of dental materials

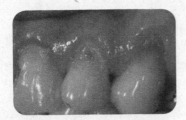

Figure 12: Abrasion.

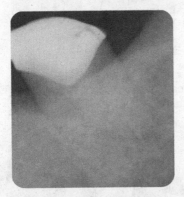

Figure 13: Thermal injury: Large uninsulated metallic restoration.

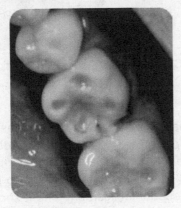

Figure 14: Chemical irritation.

3. Chemical irritation due to erosion or inappropriate use of acidic dental materials
4. Bacterial effects causing damage the pulp through toxins or directly after extension from caries or transportation via the vasculature (anachoresis) [3–5].

Communication between the periodontium and the pulp tissue can occur through many channels or pathways that might be involved in extending pulpal infections (Figures 17–20). They are apical foramina (principal route of communication), lateral and accessory canals, and dentinal tubules [1,6–8]. When

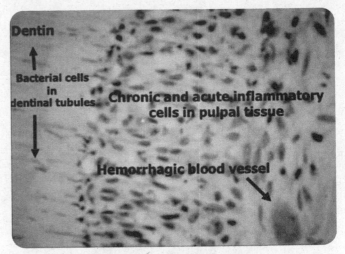

Figure 15: Bacterial effect: Caries. Courtesy of Dr. Victor Ratkus.

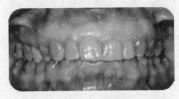

Figure 16: Bruxism (parafunctional habit).

pulp tests indicate necrosis and when a sinus tract can be traced to the lateral portion of a root, a lateral canal might be the cause of a radiolucency in the periodontal ligament (PDL) space or in the furcation [6]. It is estimated that 30–40% of all teeth have lateral canals principally in the apical third of the root. The incidence of lateral canals in the furcations of molars might vary from 23% to 76% [7].

Likewise, other possible pathways have been mentioned in the literature: lingual grooves, root/ fractures, cemental agenesis/hypoplasia, root anomalies, intermediate bifurcation ridges, and trauma-induced root resorption [8] (Figure 21).

Pulpal infection is a polymicrobial process caused mainly by endogenous opportunistic pathogens: *Eubacterium, Peptostreptococcus, Fusobacterium, Porphyromonas, Prevotella, Streptococcus, Lactobacillus, Wolinella, Actinomyces* [5], and *Spirochetes*. Acute exacerbations of chronic periapical infections are frequently associated with *Porphyromonas gingivalis* and *Porphyromonas endodontalis* [6–8]. Other microorganisms like fungus and viruses have being documented in association with endodontic infections [7].

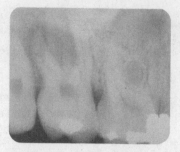

Figure 17: Apical foramen communication.

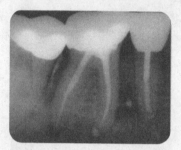

Figure 18: Lateral accessories canal. Courtesy of Dr. Victor Ratkus.

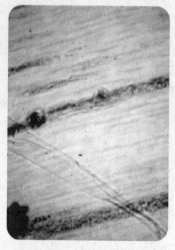

Figure 19: Dentinal tubules. Courtesy of Dr. Victor Ratkus.

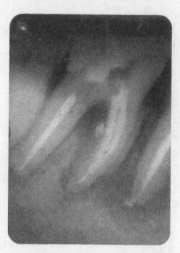

Figure 20: Furcation involvement lateral canal. Courtesy of Dr. Victor Ratkus.

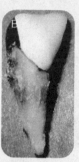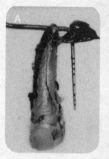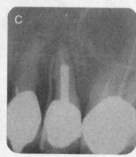

Figure 21: (A–C) Cracked teeth (roots) and vertical fracture.

The pulpal-periodontal lesion is a process that involves the interaction of diseases of the pulp and periodontium. The etiology, diagnosis, and prognosis help to classify these lesions.

- Pulpal lesions: Strictly of pulpal origin but might mimic combined lesions with signs and symptoms and will resolve with root canal treatment alone.
- Periodontal lesions: Strictly of periodontal origin but might also mimic combined lesions with signs especially with symptoms and will resolve with periodontal treatment alone.

- Combined lesions: There are three types: (1) Primary pulpal lesions, (2) primary periodontal lesions, and (3) both pulpal and periodontal lesions. The primary pulpal lesion may extend to the periapical periodontal ligament, and it shows secondary periodontal disease. The primary periodontal lesion affects the pulpal tissue due to bacterial migration through the dentinal tubules into the pulpal tissue (Figure 19). The pulpal and periodontal lesion encompasses both diseases existing independently in both tissues at the same time [1,5–8].

A pulpal lesion or a primary endodontic lesion manifests a necrotic pulp with a chronic apical periodontitis and might have a sinus tract. Usually it is asymptomatic and the suppurative process may drain along the periodontal ligament space and exit at the apical aspect of the sulcus, or it can also perforate the cortical bone close to the apex creating a sinus tract [6] (Figure 22).

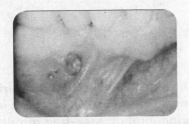

Figure 22: Draining fistula.

Likewise, multirooted teeth might have a sinus tract along the PDL space that can drain into the furcation area, creating bone loss and exiting through the sulcus (pocket) [4]. Clinically in primary pulpal lesions where there is no concomitant periodontitis, periodontal probing is within normal limits throughout the patient's mouth with the exception of the tooth in question. Also, assuming there is no associated generalized periodontal disease, radiographs will show that the osseous destruction involves this one tooth only. If a buccal or lingual swelling appears, a lateral canal should be considered. Confirmation of the diagnosis generally comes from negative pulp vitality readings. The electrical and thermal tests and a test cavity usually reveal no response [6].

The diagnosis of pulpitis might be easily correlated with a diseased tooth; however, many times the origin pulpal pain is difficult to identify. It can be referred from arch to arch on the same side, which necessitates pulp testing several teeth. Disorders such as myofascial pain, trigeminal neuralgia, atypical facial neuralgia, migraine headaches, cluster headaches, nasal or sinus pathoses, angina pectoris, and referred cardiac pain in the mandibular left have been reported

to mimic pulpitis in some patients [3]. Clinical signs and symptoms generally determine the classification of pulpal disease. Numerous investigations have shown a lack of correlation between histopathologic findings and clinical symptoms [3,5]. The percentage of spirochetes seen by darkfield microscopy might be of value in the differential diagnosis of periodontal and endodontic abscesses, with a greater number of spirochetes seen in periodontal abscesses. Coccoid cells dominate in endodontic lesions [8].

Initial treatment consists of root canal therapy, which should be performed with multiple appointments so a reevaluation of the healing process between the completion of root canal debridement and obturation visits can be made. In most of the cases, a sinus tract heals after instrumentation and irrigation of the root canal. The closure of that tract and the elimination of probing depth indicate that the root canal has been completely cleansed. No root planing should be done until the endodontic therapy is completed regardless of the original pocket depth. It is important to preserve the periodontal ligament fibers so reattachment can occur. Healing is usually accomplished within 3–6 months with complete resolution of the pocket. The prognosis is then excellent [6]. The healing of periapical lesions; however, may take up to 4 years (European Society of Endodontology 2006) [9].

When there is not periapical pathology, endodontic therapy has a success rate >96% with both vital and nonvital pulps. However, in cases with pulpal necrosis and periapical radiolucencies, only 86% show apical healing. A much lower success rate of 60% is seen with retreatment of previous root canal therapy [6].

Self-Study Questions

A. List the reasons for the mandibular left first molar feeling painful and why the patient complained of a "high sensation."

B. Why did the symptoms listed in question A disappear?

C. Which intra- and postoperative guidelines should be considered regarding the patient's medication and medical history?

D. In the differential diagnosis, why did we list periapical cyst, buccal bifurcation cyst, and metastatic breast carcinoma?

E. Explain the development of the 10-mm pocket on the facial of the mandibular first molar.

F. What is the significance of a deep periodontal pocket on one surface of a *single* tooth in a generally periodontal disease–free mouth?

G. What are the reasons that this problem is from a primary *endodontic* origin rather due to periodontitis?

H. What should be treated first, the endodontic problem or the periodontal problem, and why?

I. What is the significance of the excellent plaque control and deep pocket in determining the diagnosis?

Answers located at the end of the chapter.

ACKNOWLEDGMENT

We thank Michael A. Kahn, DDS, chairman, Department of Oral and Maxillofacial Pathology, TUSDM, and Kanchan M. Ganda, MD, director, Division of Medicine, TUSDM.

References

1. American Academy of Endodontists, Endodontics. Pulpal/periodontal relationships. Endodontics: Colleagues for Excellence, Spring/Summer 2001.
2. Armitage GC. The complete periodontal examination. Periodontology 2000;34:22–33.
3. Neville BW, Damm DD, et al. Oral and Maxillofacial Pathology. St. Louis, MO: Saunders Elsevier, 2009. Chapter 3 pp120–123, 130–132, 698–700, 669–670.
4. Lindhe J, Lang NP, et al. Clinical Periodontology and Implant Dentistry. Vol. 2. Oxford, UK: Wiley Blackwell, 2008. Chapter 40 pp848–874.
5. Carranza FA, Newman MG, et al, eds. Carranza's Clinical Periodontology. 10th ed. St. Louis, MO: Saunders Elsevier, 2006. Chapter 58 pp871–880.
6. Rose LF, Mealy BL, et al. Periodontics Medicine, Surgery and Implants. Philadelphia, PA: Mosby, 2004. Chapter 30 pp773–788.
7. Rotstein I, Simon JH. The endo-perio lesion: a critical appraisal of the disease condition. Endodontics Topics 2006;13:34–56.
8. Meng HX. Periodontic-endodontic lesions. Ann Periodontol 1999;4:84–89.
9. Walter C, Krastl G, et al. Step-wise treatment of two periodontal-endodontic lesions in a heavy smoker. Int Endodontic J 2008;41:1015–1023.
10. Levi PA, Kim DM, et al. Squamous cell carcinoma presenting as an endodontic-periodontic lesion. J Periodontology 2005;76:10:1798–1804.

TAKE-HOME POINTS

A.

1. The necrosis of the pulpal tissue allows by-products to enter the periapical space causing edema and extrusion of the tooth.
2. Periodontal ligament inflammation was due to primary occlusal trauma.

B.

1. The pressure was relieved by the drainage along the periodontal ligament space and through the sulcus.
2. With the pressure relieved, the occlusal trauma was not exacerbating the inflammation.

C. Highly protein-bound drugs like Xylocaine (lidocaine) and Valium (diazepam) should be used carefully because Evista (raloxifene) is >95% bound to plasma proteins and might affect the protein binding of these drugs. To avoid major interactions, one carpule of lidocaine was used in the case to perform the root canal therapy. Likewise, due to the history of gastric ulcer, aspirin and nonsteroidal anti-inflammatory drugs should be used with caution. These drugs inhibit the cyclooxygenase (COX)-1 that catalyzes the formation of prostaglandins from the arachidonic acid. Its reduction will cause increased gastric acid secretion, diminished bicarbonate secretion, and diminished mucus secretion. Tylenol (acetaminophen) was prescribed to the patient in case of discomfort after therapy.

D. Benign and malignant lesions can give clinical and radiographic findings similar to those described in this case. Cysts can appear as unilocular radiolucencies that are generally well defined, and malignancies can be either well or ill defined. They are usually asymptomatic; however, they can at times be painful and enlarged. They have been reported in the posterior region of the mandible, frequently associated with the molar teeth and close to the root of the tooth at the level of the bifurcation. This is similar to the periapical cyst and the buccal bifurcation cyst. Likewise, two thirds of breast carcinomas spread to bone. The skull is one of the most frequent sites involved.

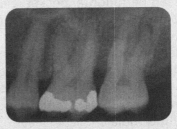

Figure 23: Radiographic image illustrating an endodontic-periodontal lesion.

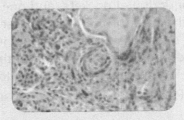

Figure 24: Histopathologic evaluation of an invasive squamous cell carcinoma [10].

However, in the jaw it is rare and has being reported in <1% of cases. In other metastatic cancers, the elderly are more affected, and 80% of reported metastases have occurred in the mandible, which usually appears like a radiolucent defect. Often it is ill defined and may resemble periodontal diseases clinically and radiographically. A definitive diagnosis is made after microscopic studies. This patient's prior breast cancer history must be considered a related factor [3] (Figures 23 and 24).

E. In an acute endodontic lesion, the pressure of the exudative process leads to tissue destruction creating a pathway for drainage (fistulous tract). The drainage in some instances may follow the periodontal ligament space along the root and exit through the sulcus creating a narrow three-walled pocket. Here the draining fistula enters into the furcation area, and the sinus tract can be traced to the apex [4].

F.

1. Periodontal disease with deep pockets is chronic and usually found associated with more than

one tooth in a mouth and commonly on more than one surface of a tooth.

2. A *single* deep periodontal pocket is an important finding that helps to generate a differential diagnosis.

3. A single deep periodontal pocket may be found associated with a tooth with a necrotic pulp, a cracked tooth, or a tooth that has sustained physical trauma such as a tooth proximal to an impacted third molar.

4. Overhanging restorations, open interproximal contacts with food impaction, enamel projections, or enamel pearls can cause deep isolated periodontal pockets, and one should evaluate the area for the findings just described. However, the pockets are usually wider at the coronal portion than if the origin of the inflammation emanated from the pulp through the PDL space.

G.

1. There was a negative pulp vitality test with electrical and thermal testing. The latter has considered the most predictable test to determine an accurate diagnosis.

2. Gingival sulcus probing revealed a single pocket on a single surface of one tooth. Otherwise, the entire mouth was periodontally healthy.

3. The clinical features were developed rapidly with dramatic changes in a short period of time.

4. Completely resolution of the endodontic–periodontal lesion was found after root canal therapy [6].

H. The diagnosis here is a primary endodontic lesion. Thus the conservative approach, treating the endodontic problem first, always should be considered for the initial treatment. Conversely, treating the periodontal problem with scaling and root planing before the endodontic therapy might prevent or lessen the amount of reattachment. Several authors have demonstrated the effectiveness of treating the endodontic problem first to achieve complete pocket reduction and allow for the restitution of a healthy periodontium without additional periodontal therapy [4–6]. In cases of combined periodontal–endodontic lesions, when the deep pocket and furcation involvement remain after endodontic therapy, the residual periodontal defect would then be addressed with resective or regenerative therapy.

I. Gingivitis and periodontitis are common inflammatory diseases strongly associated with poor oral hygiene. Patients with excellent plaque control and localized periodontitis are uncommon. Lesions such as this might occur in cases of localized aggressive periodontitis or due to trauma such as a traumatic extraction, an impacted third molar, or a fractured tooth. It is important to appreciate these concepts during the clinical examination.

Case 2

Periodontics–Prosthodontics

CASE STORY

A 50-year-old Caucasian male presented with a chief compliant of: "I have major dental problems. My previous dentist attempted to restore my bite with crowns and removable partial dentures but couldn't finish because there isn't enough space for the partials" (Figures 1–3). He was currently experiencing no dental pain but had lost faith in the dental profession as a whole. How can you help this frustrated patient reach a satisfactory outcome? What factors should you consider that your colleague overlooked in the previous attempt at diagnosis, treatment planning, and treatment execution?

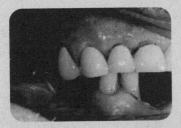

Figure 1: Preoperative right view of centric occlusion.

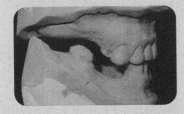

Figure 2: Preoperative photo of articulated diagnostic casts.

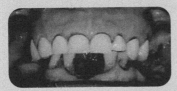

Figure 3: Preoperative frontal view of centric occlusion.

LEARNING GOALS AND OBJECTIVES

- To appreciate the necessity of diagnostic casts and treatment planning
- To evaluate vertical dimension of occlusion (VDO)
- To evaluate interarch space for restorative materials
- To evaluate occlusal planes
- To understand when crown lengthening is indicated for proper tooth preparation (retention and resistance form)
- To understand how periodontal therapy (crown lengthening, alveolectomy) and other methods can be used to create space for restorative materials
- To evaluate tooth form for aesthetics

Medical History

The patient reported a negative review of systems, other than an allergy to penicillin. There were no contraindications to elective dental treatment.

Vital Signs

- Blood pressure: 128/88 mm Hg
- Pulse rate: 84 beats/minute (regular)
- Respiration: 18 breaths/minute

Social History

The patient reported a 25 pack-year smoking history. He currently smoked half a pack of cigarettes per day. There was no reported history of alcohol or substance abuse.

Extraoral Examination

There was no history of temporomandibular joint disorder (TMD) or occlusal orthosis. TMJ examination revealed a normal range of motion with no clicking, crepitus, deviation, deflection, muscle tenderness to palpation, frequent headaches, or history of trauma to the face. The patient was unaware of clenching, bruxism, or other parafunctional habits. There was no lymphadenopathy.

Intraoral Examination

There was a negative oral cancer screen. A small epulis fissuratum was present in the edentulous area of tooth #24 from an ill-fitting interim partial denture.

Hyperkeratosis was present in the posterior mandible on the edentulous ridge crests. A small papule was noted on the left lateral tongue border, which the patient and his former dentist had been monitoring for many years. Multiple 4-mm pseudo-pockets were noted in the periodontal charting. No tooth mobility was present. Fremitus was noted on all anterior teeth. Significant atrophy of alveolar bone in the mandible could be visualized clinically. Tooth #31 had supraerupted (Figures 4–6).

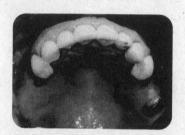

Figure 4: Preoperative occlusal view of maxilla.

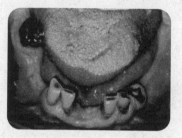

Figure 5: Preoperative occlusal view of mandible.

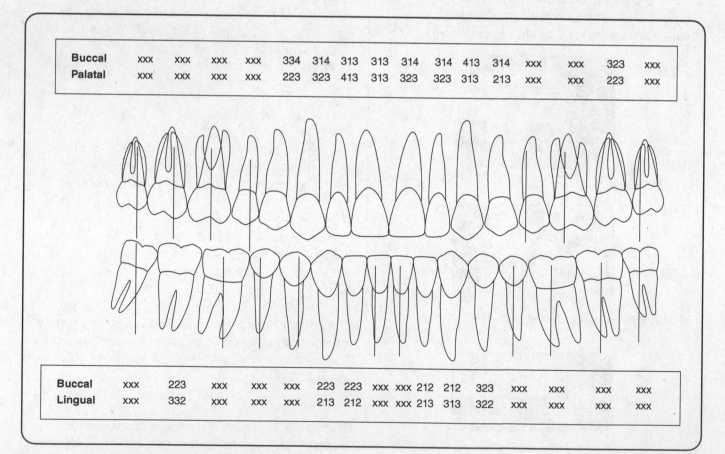

Buccal	xxx	xxx	xxx	xxx	334	314	313	313	314	314	413	314	xxx	xxx	323	xxx
Palatal	xxx	xxx	xxx	xxx	223	323	413	313	323	323	313	213	xxx	xxx	223	xxx

Buccal	xxx	223	xxx	xxx	xxx	223	223	xxx	xxx	212	212	323	xxx	xxx	xxx	xxx
Lingual	xxx	332	xxx	xxx	xxx	213	212	xxx	xxx	213	313	322	xxx	xxx	xxx	xxx

Figure 6: Initial periodontal probing measurements.

Occlusion

There were many noteworthy findings upon occlusal analysis:

- Lack of posterior occlusal contacts
- Fremitus
- Supraeruption of tooth #31 into maxillary dental space
- Loss of VDO
- Vertical maxillary excess

Aesthetics

The patient was dissatisfied with the appearance of his recently finished crowns, specifically how short and wide they appeared. The patient reported that his maxillary anterior teeth had begun to develop spacing as his bite began to collapse prior to initiating treatment. He displayed 100% of the maxillary teeth and 3 mm of gingival tissues upon maximal smiling.

Radiographic Examination

The series revealed multiple endodontically-treated teeth (Figure 7). There were favorable crown-to-root ratios on most teeth, with the exception of teeth #23 and #26, which exhibited mesial bone loss but had

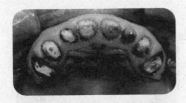

Figure 8: Occlusal view of maxillary teeth upon removal of crowns. Note short clinical crowns, caries, and high degree of total occlusal convergence.

good bony support on the distal aspect. Both of these teeth displayed widened periodontal ligament (PDL) spaces and fremitus. There was no tooth mobility. Both maxillary sinuses were pneumatized and would require elevation with bone grafting for implant placement. Significant alveolar atrophy was present in the mandibular edentulous areas.

Problem List

- Poor oral hygiene
- Smoking habit
- Gingivitis with associated pseudo-pocketing
- Fremitus
- Widened PDL spaces
- Advanced alveolar atrophy in edentulous spaces
- Loss of VDO associated with bite collapse
- Lack of posterior support
- Lack of interarch space secondary to supraeruption of tooth #31 dentoalveolar complex
- Unsatisfactory aesthetics
- Vertical maxillary excess
- Significant caries

Treatment Planning and Sequence Overview

- **Diagnostics**
  - History, examination, radiographs, clinical photographs, properly articulated diagnostic casts, diagnostic wax-up
  - Computed tomography (CT) scan with radiographic template based on wax-up
  - Present treatment options and make financial arrangements
- **Rase 1** (Figure 8)
  - Prophylaxis with localized scaling and root planing

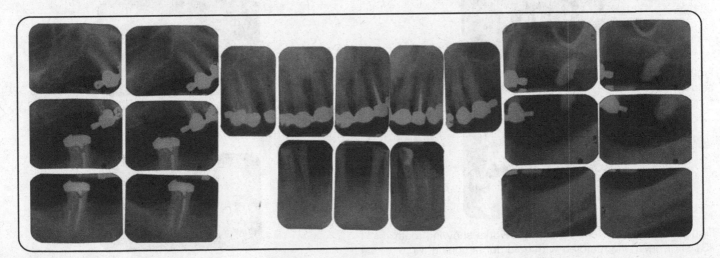

Figure 7: Preoperative full-mouth series radiographs.

- 6-week reevaluation of periodontal status and hygiene compliance
- Smoking cessation program initiated
  - ○ Aggressive caries control
    - Prepare teeth and place provisional restorations
    - Reevaluate abutment prognosis
    - Evaluate patient tolerance of restored VDO
    - Evaluate phonetics and aesthetics
    - Prescription fluoride toothpaste
- **Rase 2**
  - ○ Surgical treatment
    - Crown lengthening of all maxillary teeth to improve resistance and retention form, aesthetics, occlusal plane, interarch space, and correct total occlusal convergence (Figure 9)
  - ○ Surgical template provided by prosthodontist that follows diagnostic wax-up
- **Rase 3**
  - ○ Prosthetic rehabilitation (Figures 10–15)
- **Maintenance**
  - ○ Regular prophylaxis and periodontal reevaluation
  - ○ Regular reevaluation of removable partial denture stability with appropriate reline procedures
  - ○ Occlusal orthosis
  - ○ Fluoride trays

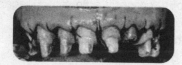

Figure 9: Maxillary teeth immediately following crown lengthening.

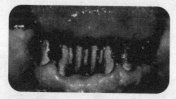

Figure 10: Clinical view of gold dome coping at time of solder relation.

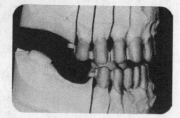

Figure 11: Right view of metal frameworks showing tooth #31 shortened and restored with gold dome coping. Note ERA attachments.

Discussion

It is not uncommon for specialists to encounter clinical situations similar to this case. In most instances, the common cause for a failure of this magnitude is inadequate treatment planning. Understanding basic principles of dentistry is essential to formulating a comprehensive problem list and treatment plan. Architects draft blueprints and assemble models before beginning any project. The same planning and attention to detail in dentistry will greatly improve the quality of dentistry in your practice and its predictability [1]. It is the responsibility of each practitioner to respect the limitations of his or her knowledge and clinical experience and refer cases to specialists when appropriate.

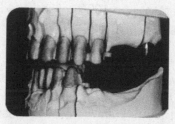

Figure 12: Left view of metal frameworks showing gold dome coping on tooth #15 for additional posterior support.

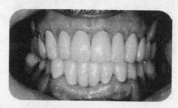

Figure 13: Facial postoperative view.

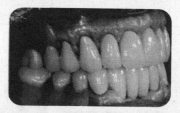

Figure 14: Right postoperative view.

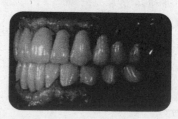

Figure 15: Left postoperative view.

Self-Study Questions

A. What information is essential when planning a complex dental treatment?

B. What steps should be performed before proceeding to definitive restorations?

C. What risks does one assume when finishing one arch of a dental rehabilitation without first placing provisional restorations in both arches?

D. Which clinical situations may require a clinician to perform crown lengthening in the course of a prosthetic treatment?

E. Other than crown lengthening, which procedures are available to create additional interarch space for restorative materials?

Answers located at the end of the chapter.

ACKNOWLEDGMENT
The presented case was completed by students in the Teaching Practice at the Harvard School of Dental Medicine, Boston, Massachusetts.

References

1. Beck CM Kaiser DA, et al. Evolution of removable partial denture design. J Prosthodont 1994;3:158–166.
2. De Van MM. The nature of the partial denture foundation: suggestions for its preservation. J Prosthet Dent 1952;2:210–218.
3. Rudd K. Making diagnostic cast is not a waste of time. J Prosthet Dent 1968;20:93–100.
4. Morgan DW, Comella MC, et al. A diagnostic wax-up technique. J Prosthet Dent 1975;33:169–177.
5. Balshi TJ, Mingledorff EB, et al. Restorative occlusion utilizing a custom incisal guide table ?J Prosthet Dent 1976;36:468–471.
6. Gargiulo A, Krajewski J, et al. Defining biologic width in crown lengthening. CDS Rev 1995;88:20–3.
7. Kois JC. The restorative-periodontal interface: biological parameters. Periodontol 2000. 1996;11:29–38.
8. Libman WJ, Nicholls JI. Load fatigue of teeth restored with cast posts and cores and complete crowns. Int J Prosthodont 1995;8:155–161.
9. Turrell AJW. Clinical assessment of vertical dimension. J Prosthet Dent 1972;28:238–246.
10. Lytle RB. Vertical dimension of occlusion by the patient's neuromusculature. J Prosthet Dent 1976;14:12.
11. Silverman MM. Accurate measurement of vertical dimension by phonetics and the speaking centric space. Dent Dig 1951;57:261–265.
12. Ismail Y, Arthur G. The consistency of the swallowing technique in determining occlusal vertical dimension in edentulous patients. J Prosthet Dent 1968;19:230.
13. Sheppard IM, Sheppard SM. Vertical dimension measurements. J Prosthet Dent 1975;34:269.
14. Wagner A. Comparison of four methods to determine rest position of the mandible. J Prosthet Dent 1971;25:506.
15. McGee G. Use of facial measurements in determining vertical dimension. JADA 1947;35:342.
16. Silverman SI. Vertical dimension record: a three dimensional phenomenon. Part I. J Prosthet Dent 1985;53:420–425.
17. Boos RH. Intermaxillary relation established by biting power. JADA 1940;27:1192.
18. Pound E. Controlling anomalies of vertical dimension and speech. J Prosthet Dent 1976;36:124.
19. Lord JL. The overdenture – patient selection, use of copings and follow-up evaluation. J Prosthet Dent 1974;32:41.
20. Morrow RM, et al. Tooth-supported complete dentures: an approach to preventive prosthodontics. J Prosthet Dent 1969;21:513–522.
21. Brewer A, Morrow R. Overdentures. St. Louis, MO: Mosby, 1975.
22. Crum RJ, Rooney GE Jr. Alveolar bone loss in overdentures: a five year study. J Prosthet Dent 1978;40:486..
23. Holmes JB. Influence of impression procedures and occlusal loading on partial denture movement. J Prosthet Dent 1965;15:474–481.
24. Leupold RJ, Kratochvil FJ. An altered cast procedure to improve tissue support for removable partial dentures. J Prosthet Dent 1965;15:672–678.
25. Leupold RJ. A comparative study of impression procedures for distal extension removable partial dentures. J Prosthet Dent 1966;16:708–720.

TAKE-HOME POINTS

A. Before any treatment begins, a thorough diagnosis must be established. This involves a comprehensive medical history, history of past dental treatment and conditions, eliciting a chief complaint, extraoral examination, oral cancer screen, periodontal examination [2], clinical dental examination with appropriate testing of pulp status, radiographic examination including full-mouth series radiographs (and panoramic radiograph and/or CT scan when appropriate), diagnostic photographs, diagnostic casts [3], diagnostic wax-up [4], and referrals to other specialists.

Prior to considering crown lengthening procedures it is essential that the practitioner assess radiologically the root length, width, and root pathology. Furthermore, soft tissue examination should include confirming the presence of adequate keratinized tissue and smile line analysis to avoid visible poor gingival contours that may result.

Once a list of diagnoses is established, a problem list is generated. This will aid in contingency planning. All possible contingencies must be anticipated. In the event that the chosen plan cannot be achieved, a smooth transition into the best possible outcome can be achieved. Your problem list will help you formulate treatment plans with the most predictable outcomes.

Always formulate an ideal treatment plan. This plan should propose the best possible outcome available within the anatomic limitations of the patient and current dental technology. Many patients cannot choose this plan because of a financial or health constraints. This ideal plan will serve as a reference for a number of secondary plans, one of which may better suit the individual goals of the patient. Once the patient is informed of all foreseeable risks and benefits, a financial arrangement is made and treatment can begin.

B. A diagnostic wax-up is a critical step in planning any complex treatment. This allows direct visualization of ideal conditions within the patient's anatomic constraints.

When the above patient presented to the clinic, it was apparent that the maxillary arch had been addressed before much attention was given to the mandible. Moving to phase 3 treatment in one arch before completing phase 1 in another is not advised, particularly in a case of this complexity. This resulted in a situation that could not be corrected without removing the definitive crowns. If provisional restorations had been placed in both arches with interim removable partial dentures, it would have been recognized that the treatment plan was in need of revision while still in phase 1. This would have saved both the dentist and the patient a considerable amount of time, expense, and frustration.

If the VDO is to be reestablished, provisional restorations allow an opportunity to ensure the proposed VDO is physiologic and tolerated by the patient. Once the clinician and the patient agree that the provisional restorations are appropriate, their form should be captured in an impression and used as a guide for the definitive restorations. Creating a custom anterior guide table on the articulator ensures that the functional guidance of the provisional restorations will be duplicated in the definitive prostheses [5].

C. When addressing a dental rehabilitation, it is sometimes advantageous to finish in segments, either for financial feasibility, for biologic reasons, or simply for the ease of the clinician. However, it can be risky to finish one segment of an extensive treatment without first placing provisional restorations on all teeth involved in the rehabilitation. One may encounter problems with aesthetics, phonetics, function, restorative space, tooth position, or a large host of other conditions that may make it difficult or impossible to finish as envisioned during the planning phase. As demonstrated in this case, an oversight like this can have devastating consequences for the patient and your practice.

D.

- **Invasion of the biologic width (BW):** If the finish line of the tooth preparation encroaches on the periodontal attachment apparatus, osseous recontouring will be required for proper soft tissue healing. Gargiulo et al determined that the biologic width included 1 mm connective tissue, 1 mm junctional epithelium, and 1 mm gingival sulcus, which then equals 3 mm from the crest to crown margin [6]. If there is a violation of the BW on the facial or lingual surface and the alveolar bone is thin, bone resorption and gingival recession develops, ultimately ending up with aesthetic problems. If violation of the BW occurs in the interproximal region (where the bone is thick), bone resorption eventually develops leading to chronically inflamed gingival tissue [7].
- **Short clinical crown:** When tooth preparation provides adequate reduction for restorative materials, there may be insufficient coronal tooth structure above the gingival crest for adequate retention and resistance form. If tooth modifications cannot compensate for these shortcomings, crown lengthening will provide additional supragingival tooth structure to fulfill restorative needs.
- **Lack of ferrule:** If ≤1.5 mm of natural tooth structure exists supragingivally, crown lengthening provides additional natural tooth structure for retention of crowns [8]. This can be supplemented by artificial tooth structure, such as a core buildup or post and core. If one forgoes this procedure, the probability of the artificial buildup material dislodging increases significantly.
- **Lack of interarch space:** If an unopposed tooth is allowed to supraerupt for a significant period of time, it can migrate to a position that makes it difficult to restore the missing tooth in its proper position. The supraerupted tooth may require crown lengthening and/or endodontic therapy to bring it back into the correct occlusal plane. This procedure can also be accomplished with orthodontic intrusion, which has been greatly facilitated in recent years with the advent of temporary anchorage devices.
- **Aesthetic considerations:** In many situations, patients may find their tooth proportions or uneven gingival margins unattractive. In these cases, an elective procedure known as aesthetic crown lengthening can be performed to provide an ideal gingival architecture. If the discrepancy is minor, this can often be done as gingivoplasty, which does not require osseous recontouring.

E. Other than crown lengthening, which procedures are available to create additional interarch space for restorative materials?

- **Orthodontic intrusion:** In most instances, an orthodontist can provide the least invasive answer to discrepancies in occlusion. Patients often decline this option because of the additional expense, the lengthy treatment time of orthodontics, or anxiety related to wearing braces as an adult. However, if this is the best option, it is our duty to educate the patient and guide him or her to the best long-term decision.
- **Alveoloplasty:** If an opposing arch is edentulous and has an abundance of alveolar bone and/or soft tissue, this tissue can be surgically recontoured to create space for restorative materials. This is frequently done in the posterior maxilla as tuberosity reduction surgery.
- **Alteration of VDO:** If other methods will not create adequate restorative space, or it is apparent that VDO has been lost over time [6–15], reestablishing VDO to an appropriate position is a very effective method for creating interarch space. This procedure should be used judiciously because it can result in catastrophe if not done within physiologic tolerance. If the freeway space is violated, a new clinical challenge will rapidly emerge because the patient will not tolerate the change. Functional, aesthetic, phonetic, and/or TMD complications may arise.
- **Extraction of supraerupted teeth with simultaneous alveoloplasty:** If an unopposed tooth is supraerupted so far out of its natural position, it may not be possible to salvage it as part of the global treatment plan. In these situations, the offending teeth are extracted and, using a surgical guide, the alveolus is recontoured to a position that will optimize implant position or removable prosthesis design. This requires careful

planning, particularly in the case of implants, where three-dimensional position is so critical to success.

- **Reduction of endodontically treated teeth:** As demonstrated in this case, a tooth can be shortened to accommodate the occlusal plane. This tooth may not function in full capacity, but it may provide vertical support with a dome coping [16,17], retention with an attachment or telescopic coping [18], or simply serve to retain bone if reduced subgingivally. These teeth can be extracted at a later date when implant placement

is planned. Planning in this capacity can help avoid bone grafting and/or sinus elevation procedures [19].

By adding support under a distal extension removable partial denture, the functional Kennedy classification of the prosthesis can be modified. Both prostheses presented earlier are considered Kennedy class II, modification I removable partial overdentures. Altered cast impressions should be made on distal extension prostheses to allow fabrication of prostheses with the most physiologic soft tissue support [20–25].

Case 3

Periodontics–Orthodontics

CASE STORY

A 14-year, 9-month-old Caucasian female presented with a chief complaint of: "I have a tooth that is rotated 180 degrees." A quick intraoral examination revealed that her maxillary left lateral incisor was severely rotated, there was spacing in the maxillary anterior segment, and both the maxillary canines were unerupted. Following the clinical examination, an appointment had been scheduled to obtain more diagnostic records including orthodontic study casts, intra- and extraoral photographs, lateral cephalogram, panoramic radiograph, and a full-mouth radiographic series to aid in treatment planning.

LEARNING GOALS AND OBJECTIVES

- To become familiar with the epidemiology and etiology of palatally displaced canines
- To know the various surgical techniques to expose palatally displaced canines
- To understand the sequencing (periodontics and orthodontics) of treating palatally displaced canines

Medical History

The patient reported no significant medical history. The patient reported no known allergies to food or drugs.

Review of Systems

- Vital signs
  - Blood pressure: 110/70 mm Hg
  - Pulse rate: 62 beats/minute (normal)
  - Respiration: 14 breaths/minute

Dental History

The patient reported that she underwent cleanings every 6 months and had been to a dentist's office for periodic scaling 3 months ago. She was currently free of caries. She had a Herbst appliance for 1 month 2 years ago.

Family History

The patient's father had a similar malocclusion. Her mother also had malocclusion and had undergone orthodontic treatment as an adolescent.

Social History

The patient reported no use of tobacco, alcohol, or recreational drugs.

Growth and Development

- The patient's height was 5 feet 7 inches (had menarche at the age of 12 years)
- Father's height was 6 feet 3 inches
- Mother's height was 5 feet 5 inches

Extraoral Examination

Extraoral examination revealed no significant pathologic findings. The patient had a round, grossly symmetric face with thin competent lips. There was no tenderness in the temporomandibular joint or of the facial muscles. There were no masses or swellings. Range of motion of the mandible was within the normal range. The centric occlusion and maximum intercuspal position were coincident. On smiling, she showed 100% of her maxillary incisors, 80% of mandibular incisors, and 2 mm of maxillary gingiva. She had a mildly convex profile, slightly retruded mandibular lip, deep mentolabial sulcus, and reduced lower facial height.

Intraoral Examination (Figures 1–5)

- Negative to oral cancer screening
- Tongue, floor of mouth, and buccal mucosa were within normal limits

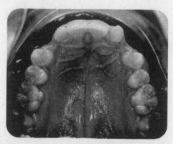
Figure 1: Maxillary occlusal view.

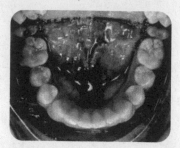
Figure 2: Mandibular occlusal view.

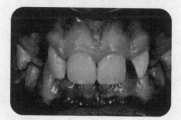
Figure 3: Intraoral frontal view.

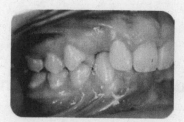
Figure 4: Intraoral right buccal view.

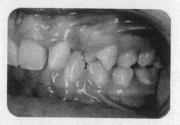
Figure 5: Intraoral left buccal view.

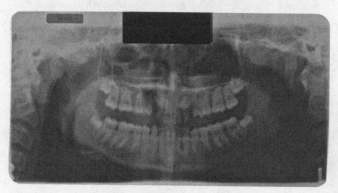
Figure 6: Panoramic radiograph.

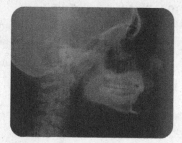
Figure 7: Lateral cephalogram.

- Enamel opacities were present in teeth #8 and 9
- Unerupted teeth #6 and 11
- Occlusion:
  - Overjet is 3 mm
  - Overbite is 6 mm (90% overlap of mandibular incisors)
  - Rotated teeth #5, 10, and 12
  - Coincident dental midlines
  - Class II molar relationship (third/fourth cusp on both sides)
  - Curve of Spee on both right and left sides was 4 mm
  - Palatally displaced canines in maxillary arch
  - Presence of torus palatinus in maxillary arch
- Periodontal examination:
  - Gingival color: Localized erythema
  - Gingival contour: Generalized scalloped
  - Consistency: Generalized firm, stippling present
  - Plaque and calculus: Generalized mild supragingival and subgingival plaque
  - Table 1 shows the periodontal chart.

Radiographic Examination

Panoramic radiograph (Figure 6), lateral cephalogram (Figure 7), and a full-mouth series were requested.
  Summary of findings from panoramic radiograph:
- Bone level was within normal limits
- Palatally displaced canines in maxillary arch
- There was no resorption of roots of teeth #7, 8, 9, and 10
- There was a slight anterior flattening of left condyle

Table 1: Periodontal Charting

Tooth #	1	2	3	4	5	6	7	8	9	10	11	12	13	14	15	16
Facial probing	X	213	222	323	222	X	312	212	212	222	X	312	211	222	312	X
Lingual probing	X	212	212	212	212	X	212	213	222	211	X	213	322	222	212	X
Attached gingival	X	5	3.5	3	1.5	X	4	4	4	3	X	1.5	4	3.5	4	X
Recession	X	0	0	0	0	X	0	0	0	0	X	0	0	0	0	X
Mobility	X	0	0	0	0	X	0	0	0	0	X	0	0	0	0	X

Tooth #	32	31	30	29	28	27	26	25	24	23	22	21	20	19	18	17
Facial probing	X	323	323	312	212	213	212	212	212	212	212	212	312	222	314	X
Lingual probing	X	323	323	323	312	212	212	212	212	212	212	222	323	323	323	X
Attached gingival	X	2	2	2.5	2	2	3	3	2.5	2.5	1.5	1.5	1.5	2	2	X
Recession	X	0	0	0	0	0	0	0	0	0	0	0	0	0	0	X
Mobility	X	0	0	0	0	1	1	1	1	1	0	0	0	0	0	X

- Third molars in maxillary and mandibular arches were developing
  Summary of lateral cephalogram findings:
- Mild skeletal class II pattern
- Hypodivergent mandible
- Retruded mandible
- Retroclined maxillary incisors

Diagnosis

Class II, division 2 malocclusion with palatally displaced maxillary canines.

Treatment Plan

Comprehensive orthodontic treatment plan with extractions of teeth #5 and 12 and surgical exposure of teeth #6 and 11.
    Treatment objectives:
- Erupt palatally displaced canines and achieve healthy periodontium around them
- Establish mutually protected occlusion
- Achieve class I canine and class II molar occlusion
- Resolve deep bite
- Align teeth
    The treatment was phased as follows:
- Phase 1
  - Oral hygiene instructions
  - Prophylaxis
  - Reevaluation
- Phase 2
  - Initiate orthodontic treatment
  - Maxillary canines exposure
  - Extraction of teeth #5 and 12

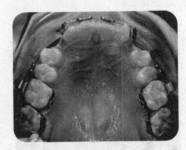

Figure 8: Start of orthodontic treatment.

- Phase 3
  - Complete orthodontic treatment
  - Retention
- Phase 4
  - Periodontal and oral hygiene maintenance

Treatment

The relative advantages and disadvantages of the various treatment plans were discussed. The patient opted for comprehensive orthodontic treatment plan with extraction of teeth #5 and 12 and surgical exposure of teeth #6 and 11. Following informed consent from the patient, the first phase of treatment that included oral hygiene instructions and prophylaxis was initiated (Figure 8). Then orthodontic treatment was started. The first step was to place bands on the maxillary first and second molars followed by bonding of all other teeth in the maxillary arch. Nickel titanium wires were used to obtain the initial alignment of teeth (Figure 9).

    Approximately 8 weeks after the banding/bonding of the maxillary arch, the maxillary canines were

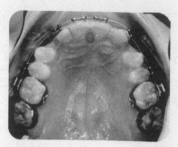

Figure 9: Four weeks later.

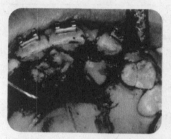
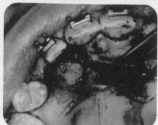

Figure 10: Canine exposure.

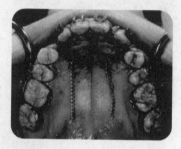

Figure 11: Gold chains attached to exposed canines.

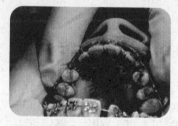

Figure 12: Gold chains ligated to the maxillary arch wires.

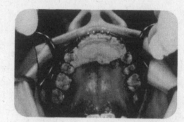

Figure 13: Periodontal pack placed over the exposure.

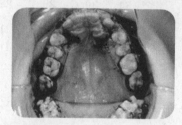

Figure 14: One-week follow-up.

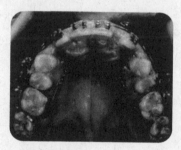

Figure 15: Two-week follow-up.

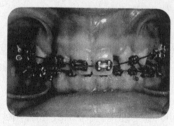

Figure 16: Both maxillary and mandibular arches are bonded.

surgically exposed by the periodontist. In this appointment, buttons were bonded to the exposed canines, and gold chains were attached to these buttons. The free ends of the gold chains were then ligated to the maxillary arch wire. The exposure site was then covered with a periodontal pack (Figures 10–15).

Four weeks after the exposure of maxillary arch canines, the mandibular arch was bonded (Figure 16).

Three weeks after the mandibular arch was bonded, the maxillary first premolars were extracted. Following

the extractions, the patient was seen periodically at 4-week intervals and the maxillary canines were retracted into the premolar extraction space using power chains. The orthodontic treatment mechanics to align and level in the mandibular arches were continued simultaneously. Periodic orthodontic treatment was continued for 16 months, at which point the canines were fully retracted into the extraction space in the maxillary arch (Figure 17).

The next step in orthodontic treatment would be to retract the maxillary anterior segment (lateral incisor to

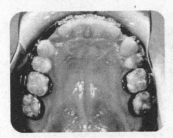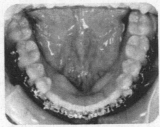

Figure 17: Retraction of palatally displaced canines and occlusal view of mandibular arch.

lateral incisor) to obtain class I canine occlusion and good intercuspation of the buccal occlusion. This would then be followed by finishing and retention phases. Following comprehensive orthodontic treatment, the patient will be debonded and then placed on periodic recall visits to follow up on retention and oral hygiene.

Discussion

In the literature, two main canine exposure techniques are discussed. The first technique is a closed technique where minimal bone removal is done and an attachment is placed on the canines at the time of exposure. Orthodontic treatment usually begins before the exposure, and traction on the canine is started soon after exposure. The advantages with this technique are the conservative bone removal and minimal surgical trauma and some degree of control over the eruption path of the canine. The

disadvantages are the limited visibility of the canine during traction and demanding moisture control during attachment placement.

The second technique involves early uncovering and spontaneous canine eruption [1]. Exposure is done before orthodontic treatment or very early on during treatment. The crown of the unerupted canine is usually fully exposed from bone and left exposed after flap closure. After the canine erupts on its own, orthodontic attachments are placed for alignment. The advantages of this technique include better visibility of the canine and better moisture control at the time of placing orthodontic attachments. The disadvantages are the aggressive bone removal and lack of precise control over the eruption path of the canine. Although it is being debated in the literature, trying to establish which technique is ultimately better is somewhat simplistic. The evidence that exists at the moment is not unequivocal. The prudent clinician realizes there is not necessarily a technique that is better in all cases. Emphasis should be placed on clinical diagnosis and individualized treatment planning. Clinical judgment should always be used to pick the best technique for every patient.

In this patient a closed eruption technique was used for two main reasons. First, precise control over the path of eruption of the canine was desired to avoid injury to the lateral incisors. Second, the orthodontist wanted to verify that the canines are moving before extraction of the first premolars. No bone removal was needed in this case.

Self-Study Questions

A. What is the difference between impacted teeth and displaced teeth?

B. What is the frequency of occurrence of impacted canines?

C. Enumerate the possible etiologies of palatally impacted canines.

D. What are some aids to determine the position of displaced canines?

E. Describe various surgical techniques to expose displaced canines.

F. Discuss the possible side effects of exposing canines and retracting them into the arch.

G. What are some possible consequences of not treating an impacted maxillary canine?

Answers located at the end of the chapter.

References

1. Schmidt AD, Kokich VG. Periodontal response to early uncovering, autonomous eruption, and orthodontic alignment of palatally impacted maxillary canines. Am J Orthod Dentofacial Orthop 2007;131:449–455.
2. Suri L, Gagari E, et al. Delayed tooth eruption: pathogenesis, diagnosis, and treatment. A literature review. Am J Orthod Dentofacial Orthop 2004;126:432–445.
3. Peck S, Peck L, et al. The palatally displaced canine as a dental anomaly of genetic origin. Angle Orthodontist 1994;64:249–256.
4. Becker A. The Orthodontic Treatment of Impacted Teeth. 2nd ed. Abington, UK: Informa Healthcare, 2007. Chapter 6, pp 93–142.
5. Becker A. Etiology of maxillary canine impactions. Am J Orthodontics 1984;37:437–438.
6. Brin I, Solomon Y, et al. Trauma as a possible etiologic factor in maxillary canine impaction. Am J Orthod Dentofacial Orthop 1993;104:132–137.
7. Wisth PJ, Nordervall K, et al. Periodontal status of orthodontically treated impacted maxillary canines. Angle Orthodontist 1976;46:69–76.
8. Woloshyn H, Artun J, et al. Pulpal and periodontal reactions to orthodontic alignment of palatally impacted canines. Angle Orthodontist 1994;64:257–264.

TAKE-HOME POINTS

A. Impacted teeth are those that are prevented from erupting due to the presence of a physical barrier in their path of eruption [2]. Displacement refers to positional variation of teeth. Displacement may lead to impaction if corrective measures are not taken [3].

B. Depending on the population studied, prevalence rates of palatally impacted canines range from 0.27% to 3% [2,3]. There is a stronger preponderance toward females compared with males [2,3].

C. A considerable body of evidence suggests an association between palatally displaced canines and the following factors [2–5]:
- Severe tooth size and arch length discrepancy
- Heredity (familial tendency)
- Retained deciduous canines
- Missing or anomalous lateral incisors
- Nonresorption deciduous canine roots
- Trauma

D. Maxillary canines should erupt in the oral cavity around 11–12 years of age. They can be palpated labially over the deciduous canines usually at 8–9 years of age [4]. Nonemergence of maxillary canine beyond 11–12 years of age should warrant further examination using tools such as periapical, occlusal

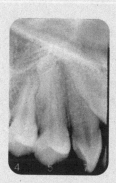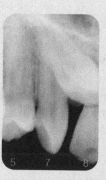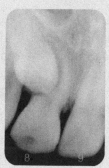

Figure 18: Periapical radiographs showing a displaced right maxillary canine.

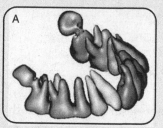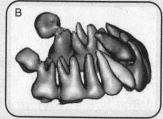

Figure 19: A three-dimensional reconstructed image of the patient's teeth from Figure 18 with and without the canine in view.

radiographs, and panoramic radiographs. Currently cone beam computed tomography is used to accurately determine the position of canines and also to examine any effects of the displaced canines on the adjacent teeth (Figures 18 and 19).

E. *Closed eruption technique* involves partial exposure of the crown, immediate attachment placement, and early application of orthodontic force. *Open eruption technique* involves early uncovering, complete exposure of the clinical crown, and spontaneous eruption. Orthodontic force is applied late, after autonomous eruption.

F. Trauma due to surgery [6]:
- Infections at the exposed sites are common.
- Etching materials used during the bonding procedure may spill over onto the surrounding soft tissues and cause localized reactions.
- Bonding failure of attachments (including buttons and brackets) to the exposed canines.

- Poor biomechanics during orthodontic retraction into the arch may lead to resorption of the roots of adjacent teeth.
- Periodontal health of the retracted canines maybe compromised. Retracted canines have shown to exhibit bone loss and increased pocket depths [7].
- Pulpal changes and discoloration of retracted canines have also been reported in the literature [8].

G. Nontreatment of impacted maxillary canine may lead to several adverse consequences including cystic changes leading to dentigerous cysts, replacement resorption of the crowns of impacted canines, and resorption of roots of adjacent permanent teeth [4].

Case 4

Occlusion–Periodontology

CASE STORY

A 50-year-old Caucasian male presented and stated that he brushed twice a day and flossed occasionally and had never seen a periodontist before. The patient complained of bleeding gums on brushing and bad breath. The patient had been referred from his general dentist's office for a comprehensive periodontal evaluation.

LEARNING GOALS AND OBJECTIVES

■ Diagnose the periodontal condition properly
■ Identify whether there are possible occlusal contributing factors
■ Treat the periodontal condition
■ Manage the occlusal element
■ Determine proper timing of occlusal management

Medical History

There were no significant medical conditions and the patient reported never having been hospitalized. The patient reported taking multivitamins but no other medications, and he had no allergies.

Review of Systems

Vital signs
- Blood pressure: 140/85 mm Hg
- Pulse rate: 75 beat/minute and regular
- Respiration: 15 breaths/minute

Social History

The patient was a nonsmoker and never smoked before. He had a habit of chewing tobacco for 15 years and stopped about 10 years ago. The patient drank socially.

Extraoral Examination

There were no significant negative findings. The patient had no masses or swelling, he had a symmetrical facial appearance, pointy chin, even and rounded shoulder points, and the temporomandibular joints (TMJs) were within normal limits.

Intraoral Examination

The soft tissues and tongue appeared normal (Figure 1). There was an adequate zone of keratinized gingiva, except on tooth #22. There was presence of significant local factors. There was mild gingival recession in relation to maxillary molars.
- A periodontal probing was completed
- The patient had partial edentulism and he was missing #17, 18, and 32.

Radiographic Examination

A full-mouth set of radiographs was ordered with a panoramic radiograph to evaluate the bone level and the temporomandibular joints through the panoramic view. An evaluation of the radiographs revealed that the patient had generalized bone loss with localized moderate to severe bone loss around teeth #1–3, 14–16 (Figure 2).

Occlusion

The patient had occlusal interferences on lateral excursions on both sides. The patient reported that his wife told him he grinds his teeth while sleeping. The patient had bilateral edge-to-edge occlusion on his posterior teeth.

Figure 1: Pretreatment periodontal charting.

Maxillary (teeth 1–16)

Facial

Row	1	2	3	4	5	6	7	8	9	10	11	12	13	14	15	16
P.D.	4 4 4	9 3 5	9 3 4	4 2 3	3 3 5	5 3 5	5 2 4	4 3 5	5 2 4	5 1 5	4 1 5	5 2 6	6 2 5	5 7 9	5 1 5	4 4 4
FGM					2 2 2									2 2 2	4 4 4	
ATTACH	4 4 4	9 3 5	9 3 4	4 2 3	5 5 7	5 3 5	5 2 4	4 3 5	5 2 4	5 1 5	4 1 5	5 2 6	6 2 5	7 9 11	9 5 9	4 4 4
FURCA																
PLAQUE																
Calculus																
MGDEF														2		

Palatal

Row	1	2	3	4	5	6	7	8	9	10	11	12	13	14	15	16
P.D.	4 1 7	7 1 6	8 11 5	4 1 5	5 1 5	5 1 4	5 1 4	3 1 5	5 1 4	4 1 4	5 1 5	5 1 7	7 1 4	4 2 6	7 1 6	6 3 5
FGM			4 4 4											4 4 4 4 4 4		
ATTACH	4 1 7	7 1 6	10 11 9	4 1 5	5 1 5	5 1 4	5 1 4	3 1 5	5 1 4	4 1 4	5 1 5	5 1 7	7 1 4	8 6 10	11 5 10	6 3 5
FURCA																
PLAQUE																
Calculus																
MOBILITY	2	2	2	1	1					1		1		2	2	2

Mandibular (teeth 32–17)

Lingual

Row	32	31	30	29	28	27	26	25	24	23	22	21	20	19	18	17
MOBILITY														2		
Calculus																
PLAQUE																
FURCA		1	1													
ATTACH	3 4 4	5 4 5	4 2 5	5 2 3	3 2 3	4 2 4	3 3 3	3 3 3	3 2 4	4 2 4	4 2 4	4 2 5	6 4 4			
FGM			1 1 1													
P.D.	3 4 4	4 3 4	4 2 5	5 2 3	3 2 3	4 2 4	3 3 3	3 3 3	3 2 4	4 2 4	4 2 4	4 2 5	6 4 4			

Facial

Row	32	31	30	29	28	27	26	25	24	23	22	21	20	19	18	17
MGDEF																
Calculus																
PLAQUE																
FURCA		1														
ATTACH	6 3 7	9 4 6	4 2 4	3 2 4	4 4 6	6 3 9	7 2 9	8 2 5	4 2 5	5 3 5	4 2 4	4 2 4	4 2 3			
FGM			2 2 2													
P.D.	6 3 7	7 2 4	4 2 4	3 2 4	4 4 6	6 3 9	7 2 9	8 2 5	4 2 5	5 3 5	4 2 4	4 2 4	4 2 3			

Figure 1: Pretreatment periodontal charting.

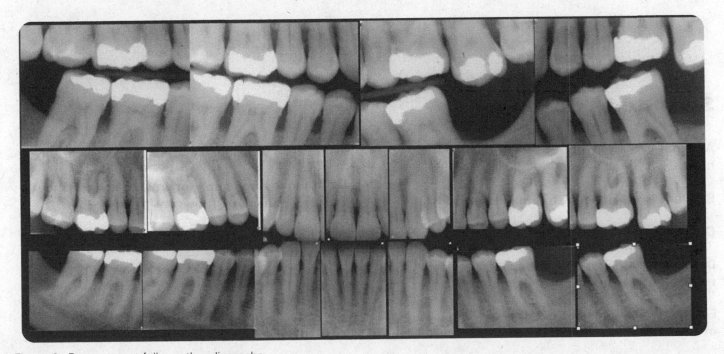

Figure 2: Pretreatment full-mouth radiographs.

Diagnosis

- Generalized plaque-induced gingivitis
- Localized moderate to severe chronic periodontitis on teeth #1–3, 14–16, 19, and 31.

Treatment Plan

- Phase 1: generalized scaling and root planing
- Reevaluation
- Phase 2: open flap debridement and osseous resection
- Occlusal management

Figure 3 shows maxillary and mandibular occlusal views.

Discussion

When the patient presents for periodontal evaluation and diagnosis, occlusion should be examined as a routine part of the periodontal evaluation. If it is determined that occlusion may contribute to the periodontal disease, the periodontist should prepare to deal with the occlusal component as part of the comprehensive periodontal treatment.

To provide guidelines about how occlusal management should be incorporated into the course of treatment, we suggest some questions to be clinically used in the treatment sequence. The role of occlusion in the etiology and progression of periodontitis as an inflammatory disease is still unclear and inconclusive. Studies show conflicting results as to whether occlusal

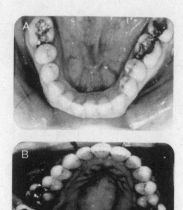

Figure 3: (A, B). Maxillary and mandibular occlusal views.

factors are significant in the process of treatment planning [1–5].

Although most studies indicate that occlusion by itself cannot induce periodontitis, most studies recommend considering occlusal management during the course of periodontal treatment and implantology.

In this case this patient had interferences on excursion and a parafunction habit that might affect the periodontal health and progress of the periodontal disease.

Treatment chosen must address the occlusal component management and its order within the overall treatment plan.

Self-Study Questions

A. What is the role of occlusion in periodontal health?

B. What is the effect of trauma from occlusion?

C. What are the stages of trauma from occlusion?

D. What is the relationship between occlusal trauma and periodontitis (inflammation)?

E. Should management of occlusal trauma be part of periodontal treatment?

F. How can we diagnose trauma from occlusion?

G. At what stage of periodontal treatment should occlusal management be considered?

H. What are the components of a full occlusal examination?

Answers located at the end of the chapter.

References

1. Svanberg G, Lindhe J. Experimental tooth hypermobility in the dog. A methodological study. Odontologisk Reby 1973;24:269–282.
2. Ericsson I, Lindhe J. Lack of effect of trauma from occlusion on the recurrence of experimental periodontitis J Clin Periodontol 1977;4:115–127.
3. Polson AM, Adams RA, et al. Osseous repair in the presence of active tooth hypermobility. J Clin Periodontol 1983;10:370–379.
4. Ericsson I, Lindhe J. Lack of significance of increased tooth mobility in experimental periodontitis. J Periodontol 1984;55:447–452.
5. Lindhe J, Ericsson I. The influence of trauma from occlusion on reduced but healthy periodontal tissues in dogs. J Clin Periodontol 1976;3:110–122.
6. Glossary of terms. J Periodontol 1986;57:20(Suppl 11).
7. Zander HA, Polson AM. Present status of occlusion and occlusal therapy in periodontics. J Periodontol 1977;48:540–544.
8. Savanberg G, Lindhe J. Influence of trauma from occlusion on progression of experimental periodontitis in beagle dogs. J Clin Periodontol 1974;1:3–13.
9. Hallmon WW. Occlusal trauma: effect and impact on the periodontium. Ann Periodontol 1999;4:102–108.
10. Parameter on occlusal traumatism in patients with chronic periodontitis. Parameters of care. J Periodontol 2000;71(Suppl 5):873–875.
11. Lindhe J, Ericsson I. The influence of trauma from occlusion on reduced but healthy periodontal tissues in dogs. J Clin Periodontol 1976;3:110–122.
12. Svanberg G, Lindhe J. Vascular reactions in the periodontal ligament incident to trauma from occlusion. J Clin Periodontol 1974;1:58–69.
13. Ericsson I, Lindhe J. Effect of longstanding jiggling on experimental marginal periodontitis in the beagle dog. J Clin Periodontol 1982;9:497–503.
14. Lobbezoo F. Topical review: new insights into the pathology and diagnosis of disorders of the temporomandibular joint. J Orofac Pain 2004;18:181–191.
15. Simons DC, Travell JG. Myofascial pain and dysfunction. In: The Trigger Point Manual. 2nd ed. Vol 1. Upper Half of the Body. Atlanta, GA: Emory University,1998.
16. Angle EH. Classification of malocclusion. Dental Cosmos 1899;4:248–264.

TAKE-HOME POINTS

A. The periodontal ligament anchors the teeth in the jaw. The occlusion in normal function can maintain the periodontium and stimulate the periodontal ligament. However, when the occlusal force is insufficient, the periodontal ligament atrophies. And if a tooth is taken out of occlusion, the periodontal ligament will completely disappear.

B. The periodontium has a capability to adapt, which allows the periodontal ligament to withstand some increase in occlusal forces. As a result of adaptation, the periodontal ligament may undergo changes such as thickening of the periodontal ligament. In addition there may be increased bone density and trabeculation. Once the forces exceed the adaptation limit, changes can take place in the teeth (wear and tear and/or mobility), the periodontium (PDL and bone) [6–8,12], or in the TMJ (pain, wear).

C. When the occlusal forces exceed the functional level of the periodontal ligament, injury may take place. The damage can be repaired if the excessive forces are eliminated or if the tooth drifts away from the forces. But if excessive occlusal forces persist, the damage may become permanent in the form of the "appearance" of angular bone loss on radiograph. In such a case, the tooth would become loose without pocket formation. If the excessive forces are removed, the defect will tend to heal [9].

D. If there is excessive force without gingival/periodontal inflammation, there may be signs/symptoms that appear, but the bone loss will not proceed at a faster rate (i.e., excessive forces alone do not cause periodontitis). If there is excessive force in the presence of gingival/periodontal inflammation, the loss of bone can occur at a relatively faster rate.

E. Occlusal trauma can alter the periodontium (bone, gingival connective tissue, and PDL). Due to this effect, it is ideal to manage occlusal trauma prior to any definitive periodontal therapy. For example, splinting teeth or delivering an appliance before surgery will reduce the micro-movements that might affect any kind of resective, regenerative, or mucogingival surgeries [7,10].

F. To answer that question, we have first to define occlusal trauma [11].
- *Occlusal trauma:* When the attachment apparatus manifests destruction due to excessive occlusal forces; generally, occlusal trauma can be classified as follows:
  - *Primary occlusal trauma:* Normal attachment apparatus of tooth subjected to occlusal forces that exceed the limits of adaptability (e.g., parafunctions or orthodontics)
  - *Secondary occlusal trauma:* Normal occlusal forces applied to a compromised periodontal apparatus
  - *Combined occlusal traumas:* The combination of primary and secondary occlusal traumas
- *Traumatogenic occlusion:* Any occlusion that produces what may lead to injuries of the periodontal apparatus
- *Occlusal traumatism:* Process by which destruction may take place

Several clinical/radiographic signs and symptoms can be present to help diagnose trauma from occlusion.
- Clinical:
  - Mobility (progressive)
  - Pain on chewing or percussion
  - Fremitus
  - Occlusal prematurities/discrepancies
  - Wear facets in the presence of other clinical indicators
  - Tooth migration
  - Chipped or fractured tooth (teeth)
  - Thermal sensitivity
- Radiographic:
  - Widened PDL space
  - Bone loss
  - Root resorption

G.
- Because immobile teeth respond better to treatment, teeth fixation should be considered before treatment

- Occlusal management alone does not produce regeneration or reattachment
- Decreased mobility would improve periodontal treatment outcomes
- Increased mobility does not influence the rate of disease progression
- Occlusal management after treatment would help to ensure long-term improvement
- Appliance therapy could be incorporated as a modality for periodontal management [13]

H. TMJ pain and symptoms may need to be checked by more than one medical specialist, such as a primary care provider, a dentist, or an ear, nose, and throat doctor, depending on symptoms. Some dentists specialize in TMJ diagnosis and treatment [14,15].

A thorough examination may involve these steps:
- Dental examination to show poor bite alignment
- Magnetic resonance imaging of the jaw area
- Feeling the joint and connecting muscles for tenderness
- Pressing around the head for areas that are sensitive or painful
- Sliding the teeth from side to side
- Watching, feeling, and listening to the jaw open and close
- X-rays to show abnormalities
- Detecting malocclusion using Angle's classification, introduced by Edward Angle in 1899 based on mesiodistal relationship of the teeth, dental arches, and jaws. Maxillary first molar is taken as the key to occlusion:
  - **Class I:** The molar relationship of the occlusion is normal or as described for the maxillary first molar, but the other teeth have problems like spacing, crowding, over- or undereruption, and so on.
  - **Class II** ("overbite"): In this situation, the upper molars are placed not in the mesiobuccal groove but anteriorly to it. Usually the mesiobuccal cusp rests in between the first mandibular molars and second premolars. There are two subtypes:
    - **Class II, division 1:** The molar relationships are like that of class II and the anterior teeth are protruded.

- ■ **Class II, division 2:** The molar relationships are class II but the centrals are retroclined and the lateral teeth are seen overlapping the centrals.
- • **Class III** (prognathism, "underbite," or "negative overjet"): Lower front teeth are more prominent than the upper front teeth. In this case the patient has very often a large mandible or a short maxillary bone [16].

Using appliance therapy will help eliminate occlusal interferences and reduce traumatic occlusion (Figure 4).

In conclusion, excessive and chronic occlusal forces produce adaptive changes in the morphology of periodontium: a widened V-shaped periodontal ligament, a thickening of bone trabeculae, and bone resorption in the gingival portion of the periodontium.

Glickman introduced a terminology called *buttressing bone* that manifests itself in the form of increasing bone trabeculae on the affected area(s).

- • This bone formation occurs both in pressure as well as in tension side and both internally (marrow) or on the external surface (surface).
- • If it occurs externally, it leads to cervical bulge; if it occurs internally, it will not lead to obvious change in the morphology but to an increase in the radio-opacity close to the affected PDL (thickening of the lamina dura).
- • Intrabony pocket formation can occur due to the interaction between bone resorption and bone formation, which is a result of traumatic occlusion (Figure 5).

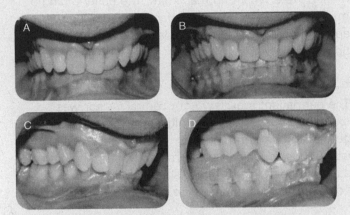

Figure 4: (A–D) Splint therapy can eliminate occlusal interferences.

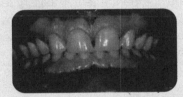

Figure 5: Buttressing bone formation due to parafunction habits.

Case 5

Periodontics–Pediatric Dentistry

CASE STORY

An 11-year-old female was brought to the Emergency Department of Children's Hospital Boston (CHB) in September 2008 for a dental injury. She had fallen off a bicycle and injured her maxillary dentition 4 hours prior and was sent to a local hospital for treatment. Her permanent maxillary right central incisor was extruded and the permanent maxillary left central incisor was avulsed. The emergency physician at the local hospital reimplanted the avulsed tooth immediately. The girl was then transferred to CHB for further evaluation. According to the parent's history, the extraoral dry time was approximately 15 minutes, and the tooth was not transported in any medium.

LEARNING GOALS AND OBJECTIVES

■ To be able to diagnose traumatic dental injuries and consider appropriate immediate acute and long- term dental management of such injuries.

Medical History

The girl's medical history was significant for asthma and attention deficit hyperactivity disorder for which she was taking Ritalin.

Social History

The patient was an only child and her parents were married. Both parents had a history of dental caries.

Extraoral Examination

The temporomandibular joint and mandibular ranges of motion were within normal limits. The patient had no masses or swelling in the orofacial region. Superficial abrasions were noted on the patient's forehead and upper and lower lip.

Intraoral Examination

The permanent maxillary right central incisor was extruded 2 mm and palatally luxated. The reimplanted permanent left central incisor was extruded 4 mm and labially positioned by approximately 1 mm. The gingiva surrounding both central incisors was bleeding; however, no lacerations were present.

Occlusion

There were no occlusal discrepancies or interferences.

Radiographic Examination

The radiographic examination was significant for a well-approximated root fracture in the apical third of the permanent maxillary right central incisor. The permanent left central incisor was extruded by 4 mm. Both central incisors had complete root formation (Figure 1).

Diagnosis

Apical root fracture of the permanent maxillary right central incisor and a partially reimplanted avulsed permanent left central incisor.

Treatment

After administering local anesthesia, the two permanent maxillary central incisors were repositioned and splinted using Ortho-Flex wire (Reliance Orthodontic Products, Inc., Itasca, IL, USA) and light-cured composite resin (Figure 2). Postoperative

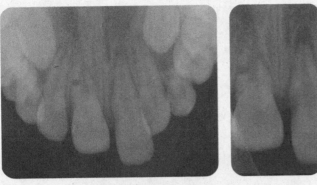

Figure 1: (A) Occlusal radiograph: maxilla; (B) periapical radiograph.

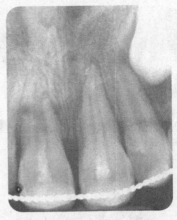

Figure 3: Periapical radiograph after root canal therapy.

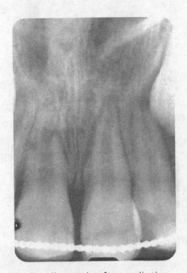

Figure 2: Periapical radiograph after splinting.

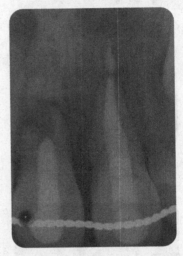

Figure 4: Periapical radiograph.

instructions were given. One week after the incident, endodontic therapy was initiated on both central incisors (Figure 3). The pulpal contents were extirpated and the canals were instrumented and irrigated with sodium hypochlorite. After drying with sterile paper points, the canals were filled with calcium hydroxide paste (Pulpdent; Pulpdent Corporation of America, Watertown, MA, USA) and the coronal access was sealed with a resin modified glass ionomer (Vitrebond).

Four weeks after the incident, the splint was removed. At 8 weeks after splinting, the right central incisor was still excessively mobile. The tooth was restabilized with the new splint. Four weeks later the canals of both teeth were obturated with zinc oxide-eugenol cement. The root canal of the left central incisor was obturated to the apex; the root canal of the right central incisor was obturated up to the apical root fracture site (Figure 4). At that time a periodontist was consulted to evaluate the excessive and chronic

mobility of the right central incisor. After all the treatment options were considered, extraction of the right central incisor and placement of a bone graft were chosen as the preferred treatment option. Five months after the accident, the right central incisor was extracted (both apical and coronal segments) and Bio-Oss Collagen bone graft was placed in the socket (Figures 5A, B, and C). The extracted tooth was decoronated and added to the splint as a provisional pontic (Figures 6 and 7). Eight weeks after the bone graft was placed, the patient returned for an impression and the removable prosthesis was delivered shortly thereafter (Figure 8).

A radiographic examination (Figure 9) and clinical examination (Figure 10) 5 months postoperative bone graft revealed that the bone graft site was healing well.

Fourteen months after the incident, the left central incisor showed no sign of ankylosis and the probing depths were all within normal limits. The removable

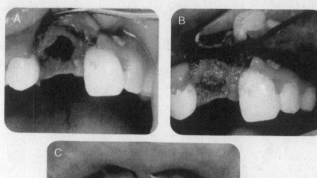

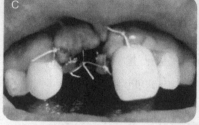

Figure 5: (A) Extraction; (B) bone graft; (C) suturing.

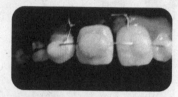

Figure 6: Temporary prostheses.

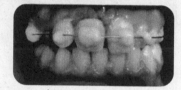

Figure 7: Postoperative view at 1 week.

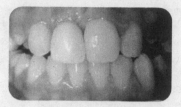

Figure 8: Temporary prosthesis.

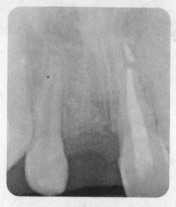

Figure 9: Five-month postoperative radiograph.

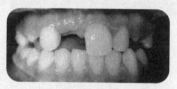

Figure 10: Fourteen-month postoperative view.

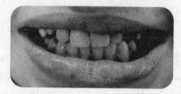

Figure 11: Fourteen-month postoperative view.

prosthesis with pontic was functionally acceptable and satisfied the patient's aesthetics (Figure 11).

Discussion

The primary goals for managing this patient's dental trauma include both acute as well as long-term endodontic, periodontal, and cosmetic considerations. The immediate goals included the repositioning and stabilization of the traumatized teeth. Long-term considerations included prevention of inflammatory root resorption, observation for potential ankylosis, and preservation of alveolar bone. The potential poor prognosis and possible need for extraction of both central incisors was explained to the child's parents on the day of the accident. Due to the right central incisor's failure to adequately stabilize after 4 months, it was extracted and a bone graft was placed. To satisfy aesthetic considerations for this child, a bone graft allowed for preservation of the alveolar bone height. The parents were informed that a second bone graft might be needed when the child was old enough for placement of a dental implant.

Special Considerations

One week after the accident, both maxillary central incisors were filled with calcium hydroxide paste. The obturation for the maxillary right central incisor appeared to be short and may have been a contribution factor to its failure. The canal of the maxillary left central incisor was not completely obturated laterally.

Self-Study Questions

A. What are the immediate, acute dental management considerations?

1. How does the extra oral time affect the prognosis and what are the ideal transport media for an avulsed tooth?
2. What criteria would preclude reimplantation of the avulsed tooth?
3. What are the procedures for repositioning and splinting luxated permanent teeth?
4. How would you manage the soft tissue injuries?

B. Does the child's medial diagnoses affect the dental management of these injuries?

C. When and what type of radiographs should be taken?

D. Should antibiotics be prescribed and if so, which type?

E. What are the appropriate splinting times for luxations and root fractures?

F. When should endodontic intervention begin for avulsions and root fractures of permanent teeth?

G. What types of pathologic sequelae can be expected after avulsions and root fractures?

H. What are the various options for endodontic therapy for root fractures?

I. What follow-up regimen should followed in traumatic dental cases?

J. What considerations should be taken into account if the patient in this case was 6 years old with open apices of the involved central incisors?

K. What is the earliest age that dental implants should be considered?

Answers located at the end of the chapter.

References

1. Sagalas E, et al. Survival of human periodontal ligament cells in media proposed for transport of avulsed teeth. Endod Dent Traumatol 2004;20:21–28.
2. Grossman LI. Origin of microorganisms in traumatized, pulpless, sound teeth. J Dent Res 1967;46:551.
3. Flores MT, et al. Guidelines for the management of traumatic dental injuries. I. Fractures and luxations of permanent teeth. Dent Traumatol 2007;23:66–71.
4. Flores MT, et al. Guidelines for the management of traumatic dental injuries. II Avulsion of permanent teeth. Dent Traumatol 2007;23:130–136.
5. Welbury R, et al. Outcomes for root-fractured permanent incisors: a retrospective study. Pediatr Dent 2002;24:98–102.
6. Andreasen JO, et al. Prognosis of root-fractured permanent incisors – prediction of healing modalities. Endod Dent Traumatol 1989;5:11–22.

TAKE-HOME POINTS

A.

1. The speed of reimplantation is essential. Immediate on-site immediate reimplantation yields the best prognosis. If the tooth's root surface is contaminated, it is important to gently cleanse it with running water or ideal storage media if available. The tooth should be held by the crown, thus minimizing contact with the root surface that could further damage the periodontal ligament. If immediate reimplantation is not possible, it is important to place the avulsed tooth as soon as possible in Hanks Balanced Salt Solution (HBSS), which is the ideal storage medium [1]. If HBSS is not available, milk is a good alternative storage medium [1]. The socket should be rinsed with saline prior to reimplantation.

2. Reimplantation is usually not indicated if the avulsed tooth has been extraoral and dry >60 minutes because the periodontal ligaments cells do not survive and ankylosis is inevitable. If the patient has special medical, emotional, or behavioral issues that would make essential follow-up examinations, radiographs, and/or potential treatment difficult, reimplantation may not be indicated. However, if reimplantation of a tooth with a closed apex is performed in this situation, the goal is to promote alveolar bone growth that will eventually encapsulate the reimplanted tooth. To reimplant a permanent tooth with an extraoral dry time of >60 minutes, the root should be debrided to remove the PDL with pumice prophylaxis, gauze, gentle scaling/root planing, or 3% citric acid for 3 minutes. The root should then be rinsed and placed in 1.23% sodium fluoride for 5–20 minutes.

3. A luxated tooth must be repositioned back into its original position using finger pressure. Local anesthesia should be used to maximize patient comfort. Teeth with >2 mm of mobility buccally or lingually must be stabilized with a splint to allow for optimal healing, most commonly fabricated with wire and composite material. The splint should be passive, flexible, without occlusal interferences,
and allow for optimal oral hygiene, thus allowing for optimal physiologic, functional mobility, and ideal healing.

4. The gingival tissues must be allowed to heal with normal reattachment after a luxation or avulsion injury. During the reattachment process, there is potential for ingress of bacteria via the gingival sulcus that can lead to ingress into the pulpal tissues with eventual devitalization [2]. Thus optimal oral hygiene, daily chlorhexidine rinses, soft diet without heavy incising, and the use of systemic antibiotics with avulsions will minimize the chances of future endodontic intervention.

B. Follow-up dental management of traumatic injuries such as avulsions require multiple and often complex dental management. Therefore, embarking on complex dental treatment such as reimplanting an avulsed tooth in individuals with serious medical and/or behavior issues may be contraindicated.

C. As soon as possible after the traumatic incident, several radiographic projections and angulations are recommended. The International Association of Dental Traumatology (IADT) guidelines are as follows [3]: (1) 90-degree horizontal angle with the central beam through the tooth in question, (2) occlusal view, and (3) lateral view from the mesial or distal aspect.

Additional radiographs should be exposed at the 1-month follow-up because pulp necrosis can occur within 2 weeks and internal resorption within 3 weeks of an accident. Close follow-up is essential because inflammatory root resorption can occur quickly leading to extensive root resorption and perforation, especially in immature teeth with large pulp canals and thin dentinal walls. Additional radiographs after 1 month should be exposed as needed.

D. Systemic antibiotics should be administered after reimplantation for avulsed teeth. Tetracycline is the antibiotic of choice for patients >12 years of age (doxycycline bid for 1 week at the appropriate dose for patient weight and age). If the child is <12 years of age, amoxicillin or penicillin should be prescribed rather than the tetracycline, which can stain calcifying teeth.

E. Splinting times vary depending on the type of injury [4]. Subluxations, extrusive luxations, and avulsions with an extraoral dry time <60 minutes require splinting for 2 weeks. Lateral luxations, avulsions with an extraoral dry time >60 minutes, root fractures (middle third), and alveolar fractures require splinting times of 4 weeks. A root fracture in the cervical third requires splinting for up to 4 months. Splinting for longer than recommended and/or splinting with rigid fixation promotes ankylosis by decreasing physiologic function, which is important to allow for normal healing.

F. For a mature, closed apex tooth with an extraoral dry time <60 minutes, endodontic therapy should be initiated 7–10 days after reimplantation and before the splint is removed. Calcium hydroxide should be used to temporarily obturate the root canal prior to final root canal therapy. For a mature, closed apex tooth with an extraoral dry time >60 minutes, endodontic therapy can be initiated prior to reimplantation or delayed to no longer than 7–10 days after replantation. For root fractures, the pulp status should be monitored for at least 1 year. If necrosis develops, endodontic therapy is usually only necessary to the fracture line where the periradicular pathology is located. Calcium hydroxide is the ideal intracanal medicament. The apical fragment usually remains vital and thus rarely exhibits periapical pathology [5]. The calcium hydroxide should be left in place for 1 year, followed by definitive obturation.

G. Pathologic sequelae that may result after an avulsion of a closed apex tooth include inflammatory external root resorption (IRR) or replacement external root resorption (RRR). Teeth with IRR can present clinically with excessive mobility and symptoms of periradicular pathology. Teeth with RRR present with limited or no mobility

when percussed have a dull sound and do not respond to orthodontic forces. With time these teeth appear to submerge below the plane of occlusion as the alveolar bone increases in height either actively during growth or passively throughout life. Once the crown submerges significantly below the occlusal plan, one should consider decoronation of the tooth to preserve the contour of the alveolar ridge.

For root fractures, prognosis improves as the fracture line approaches the apex. In addition, a horizontal fracture has a more favorable prognosis than vertical fracture, and a nondisplaced fracture is better than a displaced fracture. Healing can occur with either connective tissue (periodontal ligament-like), calcified tissue (cementum-like) or bone and connective tissue [6]. Nonhealing with granulation tissue results in areas of radiographic pathology adjacent to the fracture line and requires endodontic intervention.

H. Pulp necrosis usually affects only the coronal fracture because the apical fragment remains vital; thus apical endodontic therapy is usually not necessary.

I. The postoperative instructions are vital and must include optimal oral hygiene with emphasis on the gingival sulcus of affect teeth and a soft diet for up to 2 weeks with no incising of affected teeth until the teeth are stable. Chlorhexidine oral rinses should be used during the initially healing period (0.12%, 15 ml swish for 30 seconds bid for 1 week). If the tetanus coverage is uncertain, the patient should be referred to a physician for evaluation. Post-trauma follow-up appointments generally should be at 1 week, 1 month, 3 months, 6 months, and yearly thereafter for 5 years.

J. For an avulsed permanent tooth with open apex, the goal is to promote revascularization of the pulpal tissue. If the extraoral dry time is within 60 minutes, the root surface should be covered either with Arestin (minocycline hydrochloride microspheres) or soaked in a 1% solution of doxycycline for 5 minutes before reimplanting the tooth. If neither is readily available, the tooth should be reimplanted as soon as possible. The tooth should be monitored closely because periapical pathology and IRR can progress quickly with severe destruction of the root. Endodontic therapy should be avoided unless there is evidence of pulpal necrosis, in which case it must be initiated immediately with extirpation of the pulp contents and obturation with calcium hydroxide.

For a root fractured tooth with an open apex, the goal is also to promote revascularization of the pulpal tissue. Immature teeth generally have a better prognosis of healing compared with mature teeth. The tooth should be monitored closely and endodontic therapy should be avoided unless there is evidence of pulpal necrosis.

K. Dental implants should only be placed once skeletal growth is complete. In a few cases where dental implants have been placed in children, the implants have either submerged due to alveolar bone growth or displaced into the sinus. The goals in children who are still growing and require implants should be the best permanent prosthetic treatment. In the cases where dental implants should be considered, the preservation of soft and hard tissue should be considered. In this case because a dental implant was considered, a decision was made to "preserve" the socket and bone by placing Bio-Oss in the socket.

7

Implant Site Preparation

Clinical Cases in Periodontics, First Edition. Nadeem Karimbux.
© 2012 John Wiley & Sons, Inc. Published 2012 by John Wiley & Sons, Inc.

Case 1

Sinus Grafting: Lateral

CASE STORY

The patient was a 52-year-old male who presented to the Department of Periodontology for a consultation regarding the edentulous space in the maxillary right quadrant. His chief complaint was to have fixed restorations to replace the missing teeth. Figures 1 and 2 illustrate the initial clinical examination.

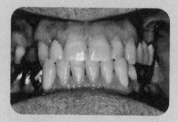

Figure 1: Facial view of the maxilla and the mandible.

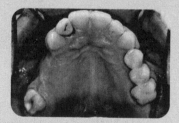

Figure 2: Occlusal view of the maxilla.

LEARNING GOALS AND OBJECTIVES

- To identify the indications for a sinus elevation
- To understand the preoperative considerations
- To be introduced to a surgical technique and biomaterial used to perform a sinus elevation

Medical History

The patient was in good health and had regular physical examinations. He did not report any allergies or sinus-related pathology.

Review of Systems

- Vital signs
  - Blood pressure: 120/65 mm Hg
  - Pulse rate: 65 beats/minute (regular)

Social History

The patient did not drink alcohol and did not consume recreational drugs. He had been smoking 10 cigarettes per day for the last 25 years.

Extraoral Examination

No significant findings were noted. The patient had no masses or swelling, no trismus. No palpable lymphadenopathy and the temporomandibular joints were within normal limits (Figure 3).

Intraoral Examination

- The soft tissues of the mouth including tongue appeared normal. The oral cancer screen was negative.
- The gingival examination revealed a generalized mild marginal erythema and a melanotic macule in the gingiva (site #5) consistent with an amalgam tattoo (Figure 2).
- A hard tissue examination was completed by the referring general dentist.
- The edentulous ridge in the maxillary right quadrant had deformities in the buccolingual and apico-coronal directions (Seibert class 3) (Figure 1).

Occlusion

Lack of posterior support, unprotected occlusion, cross-bite occlusion #22 and 27.

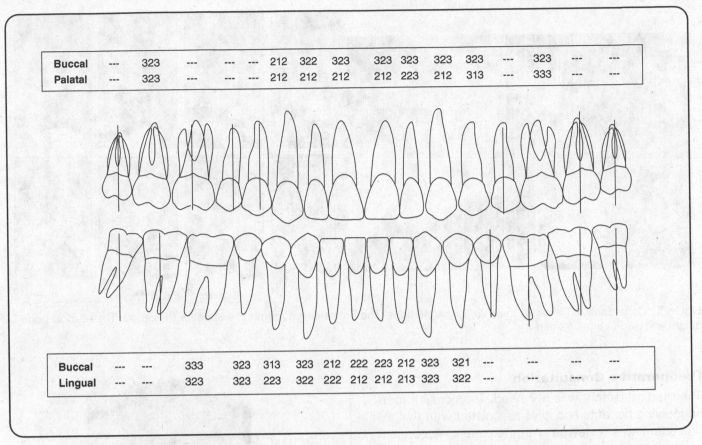

| Buccal | --- | 323 | --- | --- | --- | 212 | 322 | 323 | 323 | 323 | 323 | 323 | --- | 323 | --- | --- |
| Palatal | --- | 323 | --- | --- | --- | 212 | 212 | 212 | 212 | 223 | 212 | 313 | --- | 333 | --- | --- |

| Buccal | --- | --- | 333 | 323 | 313 | 323 | 212 | 222 | 223 | 212 | 323 | 321 | --- | --- | --- | --- |
| Lingual | --- | --- | 323 | 323 | 223 | 322 | 222 | 212 | 212 | 213 | 323 | 322 | --- | --- | --- | --- |

Figure 3: Probing pocket depth measurements.

Radiographic Examination

A periapical radiograph of the right posterior maxillary sextant showed that the maxillary right sinus was pneumatized and the height of bone mesial to tooth #2 was about 1 mm (Figure 4).

Treatment Plan

Prosthodontic, endodontic, and orthodontic consultations are required to establish a comprehensive treatment plan. A cone beam computed tomography (CT) scan is ordered for the maxillary arch to get further information on the anatomy and the condition of the sinus (Figure 5).

A thickening of the Schneiderian membrane is observed in the maxillary right sinus (Figure 5). A consultation with an otolaryngologist is indicated to rule out any sinus pathology. He performed a nasal endoscopy and reported a "very mild edema and erythema." He diagnosed a mild sinusitis and did not consider any contraindication for the sinus elevation procedure.

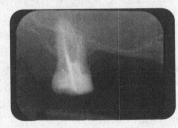

Figure 4: Radiographic evaluation: the periapical radiograph of the maxillary right quadrant shows the pneumatized sinus and the lack of bone.

The final treatment plan included a full-mouth prosthetic and occlusal rehabilitation, including an implant supported fixed partial denture #3-x-5.

Treatment

The patient received oral hygiene instructions and a prophylaxis. Tooth #2 was extracted prior to the sinus elevation.

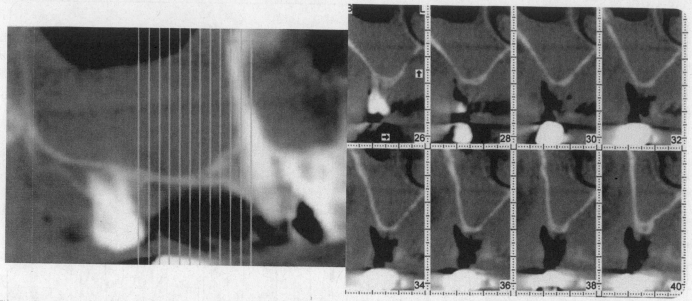

Figure 5: Cone beam CT scan of the maxillary right sinus. The Schneiderian membrane appears thickened. The residual bone height is 1 mm in sites #3 and 4.

Preoperative Consultation

The medical history was reviewed. The consent form addressing benefits and risks associated with the procedure was reviewed with the patient. Accessibility to the surgical site was clinically assessed. The CT scan showed that less than 4 mm of bone was present in the edentulous ridge area so a lateral window approach was selected to achieve 10–12 mm of bone augmentation in sites #3, 4, and 5. No evidence of the lateral branch of the posterior superior lateral artery could be seen on the CT scan (Figure 5). The following prescriptions were delivered to the patient: amoxicillin 500 mg (tid for 10 days starting 24 hours before the procedure), ibuprofen 600 mg (every 4–6 hours as needed for pain), and Peridex 0.12% (bid).

Sinus Elevation Procedure

A procedural sedation and analgesia nerve block and local infiltrations were achieved with lidocaine 2% (epinephrine 1/100,000) (Figure 6). A full-thickness flap was elevated in the maxilla right quadrant to expose the cortical bone of the lateral wall of the maxillary sinus. A lateral window (20 mm × 8 mm) was outlined with a piezotome until the Schneiderian was visible (Figure 7). The Schneiderian membrane was elevated in a medial and anterior direction so that a space could be created in between the Schneiderian membrane and the bony floor of the sinus. A collagenic membrane was placed in the sinus against the membrane (Figure 8). Bone grafting material (a mix of

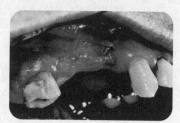

Figure 6: Preoperative condition, buccal view.

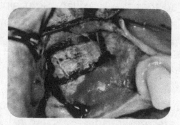

Figure 7: The lateral window is outlined with a piezotome.

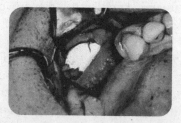

Figure 8: The Schneiderian membrane is elevated. A collagenic membrane is inserted against the membrane.

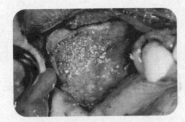

Figure 9: The bone grafting material is placed into the sinus in between the Schneiderian membrane and the floor of the sinus.

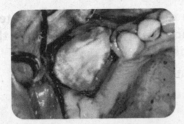

Figure 10: A collagenic membrane is placed over the lateral window.

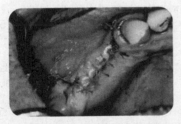

Figure 11: The flap is repositioned and sutured to achieve primary closure.

rehydrated freeze-dreid bone allograft [FDBA] and anorganic bovine bone mineral) was placed into the space created into the sinus (Figure 9). A collagenic membrane was placed over the lateral window (Figure 10) and the flap was repositioned and sutured in its initial position (Figure 11). A panoramic radiograph was taken at the end of the surgery. The bone grafting material appears well contained in the maxillary right sinus (Figure 12).

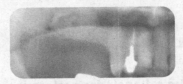

Figure 12: Panoramic radiograph the day of the procedure.

Discussion

Although a high predictability of sinus elevation procedures have been extensively reported in the literature as it relates to the regeneration of bone in a pneumatized maxillary sinus, this particular case presents some challenges that could compromise some determinants of success. One of the risk factors identified and discussed in the medical history is the smoking status of the patient, which exposes him to a more elevated risk of complications. Thus an interdisciplinary approach was necessary where a well-coordinated team including the otolaryngologist and restorative dentist worked simultaneously in their respective fields in conjunction with the periodontist to provide the maximum benefit of the therapy for the patient and to evaluate and limit the risks of complications.

The surgical procedure went as planned and the patient complied with all the postoperative instructions given. The patient was seen for postoperative visits at 1 week to remove the sutures and at 3 and 6 weeks to monitor his healing response. The allocated time for healing prior to implant placement was 6 months, which corresponds to the remodeling and maturation of newly formed bone and concurs with what is suggested in the literature. Panoramic and periapical radiographs were taken to have a preliminary assessment of the amount of newly formed bone present. However, a new CT scan if performed could have provided more information regarding the volume, the anatomy, and the irregularities of the newly formed bone. It was determined, however, that the regenerated site could allow the placement of two implant fixtures, which were placed in sites 3 and 5 and will support a three-unit fixed prosthesis (FPD 3-X-5).

Self-Study Questions

A. What is the rationale for performing a sinus elevation?

B. What are the anatomic landmarks to know to perform a sinus elevation?

C. What are the techniques used?

D. Which biomaterials can be used in a sinus elevation? Is there histologic evidence of bone formation?

E. What are the determinants of success in a sinus elevation?

F. Are implants placed in a sinus elevated site as successful as implants placed in pristine bone? Does the surgical technique have an influence on the implant survival rate in the long term?

G. What are the complications associated with sinus elevations? How do you manage these complications?

Answers located at the end of the chapter.

References

1. Mosby's Dental Dictionary. 2nd ed. Elsevier, 2008.
2. Boyne JP, James RA. Grafting the maxillary sinus floor with autogenous marrow and bone. J Oral Surg 1980;38:613–616.
3. Wood RM, Moore DL. Grafting of the maxillary sinus with intraorally harvested autogenous bone prior to implant placement. Int J Oral Maxillofac Implants 1988;3:209–214.
4. Tatum H Jr. Maxillary and implant reconstructions. Dent Clin North Am 1986;30:207–229.
5. Testori T, Del Fabbro M, et al. Maxillary Sinus Surgery and Alternatives in Treatment. Chicago, IL: Quintessence, 2006.
6. Ella B, Sédarat C, et al. Vascular connections of the lateral wall of the sinus: surgical effect in sinus augmentation. Int J Oral Maxillofac Implants 2008;23:1047–1052.
7. Uschida Y, Goto M, et al. A cadaveric study of maxillary sinus size as an aid in bone grafting of the maxillary sinus floor. J Oral Maxillofac Surg 1998;56:1158–1163.
8. Ella B, Noble Rda C, et al. Septa within the sinus: effect on elevation of the sinus floor. Br J Oral Maxillofac Surg 2008;46:464–467.
9. Kim MJ, Jung UW, et al. Maxillary sinus septa: prevalence, height, location and morphology. A reformatted CT scan analysis. J Periodontol 2006;77:903–908.
10. Summers RB. Sinus floor elevation. J Esthet Dent 1998;10:164–171.
11. Jensen OT, Shulman LB, et al. Report of the sinus consensus conference of 1996. Int J Oral Maxillofac Implants 1998;13(Suppl):11–32.
12. Del Fabbro M, Testori T, et al. Systematic review of survival rates for implants placed in the grafted maxillary sinus. Int J Periodontics Restorative Dent 2004;24:565–577.
13. Wallace SS, Froum SJ, et al. Tarnow DPSinus augmentation utilizing anorganic bovine bone (Bio-Oss) with absorbable and nonabsorbable membranes placed over the lateral window: histomorphometric and clinical analyses. Int J Periodontics Restorative Dent 2005;25:551–559.
14. Kahnberg KE, Vannas-Löfqvist L. Sinus lift procedure using a 2-stage surgical technique: I. Clinical and radiographic report up to 5 years. Int J Oral Maxillofac Implants 2008;23:876–884.
15. Wallace SS, Froum SJ. Effect of maxillary sinus augmentation on the survival of endosseous dental implants. A systematic review. Ann Periodontol 2003;8:328–343.
16. Pjetursson BE, Tan WC, et al. A systematic review of the success of sinus floor elevation and survival of implants inserted in combination with sinus floor elevation. Part I: lateral approach. J Clin Periodontol 2008;35:216–240.
17. Boyne PJ, Lilly LC, et al. De novo bone induction by recombinant human bone morphogenetic protein-2 (rhBMP-2) in maxillary sinus floor augmentation. J Oral Maxillofacial Surg 2005;63:1693–1707.
18. Boyne PJ, Marx RE, et al. A feasibility study evaluating rhBMP-2/absorbable collagen sponge for maxillary sinus floor augmentation. Int J Periodontics Restorative Dent 1997;17:11–25.
19. Valentini P, Abensur D, et al. Histological evaluation of Bio-Oss in a 2-stage sinus floor elevation and implantation procedure. A human case report [review]. Clin Oral Implants Res 1998;9:59–64.
20. Coatoam GW, Krieger JT. A four-year study examining the results of indirect sinus augmentation procedures. J Oral Implantol 1997;23:117–127.
21. Kim DM, Nevins ML, et al. The efficacy of demineralized bone matrix and cancellous bone chips for maxillary

sinus augmentation. Int J Periodontics Restorative Dent 2009;29:415–423.

22. Tarnow DP, Wallace SS, et al. Histologic and clinical comparison of bilateral sinus floor elevation with and without membrane barrier placement in 12 patients. Part 3 of an ongoing prospective study. Int J Periodontics Restorative Dent 2000;20:116–125.

23. Torella F, Pitarch J, Cabanes G, et al. Ultrasonic ostectomy for the surgical approach of the maxillary sinus: a technical note. Int J Oral Maxillofac Implants 1998;13:697.

24. Papa F, Cortese A, et al. Outcome of 50 consecutive sinus lift operations. Br J Oral Maxillofacial Surg 2005;43:309–313.

25. Valentini P, Abensur DJ. Maxillary sinus grafting with anorganic bovine bone: a clinical report of long-term results. Int J Oral Maxillofacial Implants 2003;18:556–560.

26. Fugazzotto PA, Vlassis J. Report of 1633 implants in 814 augmented sinus areas in function for up to 180 months. Implant Dent 2007;16:369–378.

27. Ferrigno N, Laureti M, et al. Dental implants placement in conjunction with osteotome sinus floor elevation: a 12-year life-table analysis from a prospective study on 588 ITI implants. Clin Oral Implants Res 2006;17:194–205.

28. Chen L, Cha J. An 8-year retrospective study: 1,100 patients receiving 1,557 implants using the minimally invasive hydraulic sinus condensing technique. J Periodontol 2005;76:482–491.

29. Rosen PS, Summers R, et al. The bone-added osteotome sinus floor elevation technique: multicenter retrospective report of consecutively treated patients. Int J Oral Maxillofac Implants 1999;14:853–858.

30. Tan WC, Lang NP, et al. A systematic review of the success of sinus floor elevation and survival of implants inserted in combination with sinus floor elevation. Part II: transalveolar technique [review]. J Clin Periodontol 2008;35(8 Suppl):241–254.

31. Tonetti MS, Hammerle CHF. Advances in bone augmentation to enable dental implant placement: Consensus Report of the Sixth European Workshop on Periodontology. J Clin Periodontol 2008;35 (Suppl 8):168–172.

32. Krennmair G, Krainhofner M, et al. Maxillary sinus lift for single implant-supported restorations: a clinical study. Int J Oral Maxillofac Implants 2007;22:351–358.

33. Khoury F. Augmentation of the sinus floor with mandibular bone block and simultaneous implantation: a 6-year clinical investigation. Int J Oral Maxillofacial Implants 1999;14:557–564.

34. Schwartz-Arad D, Herzberg R, et al. The prevalence of surgical complications of the sinus graft procedure and their impact on implant survival. J Periodontol 2004;75:511–516.

35. Zijderveld SA, van den Bergh JP, et al. Anatomical and surgical findings and complications in 100 consecutive maxillary sinus floor elevation procedures. J Oral Maxillofac Surg 2008;66:1426–1438.

36. Fugazzotto PA, Vlassis J. A simplified classification and repair system for sinus membrane perforations. J Periodontol 2003;74:1534–1541.

37. Elian N, Wallace S, et al. Distribution of the maxillary artery as it relates to sinus floor augmentation. Int J Oral Maxillofac Implants 2005;20:784–787.

TAKE-HOME POINTS

A. The absence of teeth in the posterior maxilla can become a restorative challenge when little or no alveolar bone is present. The presence of the maxillary sinus as the basis of the maxillary alveolar process can be an obstacle to the placement of an implant. In addition, sinus pneumatization, described as an enlargement of the maxillary sinus due to the aging process and as a result of the loss of maxillary teeth [1], tends to reduce the amount of bone available over time. As a consequence, there is usually a need to increase the bone volume in the posterior maxilla prior to implant placement. The goal of a sinus elevation procedure is to surgically increase the alveolar bone height by grafting bone in the floor of the maxillary sinus [2]. Evidence has shown that the imposition of an appropriate grafting material placed along the antral floor and below the Schneiderian membrane can successfully lead to viable antral bone formation and remodeling [2–4]. After a healing period of time needed for bone formation and maturation, an implant can be placed with adequate primary stability, osseointegrate, and eventually be restored with high rates of success [5].

B. The maxillary sinus is an air-filled space located in the body of the maxilla. It is a pyramid with a nasal wall (its base), an anterior wall, a superior wall (the orbital floor), a lateral wall, and an inferior wall (the maxillary alveolar process). It is innervated by branches of V2 and is supplied by branches of the internal maxillary artery: the infraorbital artery, the posterior lateral artery, and the posterior superior alveolar artery that have inconsistent branches running along the lateral wall of the sinus [6]. Evaluation for the presence of these branches in CT scans is necessary prior to surgery to prevent perioperative hemorrhage if a lateral window approach is selected. The presence of these branches needs to be evaluated prior to surgery to prevent preoperative hemorrhage if a lateral window approach is selected. The sinus drains in the nasal cavity through an ostium located at the superior aspect of its medial wall (nasal wall), about 28.5 mm above the sinus floor [7]. A sinus elevation should never obliterate the ostium as to not compromise the sinus drainage. Sinus septa are commonly present in the apical third of the sinus. They represent a challenge during sinus elevations. Ella et al [8] report that 40% of patients have bony septa that can partly or totally compartmentalize the sinus. Septa would be more present in the middle region of the sinus (50%) and would be highest on the medial area [9]. The radiographic examination with a CT scan will help identify them and better evaluate the anatomic challenges faced during the procedure.

C. There are two main approaches to performing a sinus elevation:

1. **The crestal approach:** This technique gives access to the sinus floor through the ridge crest. Tatum [4] first described a technique involving the following sequence: flap elevation, removal of the bone until the cortical bone of the sinus floor is exposed, greenstick fracture of the cortical bone with osteotomes and burs, elevation of the Schneiderian membrane, and placement of the bone grafting material. Summers [10] described a variation of Tatum's technique called the "osteotome sinus floor elevation technique." Osteotomes of increasing diameters with concave tips are used to relocate the existing alveolar bone apically and laterally toward the antral floor. Some bone grafting material can be added to the procedure ("bone-added osteotome sinus floor elevation technique") to decrease the risk of membrane

perforation and better control the ultimate height of the grafted space.

2. **The lateral window approach:** This technique gives access through the lateral wall of the sinus [3,4]. A full-thickness flap is elevated to expose the lateral antral wall, a window is made in the bony wall using rotary or hand instruments, and then it is displaced medially. The membrane is carefully elevated, and the bone is placed in the space located below the Schneiderian membrane and above the sinus floor.

D. Autografts (extraoral and intraoral), allografts (FDBA, decalcified freeze-dried bone allograft [DFDBA]), xenografts (anorganic bovine bone mineral), and alloplasts (calcium phosphate) have been used for bone grafting materials for more than 20 years. The sinus consensus conference of 1996 [11] approved autogenous bone as an acceptable grafting material. Other studies proved that bone substitutes including allografts and xenografts could be successfully used for sinus elevation [12,13]. Further evidence [14] has shown that autogenous bone is a viable option, although a higher rate of complications (including infections, bone resorption) was observed when compared with xenografts and allografts. Recent systematic reviews have shown that sinus elevation using bone substitutes alone or in combination with autogenous bone had a similar or even a better implant survival rate when compared with studies using autogenous bone only [15,16]. New materials such as bone morphogenic proteins (BMP-2) used with a collagenic sponge carrier have proved their efficacy and got Food and Drug Administration approval for sinus elevation procedures [17,18].

A few studies have provided histologic evidence of bone formation in a grafted sinus. Histology of an explant from the maxillary sinus showed new bone formation around the implant and the xenograft particulates [19]. Another study showed evidence of bone formation when autogenous bone alone or a mix of DFDBA and autogenous bone were initially used [20].

Boyne et al [17] and Kim et al [21] showed evidence of normal bone formation in an elevated sinus, respectively, when rhBMP-2 (Infuse) and demineralized bone matrix and cancellous bone chips (DynaBlast) were used as grafting material.

The placement of a membrane over the window is usually recommended to enhance the bone formation [22]. Both resorbable (collagenic) and nonresorbable (expandable polytetrafluoroethylene [ePTFE]) membranes can be used, although the resorbable one is more commonly used to avoid a surgical reentry.

E. The success of a sinus elevation procedure depends on a series of parameters that include chronologically an uneventful surgical procedure, minimal or no postoperative pain and complications, bone formation, osseointegration of implants, and their survival under functional load.

Some determinants promoting success have been reported in the literature. They include the following:

1. Absence of medical conditions (including systemic diseases, bisphosphonate, and irradiation), sinus pathology, and smoking. The patient should be referred to a physician if there is any significant medical condition reported during the preoperative examination.
2. The use of rough surfaced implants as opposed to machined surface implants to enhance the survival rate [15,16].
3. The use of particulates grafts or BMP-2 as opposed to block graft to decrease complications. However, autogenous block grafts remain a viable option [15,16].
4. The use of a membrane when a lateral window approach is selected [15,16].
5. The use of piezo surgical instruments to decrease the rate of complications at the time of osteotomy [23].

The surgeon should deliver regular postoperative instructions emphasizing these points:

1. Do not blow your nose
2. Do not sneeze
3. Do not travel by plane or scuba dive for the next 15 days
4. Do not engage in physical activity for a few days (i.e., strenuous exercise)

F. Implants placed in a sinus elevated site have a very high rate of success (>90%), which is comparable with implants placed in pristine bone [15]. Multiple studies have proved that the lateral approach is a predictable technique and allows implants survival rates of ≥95% over the long term [24–26]. Similar results can be found when a crestal approach is used [27,28]. Nevertheless, the amount of residual bone seems to have a significant impact on the implant survival rate with this technique; a minimum of 5 mm would be necessary to achieve a high success rate [29].

Evidence has shown that there are no statistically differences in implants survival rates when a lateral approach is used as opposed to a crestal approach. A recent meta-analysis reporting on 12,020 implants placed in sinus elevated sites with a lateral approach indicated an implant survival rate at 3 years of 90.1% [16], whereas the survival rate over the same period of time was 92.8% when a crestal approach was used [30]. If both surgical techniques are compatible with success, the Consensus Report of the Sixth European Workshop on Periodontology [31] stated that the question regarding the choice of the most appropriate procedure still needed to be addressed.

G. Complications associated with sinus elevation procedure can be divided into two categories:

1. The operative complications:
   a. The perforation of the Schneiderian membrane is reported to be the most common complication and happens on average in 19.5% [16] and up to 58% [32] of the procedures. There is some controversy with regard to its impact on the implant survival [33,34].
   b. Hemorrhage at the time of the osteotomy with the lateral approach, which is the consequence of the section of a branch of the posterior lateral artery running along the lateral wall of the sinus. Zijderveld et al [35] reported it happening in 2% of the cases.
   c. Inadvertent implant migration in the sinus cavity and injury of the infraorbital neurovascular bundle have been rarely reported.
2. The postoperative complications:
   a. Infection as a direct consequence of the procedure or as a result of an overfill of the

sinus resulting in the absence of its drainage in the nasal cavity. Infections occur 2.9% of the time and would be correlated to membrane perforations [16].

b. Absence of adequate bone volume. It would be more common with autogenous bone [14].

c. Hematoma and wound dehiscence have also been reported.

3. Management of perioperative complications:

a. Perforation of the Schneiderian membrane: a resorbable membrane can be placed against the Schneiderian membrane and over the perforated area. If the perforation is small, Fugazzotto advocates not to try to repair it as long as it "folds over itself" [36]. If the perforation is large and cannot be repaired, the sinus elevation should be postponed after complete healing of the Schneiderian membrane.

b. Hemorrhage [37]: Pressure can be applied on the bleeding point with gauze until hemostasis is observed. If the severed vessel is located in a bony crypt, bone wax can be placed in it to act as a plug that encourages clot formation. One can also inject some local anesthetic with epinephrine 1/50,000 to enhance vasoconstriction. Vessel ligature and electrocautery have also been reported, although they need to be used with caution.

c. Inadvertent implant migration: The implant should be retrieved as soon as possible. An emergency consultation with an ORL should be scheduled.

4. Management of postoperative complications:

a. Infections: The first choice of therapy is the use of antibiotics and choosing the appropriate one for the specificity of the sinus infection. In that regard, Augmentin could be considered as the first choice followed by DNA gyrase inhibitors such as ofloxacin, levofloxacin, and so on. In addition, one could consider the use of broader spectrum antibiotics such as amoxicillin or clindamycin for penicillin-allergic patients. If the infection cannot be controlled with antibiotics, the removal of the bone graft might be necessary.

b. Inadequate bone volume: The clinical situation should be reevaluated. The options of placing shorter implants or performing a complementary sinus elevation can be discussed.

Case 2

Sinus Grafting: Crestal

CASE STORY

A 32-year-old Korean female who had had extensive restorative treatment by her general dentist came in for an implant consultation. However, many of her restorations had recurrent decay, and several restorations had failed continually. Her main goal for visiting the clinic was to have fixed implant restorations to replace missing teeth #14 and 15. Figures 1 and 2 illustrate the initial clinical examination.

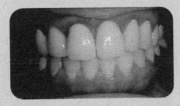

Figure 1: Facial view of the maxilla and the mandible.

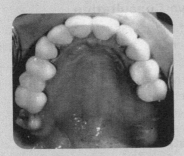

Figure 2: Occlusal view of the maxilla.

LEARNING GOALS AND OBJECTIVES

- To understand the indications/contraindications for the crestal approach and what diagnostic information is needed to make this decision
- To understand the advantages and disadvantages of the crestal approach, including the sequence of treatment (internal sinus lift/graft/implant all at same time vs. internal sinus lift/wait for healing and then implant)
- To learn how to achieve good initial stability in situations with weak and a low amount of bone
- To understand the advantages/disadvantages of the Crestal Window Technique, Summer's osteotome, balloon technique, hydraulic sinus condensing, use of bone condensing drills, and use of piezo tips

Medical History

The patient was in good health and had had regular physical examinations (she was a nurse in the Emergency Department). She did not report any allergies or sinus-related pathology.

Review of Systems

- Vital signs
  - Blood pressure: 135/85 mm Hg
  - Pulse rate: 65 beats/minute (regular)

Social History

The patient did drink alcohol, and she smoked 10 cigarettes per day. This habit had been shown to

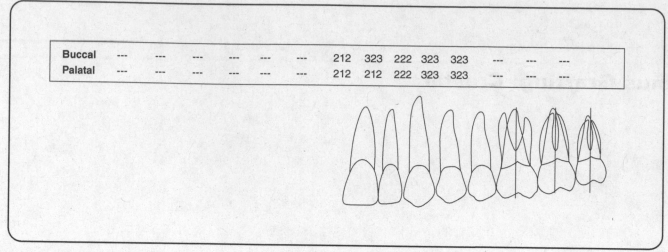

Buccal	---	---	---	---	---	---	212	323	222	323	323	---	---	---
Palatal	---	---	---	---	---	---	212	212	222	323	323	---	---	---

Figure 3: Probing pocket depth measurements of the maxillary left quadrant.

impact the survival rates of endosseous dental implants, according to research. Therefore, the patient was asked to stop smoking at least for 1 month before dental implant surgery.

Extraoral Examination

No significant findings were noted. The patient had no masses or swelling, and no trismus. No palpable lymphadenopathy was observed, and the temporomandibular joints were within normal limits (Figure 3).

Intraoral Examination

- The soft tissues of the mouth including the tongue appeared normal. The oral cancer screening was negative.
- The gingival examination revealed a generalized mild marginal erythema.
- A hard tissue examination was completed by the referring general dentist.
- The edentulous ridge in the maxillary left quadrant had slight deformities in the buccolingual and apico-coronal directions (Seibert class 3) (Figure 1).

Occlusion

Lack of posterior support, unprotected occlusion, group function was noted.

Radiographic Examination

A digital panoramic radiograph showed a pneumatized left maxillary sinus. Cross-sectional computed tomography (CT) showed about 4.1 mm of initial bone height with a buccal lingual dimension of 7.5 mm. There was slight septum on distal of #15 area, and

#14, 15 area was a concave shape, making transalveolar technique favorable (Figure 4).

Good patency of the natural ostium of the maxillary sinus was observed on cross section of the CT scan. This is important because it allows drainage of mucus and foreign material out of the maxillary sinus [1]. If this opening is obliterated, sinusitis will develop with the patient having symptoms of "pressure in the sinus." CT shows that sinus membrane is not thickened, which indicates a healthy sinus. The cavity of maxillary sinus is clear and free of sinus pathogenesis.

Treatment

Although a comprehensive treatment plan was presented to the patient to address all of the issues, the patient only sought #14, 15 fixed implant prosthesis for now. All active disease was treated.

The patient received oral hygiene instructions and a prophylaxis. She was premedicated with amoxicillin 500 mg tid, metronidazole 500 mg tid, and Sudafed 30 mg [1].

Preoperative Consultation

The medical history was reviewed. The consent form addressing benefits and risks associated with the procedure was reviewed with the patient. The patient emphasized that she could not afford to miss work and the procedure must be atraumatic. Therefore, we offered a crestal approach to reduce morbidity.

Sinus Elevation Procedure

A posterior superior alveolar nerve block, greater palatine nerve block, and local infiltrations were

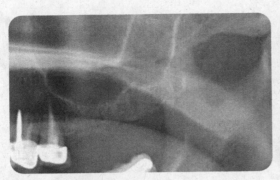

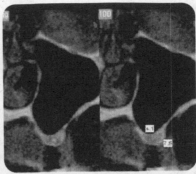

Figure 4: Cone beam CT scan of the maxillary right sinus. The Schneiderian membrane appears healthy and thin. The residual bone height is 4.1 mm in sites #14 and 15. The septum present on the distal of #15 area with a concave shape in #14, 15 area makes transalveolar technique favorable.

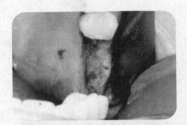

Figure 5: Full-thickness palatal flap raised on #14, 15 site.

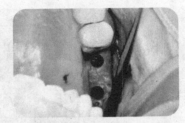

Figure 7: After the removal of bone core using ASBE trephine.

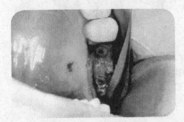

Figure 6: Pointed trephine to mark osteotomy site.

has a tendency to glide out of the intended site. The pointed trephine engages the center point first, thus preventing sliding of the trephine bur from the intended site (Figure 6). The height of bone to sinus floor was estimated from radiographs: 1 mm was subtracted from the height of bone and stopper was set on an adjustable stopper and bone ejector (ASBE) trephine. Slow 30 rpm with 50 Ncm was used to go 1 mm short of the sinus floor. When the trephine depth was close to the sinus floor, a slight tilt of trephine was used to fracture off the bone core. After removal of this bone core, the sinus membrane could be visualized as seen on Figure 7. Note that because the sinus floor was not flat, some parts of it were still intact, and manual enlargement of the sinus window was needed. A small instrument called a "mushroom elevator" was used to elevate the membrane (Figure 8) and pry away the remaining bone of the sinus floor (Figure 9). A bone graft (rehydrated freeze-dried bone allograft [FDBA]) was placed into the space created in the sinus (Figure 10). It is important to laterally condense the bone graft to spread the bone graft mesial-distally as well as buccal lingually using the "spreader instrument" (Figure 11 shows before; Figure

achieved with two carpules of Septocaine 4% with epinephrine 1:100,000) (Figure 5). A full-thickness palatal flap was elevated in the maxillary left quadrant to expose the crestal ridge of #14, 15 site. The palatal flap was used for three reasons: unilateral retraction of flap, less postoperative pain (all incisions in keratinized tissue, and prevention of oral antral communication (due to window present on crestal). In this case a novel Crestal Window Technique using specific drill bits was used. The osteotomy site was marked with "pointed trephine" (Figure 6). The use of a regular trephine is very technique sensitive because trephine

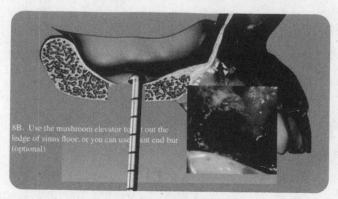

Figure 8: Mushroom elevator is used to identify and lift sinus membrane.

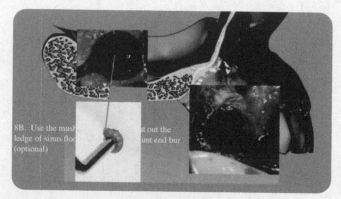

Figure 9: Mushroom elevator is used to pull out sinus floor (bone).

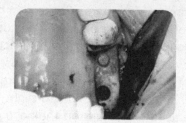

Figure 10: FDBA is inserted via osteotomy.

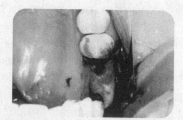

Figure 11: Use of spreader to condense bone laterally as well as mesial-distally.

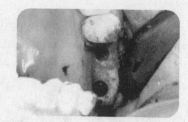

Figure 12: After use of spreader.

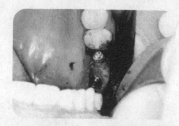

Figure 13: Two MegaGen EZ Plus implants placed 5 × 10 mm with good initial stability 45 Ncm.

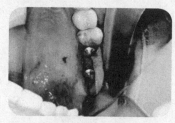

Figure 14: Healing abutment measuring 6 mm in diameter and 3 mm in height is used.

12, after). About 1.5 ml of FDBA was used to graft the sinus transalveolarly. Then 5 × 10 mm MegaGen EZ Plus implants were inserted on the #14, 15 site (Figure 13). To get good initial stability, clinician should keep three things in mind: (1) Selection of implant (crestal portion should be wider than body of implant); (2) Slow insertion to expand the bone (<20 rpm), and (3) Skipping last drill in case of very poor quality. In this case, >45 Ncm was achieved, and healing abutment was inserted making this a one-stage surgery (Figure 14). A papillary finger flap was used to gain primary closure around the healing abutment (Figure 15). Digital panoramic (Figure 16) as well as a CT scan was taken at the end of the surgery (Figure 17) to verify an intact sinus membrane. The bone grafting material appears well contained in the maxillary right sinus (Figure 17).

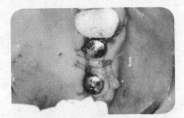

Figure 15: Papillary rotation flap used to close around healing abutment.

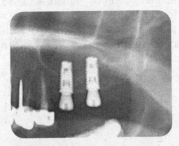

Figure 16: Panoramic X-ray after implant and sinus lift.

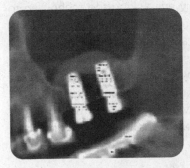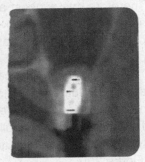

Figure 17: CT scan the day of the procedure.

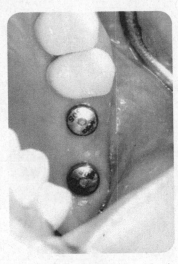

Figure 18: Healing of #14, 15 implant with simultaneous sinus lift after 6 months.

Discussion

Most crestal approaches are "blind techniques" [2]. Therefore, visualization of the Schneiderian membrane is impossible with conventional crestal approaches. With this new Crestal Window Technique, the membrane can be visualized and elevation of sinus can be achieved in a more controlled fashion [3] (Figures 7–9). Summer's osteotome technique requires the use of malleting, and improper use of forceful malleting can lead to complications [4]. The Crestal Window Technique described here does not use any mallet, which enhances both the patient's comfort and the clinician's confidence.

One of the main limitations of conventional crestal approaches is that they require a minimal bone height of 5 mm [5]. In contrast, the Crestal Window Technique is easier on bone that is <5 mm in height.

Visualization and access to the sinus with Crestal Window's instruments are improved if bone height to sinus floor is within 1–4 mm. Therefore, with a combination of conventional crestal techniques and the Crestal Window Technique, all sinus cases can be successfully augmented without limitation of initial bone height [3].

Although debatable, it is our clinical opinion that a good amount of attached gingival should be present around the implant. This will aid in the patient's comfort performing oral hygiene and eliminate the sulcus opening when the patient functions (muscle pull). Therefore, whenever possible, insertion of healing abutment is recommended to aid in gaining keratinized tissue in one-stage surgery. However, if the initial stability is <20 Ncm or if poor bone quality is suspected, two-stage surgery is recommended to prevent movement of the implant during the healing phase [6]. But too much torque on the implant is not recommended. In this case, stability was too tight (>50 Ncm) and could lead to slight pressure necrosis of the crestal bone on the distal of #14 (Figures 18–21). During the surgery, the 4.3-mm drill was skipped and the final drill was 3.6 mm (for a 5-mm implant). This achieved great initial stability, but perhaps it was overtightened and reduced blood supply to the bone surrounding the implant.

One of the most common prosthetic failures of an implant is fractured porcelain. Although it can happen due to multiple factors, the main factor in our opinion is poor metal design [7]. A cutback from a full-contour wax-up guarantees uniform thickness of porcelain.

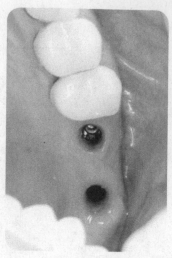

Figure 19: Removal of healing abutment from implant #14, 15.

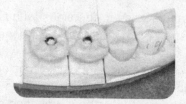

Figure 20: Full contour of wax-up to verify that technician will cut back to get uniform thickness of porcelain.

However, due to time constraints, many laboratory technicians use a "dipping technique" to wax up metal support for a PFM. This "dipping wax technique"

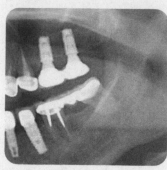

Figure 21: Digital panograph of implant #14, 15. Notice the satisfactory uniform thickness of porcelain on #14, 15 versus poor (too thick and irregular) on tooth #20. Note new sinus floor (new cortical bone) formation on top of implants and the disappearance of old cortical bone.

results in uneven thickness of porcelain and often very thick porcelain, which results in a crack/fracture. Therefore, we suggest always asking the technician to show a full-contour wax-up to verify that cutback is performed and thus guarantee uniform thickness of porcelain (Figure 20).

Radiographic evidence of successful sinus grafting can be evaluated 6–9 months after the surgery. The new sinus floor will be evident on a new radiograph. This represents a medullary bone sandwiched by two cortical bones (sinus floor and crestal bone) (Figure 20).

Self-Study Questions

A. What is the minimum bone height needed for the crestal technique?

B. What anatomic landmarks should be evaluated on a preoperative sinus CT scan?

C. What are the advantages/disadvantages of the Crestal Window Technique, Summer's osteotome, balloon technique, hydraulic sinus condensing, use of bone condensing drills, and the use of piezo tips?

D. How can you achieve good initial stability in maxillary posterior bone?

E. Why is the cutback technique so important in PM fabrication?

F. What is pressure necrosis of crestal bone, and how can you avoid it?

G. What is the radiographic evidence of successful sinus grafting?

Answers located at the end of the chapter.

References

1. Garg JN, Quinones CR. Augmentation of the maxillary sinus. A surgical technique. Pract Periodontics Aesthet Dent 1997;9:211–219.
2. Chen L, Cha J. An 8-year retrospective study: 1,100 patients receiving 1,557 implants using the minimally invasive hydraulic sinus condensing technique. J Periodontol 2005;76:482–491.
3. Lee S, Kang G, et al. Crestal sinus lift: a minimally invasive and systematic approach to sinus grafting. J Implant Adv Clin Dent 2009;1.
4. Sammartino G, Mariniello M, et al. Benign paroxysmal positional vertigo following closed sinus floor elevation procedure: mallet osteotomes vs screwable osteotomes. A triple blind randomized controlled trial. Clin Oral Implants Res 2011;22:669–692.
5. Bruschi GB, Scipioni A, et al. Localized management of the sinus floor with simultaneous implant placement: a clinical report. Int J Oral Maxillofac Implants 1998;13:219–226.
6. Torelli S, Bercy P. Incidence and primary prevention of complications related to the placement of dental implants. Rev Belge Med Dent (1984); 2001;56:35–61.
7. Cranham JC. Why porcelain breaks: ten factors to consider in the restorative process. Dawson Acad Vistas 2008;1:22–27.
8. Jensen OT. The Sinus Bone Graft Book. 2nd ed. Hanover Park, IL: Quintessence, 2006.

TAKE-HOME POINTS

A. In general, crestal or internal sinus lifts need at least 5 mm of initial bone height [8]. A minimum of 5 mm of bone is necessary due to poor access of an instrument into the sinus cavity, and clinicians must rely on the "bone pressure elevation" of the Schneiderian membrane. In contrast to conventional crestal approaches, the Crestal Window Technique described here requires *less* than 5 mm of initial bone height [3]. More than 5 mm of bone height reduces visibility to the sinus membrane and decreases access to the sinus cavity due to increased hindrance of instruments reaching the sinus walls. Figure 22 shows examples of 1-mm initial bone height versus 6 mm of initial bone height. Note that visibility and access to sinus is much easier for 1 mm of initial bone height.

B. A CT scan should be the standard of care before performing any sinus grafting procedures. Four anatomic landmarks should be evaluated prior to sinus surgery: (1) Patency of natural ostium, to make sure sinus is self-draining; (2) Thickness of sinus membrane or any pathology associated with it (polyp, cyst, inflammation); (3) location of intraosseous anastomosis of posterior superior alveolar artery; and (4) thickness of lateral wall, buccal-lingual dimension of alveolar bone, and initial bone height and quality of alveolar bone.

C. The Crestal Window Technique is not a blind technique in contrast to all other transalveolar techniques. The use of an osteotome can lead

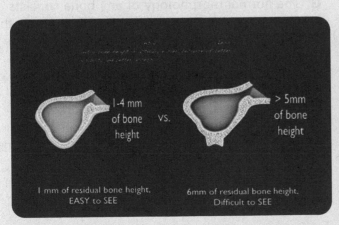
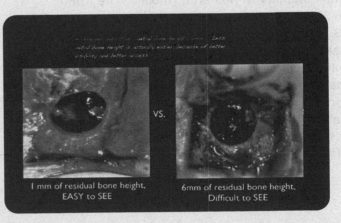

Figure 22: Crestal Window Technique is easier if initial bone height is less.

Table 1: Advantages and Disadvantages of all Internal Sinus Techniques

	Minimum Bone Height	Visibility of Sinus membrane	Access to Sinus	Cost	Vertigo Incidence
Crestal Window	<5mm	Good	Good	Moderate	None
Summer's osteotome	>5mm	Poor	Poor	Moderate	Low
Balloon	N/A	Poor	Poor	High	None
Hydraulic sinus condensing	N/A	Good	Poor	Moderate	None
Bone condensing drills	>5mm	Poor	Poor	moderate	None
Piezo tips	>5mm	Poor	Poor	High	None

to complications due to use of a mallet [4]. In contrast, the Crestal Window Technique uses a large diamond drill and the chances of benign vertigo are eliminated. Osteotome or other transalveolar techniques requires a minimum of 5mm initial bone height versus the Crestal Window Technique where it is easily achieved with only 1–4mm of initial bone height. The use of an osteotome or other transalveolar techniques relies on "bone pressure elevation" of membrane; therefore it is very difficult to fully elevate the buccal and palatal wall of the sinus. In contrast, the Crestal Window Technique uses small "cobra elevators" to manually lift the buccal and palatal wall of sinus (Table 1).

D. Three clinical tips are useful in achieving good initial stability in posterior maxilla. The bone quality in posterior maxilla is often very poor, D4 or D3. Therefore, a clinician should skip a drill (making a smaller osteotomy than he or she would in a mandibular bone). Second, selection of implant shape is very important. A wider platform than the body of implant is essential to get excellent initial stability from crestal bone. Third, a slow insertion of implant at a speed <20rpm is recommended to allow alveolar bone to expand.

E. The most common complication after implant therapy is porcelain fracture. It is usually due to poor metal design in a PFM restoration and a lack of sensation (feedback) upon biting hard substances. Uniform thickness of porcelain is crucial to ensure hardness of porcelain during function. Full-contour wax-up is necessary to do cutback, and clinicians should verify this prior to casting of metal framework [7].

F. Cortical bone (crestal bone) consists of Haversian canals to provide nutrients to osteocytes. If too much torque is applied during insertion of the implant, pressure necrosis will occur around the implant. You can avoid this by making proper osteotomy size to achieve 15–45 Ncm.

G. The normal morphology of any bone consists of medullary bone surrounded by cortical bone. In the case of maxillary alveolar bone, there is the sinus floor and the alveolar crest (two cortical plates). Disappearance of old sinus floor and appearance of new sinus floor after a sinus elevation procedure indicates success. This happens on average 6–9 months postsurgery depending on the shape of sinus, rate of healing of individuals, choice of bone graft materials, and initial bone height.

Case 3

Socket Grafting

CASE STORY

A 63-year-old Caucasian male presented with a chief compliant of: "My dentist referred me for periodontal treatment." The patient's dentist had observed 7- to 8-mm probing depths in a few teeth and referred him to the clinic for a periodontal consultation. The tooth (#5) had grade I mobility but exhibited no signs or symptoms (Figures 1–3).

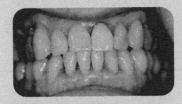

Figure 1: Preoperative presentation.

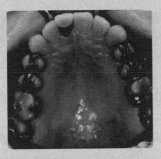

Figure 2: Preoperative maxillary dentition.

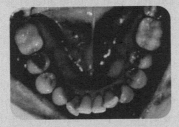

Figure 3: Preoperative mandibular dentition.

LEARNING GOALS AND OBJECTIVES

■ To understand the normal physiologic healing events after tooth extraction
■ To know the indications and contraindications for socket preservation
■ To understand the clinical procedures involved in socket preservation

Medical History

The patient had been diagnosed with osteoarthritis, and he took naproxen whenever he was in pain. He had undergone knee joint arthroscopy 4 years ago. On questioning, the patient reported no allergies to food or to drugs.

Review of Systems

- Vital signs
  - Blood pressure: 130/80 mm Hg
  - Pulse rate: 75 beats/minute (regular)
  - Respiration: 14 breaths/minute

Social History

The patient used to smoke tobacco and drink alcohol but quit smoking 20 years ago and quit drinking 30 years ago.

Extraoral Examination

No significant findings were noted. The patient had no masses or swelling, and the temporomandibular joint was within normal limits (Figure 4).

Intraoral Examination

- No abnormal findings with respect to tongue, floor of the mouth, palate, or buccal mucosa were observed.

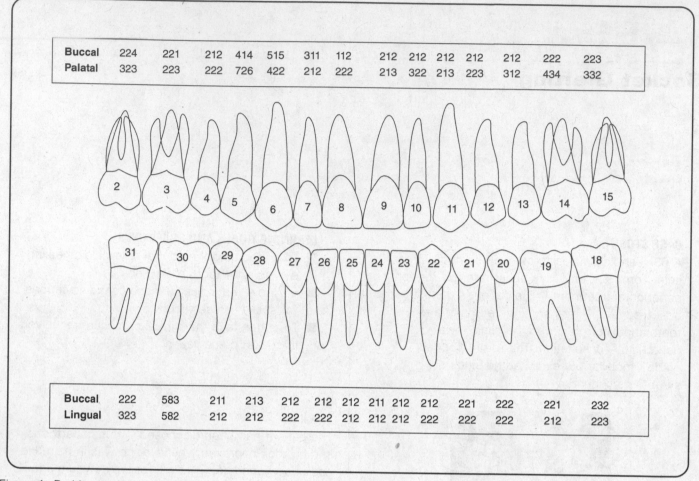

Buccal	224	221	212	414	515	311	112	212	212	212	212	212	222	223
Palatal	323	223	222	726	422	212	222	213	322	213	223	312	434	332

Teeth (upper): 2 3 4 5 6 7 8 9 10 11 12 13 14 15

Teeth (lower): 31 30 29 28 27 26 25 24 23 22 21 20 19 18

Buccal	222	583	211	213	212	212	212	211	212	212	221	222	221	232
Lingual	323	582	212	212	222	222	212	212	212	222	222	222	212	223

Figure 4: Probing pocket depth measurements during phase 1 revaluation.

- A gingival examination revealed mild marginal erythema, with localized areas of rolled margins and swollen papillae (Figures 1, 2, and 3).
- Periodontal charting was recorded (Figure 4). Teeth #5 and 30 exhibited probing pocket depths >6 mm. Tooth #5 exhibited furcation involvement and tooth #30 had class III furcation involvement.
- Grade 1 mobility was observed in tooth #5.
- The patient had generalized recessions that were asymptomatic, and the patient exhibited adequate attached gingiva.

Occlusion

There were no occlusal discrepancies or interferences.

Radiographic Examination

A full-mouth set of radiographs was ordered. Periapical radiographs of the involved area before and after the treatment are shown in Figure 5.

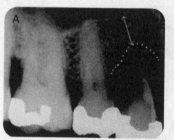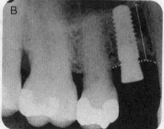

Figure 5: Periapical radiographs depicting severe bone loss (white dotted line) extending to the apical third of the root (left) and the improved bone volume after regenerating bone and the subsequent implant placement (right).

Diagnosis

The patient's history and his clinical and radiographic examinations clearly pointed to the diagnosis of localized severe chronic periodontitis. The bone loss in the proximal aspect of #5 was severe enough to involve the furcation. It was considered to have a hopeless prognosis and therefore was planned for extraction.

Treatment Plan

The treatment was planned in the following phases.

- The diagnostic phase included a comprehensive periodontal examination, radiographs, and study models.
- Disease control phase included oral hygiene instruction and prophylaxis.
- Surgical phase consisted of extractions of #5 and 30. Socket preservation of both the sites was then carried out.
- After adequate healing of the ridge, dental implants were placed in a prosthetically driven position using surgical stents and computed tomography (CT) (Figure 6) as guides.
- After an adequate period for osseointegration, implants were then loaded with prosthetic crowns. The patient was then placed on a maintenance program.

Treatment

The patient opted for a dental implant–supported single crown. Once the patient chose the implant option prior to extraction, the importance of socket preservation was explained to the patient. The patient agreed to the socket preservation procedure. Extraction of the tooth was carried out atraumatically using periotomes. Once the tooth was extracted out of the socket, the socket was degranulated and bone grafting was performed. A membrane was used to cover the bone graft material and the flap sutured over the membrane. The patient was given postoperative antibiotics and was seen after 2 weeks for postoperative follow-up (Figure 7). Another tooth that

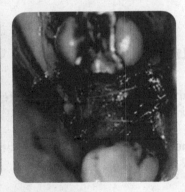

Figure 6: CT scan of the completely healed area in cross section depicting adequate bone width and height for the placement of a premolar area implant.

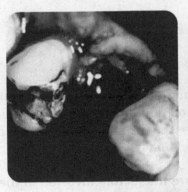
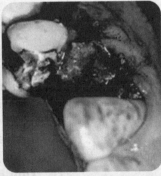
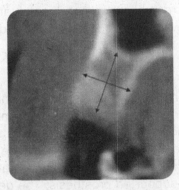
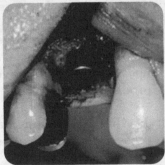
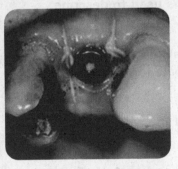

Figure 7: Socket (#5) soon after tooth extraction (top left) was packed with FDBA bone graft particles and covered with a membrane and flaps sutured on top of the membrane (top middle and top right). Implant placed after 8 months of healing (bottom left) and 10 days after surgery (bottom right).

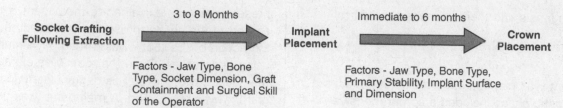

Figure 8: Treatment sequence following tooth extraction that requires implant-supported prosthesis and the factors affecting the duration of each stage.

had severe periodontal breakdown in this patient was #30. It was also extracted and the socket was also grafted with freeze-dried bone allograft (FDBA) and covered by a resorbable collagen membrane. A molar size implant was later placed in the healed bone after 7 months.

Discussion

Extraction of hopeless teeth is a very common procedure performed by dentists. Following single or multiple extractions, various options exist to replace the missing teeth including fixed partial dentures (if adjacent teeth are present), removal partial dentures, or an implant-supported prosthesis. The decision to graft the bony socket after extraction is critical and should be based on the future treatment option planned for the particular site and the location of the site. If an implant-supported prosthesis is planned for a particular site, maximum effort should be made to preserve the bone starting from atraumatic extraction to bone grafting. Apart from the bone loss that exists in a periodontally compromised tooth, the bone loss that occurs after tooth extraction will certainly impose challenges in maintaining bone for future implant placement.

Apart from aiding in implant installation in a prosthetically driven position, implant success depends highly on the peri-implant bone thickness. Another indication for socket preservation is in anterior sextants, where aesthetics is an important consideration and bone grafting in anterior sockets can help maintain the aesthetically favorable tissue bulkiness, even in cases where fixed partial dentures are planned (Figure 8).

Self-Study Questions

A. Describe the events involved in socket healing after tooth extraction.

B. What is the rationale for doing socket preservation?

C. What are the other terms used to describe socket preservation?

D. What are the biomaterials used to do socket preservation and the rationale for choosing the materials?

E. How would you perform the socket preservation procedure?

F. What are the indications and contraindications for the socket preservation procedure?

G. How long do you have to wait after socket preservation and before implant placement, and how successful are the implants placed in augmented bone?

H. What are the factors involved in the successful outcome of socket preservation procedures?

I. What are the postoperative complications associated with socket preservation and the necessary postoperative care required after the procedure?

J. What are the drawbacks of doing socket preservation procedures?

Answers located at the end of the chapter.

References

1. Araujo M, Lindhe J. The edentulous alveolar ridge. In: Clinical Periodontology and Implant Dentistry. 5th ed. Oxford, UK: Blackwell Munksgaard. Chapter 2, pp57–62.
2. Pietrokovski J, Massler M. Ridge remodeling after tooth extraction in rats. J Dent Res 1966;46:222–231.
3. Lekovic V, Camargo PM, et al. Preservation of alveolar bone in extraction sockets using bioabsorbable membranes. J Periodontol 1998;69:1044–1049.
4. Schropp L, Wenzel A, et al. Bone healing and soft tissue contour changes following single-tooth extraction: a clinical and radiographic 12-month prospective study. Int J Periodontics Restorative Dent 2003;23:313–323.
5. Trombelli L, Farina R, et al. Modeling and remodeling of human extraction sockets. J Clin Periodontol 2008;35:630–639.
6. Cardaropoli D, Cardaropoli G. Preservation of the postextraction alveolar ridge: a clinical and histologic study. Int J Periodontics Restorative Dent 2008;28:469–477.
7. Aimetti M, Pigella E, et al. Clinical and radiographic evaluation of the effects of guided tissue regeneration using resorbable membranes after extraction of impacted mandibular third molars. Int J Periodontics Restorative Dent 2007;27:51–59.
8. Nevins M, Camelo M, et al. Human histologic evaluation of mineralized collagen bone substitute and recombinant platelet-derived growth factor-BB to create bone for implant placement in extraction socket defects at 4 and 6 months: a case series. Int J Periodontics Restorative Dent 2009;29:129–139.
9. Fickl S, Zuhr O, et al. Dimensional changes of the alveolar ridge contour after different socket preservation techniques. J Clin Periodontol 2008;35:906–913.
10. Ackermann KL. Extraction site management using a natural bone mineral containing collagen: rationale and retrospective case study. Int J Periodontics Restorative Dent 2009;29:489–497.
11. Bartee BK. Extraction site reconstruction for alveolar ridge preservation. Part 1: rationale and materials selection. J Oral Implantol 2001;27(4):187–193.
12. Fowler EB, Breault LG. Ridge augmentation with a folded acellular dermal matrix allograft: a case report. J Contemp Dent Pract 2001;2:31–40.
13. Bartee BK. Extraction site reconstruction for alveolar ridge preservation. Part 2: membrane-assisted surgical technique. J Oral Implantol 2001;27(4):194–197.
14. Amler MH, Johnson PL, et al. Histological and histochemical investigation of human alveolar socket healing in undisturbed extraction wounds. J Am Dent Assoc 1960;61:32–44.
15. Boyne PJ. Osseous repair of the postextraction alveolus in man. Oral Surg Oral Med Oral Pathol 1966;21:805–813.
16. Ohta Y. Comparative changes in microvasculature and bone during healing of implant and extraction sites. J Oral Implantol 1993;19:184–198.
17. Hämmerle CH, Chen ST, et al. Consensus statements and recommended clinical procedures regarding the placement of implants in extraction sockets. Int J Oral Maxillofac Implants 2004;19(Suppl):26–28.
18. Fugazzotto PA. Success and failure rates of osseointegrated implants in function in regenerated bone for 72 to 133 months. Int J Oral Maxillofac Implants 2005;20:77–83.
19. Kohal RJ, Mellas P, et al. The effects of guided bone regeneration and grafting on implants placed into immediate extraction sockets. An experimental study in dogs. J Periodontol 1998;69:927–937.

TAKE-HOME POINTS

A. Tissue healing following extraction of a tooth is a highly orchestrated event ultimately leading to bone formation in the open bony socket. Soon after tooth extraction, blood clot formation occurs, leading to a seal of the open wound with blood coagulum. The platelets form a plug sealing the blood vessels that are damaged during tooth removal. Neutrophil and macrophages then enter the clot and engulf foreign products or bacteria and make the wound sterile. The blood clot is then subsequently replaced by granulation tissue formation. The granulation tissue is composed predominantly of collagenous extracellular matrix produced by the mesenchymal cells as well as blood vessels sprouting (angiogenesis) into the wound by a process called neovascularization. Mesenchymal cells from the periodontal ligament remnants or the surrounding bone enter the granulation tissue and get differentiated into bone-forming osteoblasts. The osteoblasts lay down the collagen (predominantly type 1) rich osteoid, which gets mineralized to form woven bone. By a process of bone remodeling, the woven bone is then replaced with mature lamellar bone and marrow. By 21 days reepithelialization begins, which will be completed in 6 weeks. It takes an average of 6 weeks for both soft tissue and hard tissue healing to complete [1].

B. One of the serious consequences of tooth extraction is the bone resorption that follows that prevents future implant placement. Studies have shown clearly that extraction of either single or multiple teeth leads to topographical changes in the alveolar ridge. It was shown that the resorption of bone in the buccal surface is significantly more pronounced than the palatal or lingual surface [2]. Without bone grafting, it was shown that in the first 6 months, 40% of the alveolar bone height and 60% of the alveolar bone width will be lost [3]. Bone resorption progresses significantly faster in maxilla, compared with mandible, and the degree of resorption is directly proportional to the time since the tooth was extracted.

Using subtraction radiography, authors [4] have shown that after extraction of the tooth, some bone loss occurs in the initial few months, with some bone gain occurring up to 6 months following extraction. Remodeling of the bone occurs between 6 and 12 months leading to an overall reduction in the amount of mineralized tissue. Moreover, there exists a considerable individual variability in the capacity to form new bone in the extraction socket [5].Therefore it is important to preserve as much bone as possible soon after extraction by doing socket preservation, which allows the placement of dental implants in the ideal prosthetically favorable positions. Doing socket preservation at the time of extraction prevents future interventions required to build bone (prior to dental implant placement) that are more invasive, expensive, and time consuming as well as having a lower degree of predictability. Socket status soon after extraction can range from a complete intact socket to the loss of one or two walls (due to surgical trauma, periodontal defect, dehiscence, or previous apical surgery). Although several studies have strongly indicated the benefits of doing bone grafting at the time of extraction in all forms of postextraction socket defects [6–8], socket preservation is shown not to avoid the postoperative contour shrinkage completely [9].

C. *Socket grafting, ridge preservation,* and *socket augmentation* are some of the terms used interchangeably to describe socket preservation.

D. Socket preservation typically uses scaffold and a membrane. Scaffolds most commonly used in this procedure are bone grafts. The bone grafts used for socket preservation can range from osteogenic autogenous bone particles and osteoconductive materials such as FDBA particles to osteoinductive materials such as demineralized version of freeze-dried bone (DFDBA) particles and morphogens such as bone morphogenetic proteins (BMPs). Alloplastic materials such as hydroxyapatite, which are poor osteoconductive materials, can be used in some clinical scenarios. Recent studies indicate that bone mineral containing collagen is a favorable material for socket preservation [10]. Currently, BMP-2 protein delivered in an absorbable collagen sponge (Infuse) is approved by the U.S. Food and Drug Administration for socket preservation procedures. Apart from BMP-2, recombinant PDGF-BB is shown to enhance bone formation in extraction sockets prior to implant placement [8].

Membranes are commonly used to prevent the highly proliferating epithelial cells to enter the defect, thereby allowing the osteogenic cells to synthesize bone in and around the scaffold used [11]. For socket preservation procedures, bioresorbable membranes such as collagen membranes (Bio-Gide, Ossix, etc.) are commonly used. Collagen with different degree of cross-linking is shown to have different resorption profiles, providing a range to membranes to choose from for different clinical situations. Other option is to use a nonresorbable membrane such as expanded polytetrafluoroethylene membrane (Gore-Tex). The extent and morphology of the defect are some of the factors that dictate the selection of nonresorbable versus resorbable membrane [11]. Recent studies have shown that acellular dermal matrix allograft (AlloDerm), which is commonly used for soft tissue procedures in periodontics, can be used as a membrane for socket preservation procedures [12].

The selection of bone graft for socket preservation should be based exclusively on the clinical situation and the established resorption profile of a graft material. Alloplastic materials such as dense hydroxyapatite (HA) or bioactive glass are generally used for long-term ridge preservation (in sites where implants are not planned) because these materials are poorly osteoconductive with a low resorption capacity. In areas where implants are planned, biomaterials that allow transitional ridge preservation with good resorption profile should be selected. Synthetic materials such as resorbable HA and xenografts such as bovine anorganic bone grafts can be used in such clinical scenarios. For short-term ridge preservation, DFDBA or a combination of autogenic bone with other graft materials like DFDBA or xenografts can be used [11].

E. Socket preservation initially was performed using hydroxyapatite in the form of the root-shaped cones. Currently, the socket preservation is mostly performed using bone grafts and a membrane. The procedure starts with atraumatic extraction, followed by complete debridement (curetting) of the socket and then grafting the socket with the bone graft particles. After the bone graft particles are placed in the socket, a barrier membrane is placed over the bone graft to contain or stabilize the graft particles and also to prevent epithelial ingrowth into the defect, which will prevent bone regeneration. After obtaining adequate anesthesia, buccal and lingual/palatal flaps are reflected to allow tugging of the membrane after bone grafting. Flap reflection also increases the clinician's visibility while doing extractions. Applications of periotomes or physics forceps and/or tooth sectioning are the commonly used techniques to remove the tooth atraumatically from the socket. Once the tooth is extracted, the socket should be inspected for any remaining granulation tissue, periodontal ligament, or periradicular cysts. The intactness of the socket walls, especially the buccal wall, which is usually thin, should be evaluated. Bone graft particles are hydrated in saline as per instructions. Once the socket is degranulated and cleaned, well-hydrated bone graft particles taken in a bone syringe or a periosteal elevator are incrementally placed into the socket and subsequently condensed. Prior to bone grafting, decortication of the socket cortical bone may be performed, to allow migration of the bone

precursors from the subcortical trabecular bone into the defect [13]. Appropriate membrane with adequate length to cover the socket should be selected and trimmed in such a way that 3–4 mm of the membrane extends beyond the socket margin into sound host bone. The membrane is then placed over the bone graft particle, tugging it underneath the buccal and lingual flaps. Any wrinkling or folding of the membrane should be avoided. The flaps are positioned to cover the membrane as much as possible and sutured in place. Complete primary closure is not an absolute requisite for this procedure. Interrupted sutures should be placed in the two adjacent interdental papilla, and a horizontal mattress suture can be used in the socket area. The patient will be seen after 2 weeks for the postoperative visit, during which remaining sutures will be removed [13].

F. As previously mentioned, socket preservation is beneficial in a variety of defects ranging from a socket lacking the buccal bone completely to a socket with all walls intact. Therefore if implant is planned in an area that requires extraction, socket preservation should be an important consideration during extraction. On the contrary, animal studies have shown that sockets with intact walls do not require bone grafting and have the inherent potential for socket defect bone formation [14–16].

Acute dental infection in the form of an abscess, sinus, or fistula associated with the tooth that needs extraction is an absolute contraindication for socket preservation. Failure rate of bone grafting procedure in the presence of active bacterial infection is very high. In such cases, extraction should precede grafting. Following extraction and debridement, the patient should be placed on antibiotics for 1–2 weeks and after initial healing, the site can be reopened and socket preservation should be performed using a similar approach to the one previously described.

G. How long the clinician has to wait following socket preservation and prior to implant placement depends on various factors that include the extent and topography of the bony defect, surgical skill of the operator, type of bone graft utilized, and the type of membrane used. For example, the type of bone graft used tends to have a huge influence on the time it takes for the bone regeneration to occur because different bone grafts tend to have different resorption profiles. A consensus report published by Hämmerele et al in 2004 [17] classifies the implant placement after extraction into four types based on the length of time from extraction to implant placement. The type 4 (>16 weeks) protocol allows the placement of dental implants in clinically healed bone. With the addition of another biomaterial such as bone grafts in the extraction socket, a wait of 6–12 months is considered adequate prior to implant placement. With respect to the predictability of dental implants, studies have clearly indicated that the success rate of implants placed on augmented bone (>95%) is highly comparable with implant placed on native bone [18]. The torque required to remove dental implants placed in bone-grafted sites versus nongrafted sites was shown to be highly comparable [19].

H. Case selection: Both site and patient selections are important to the success of any periodontal procedure. Patients with no relevant medical conditions and a negative history of smoking tend to have better outcome than a patient who is a chronic smoker as well as a person with uncontrolled diabetes.

1. Initial socket morphology: The greater the number of wall of the socket present, the greater the regeneration
2. Surgical skills of the operator: Soft tissue management and proper suturing to prevent graft loss
3. The type of bone graft used: autogenous versus osteoconducive materials

I. Flap opening due to loss of sutures:
1. Membrane exposure and loss of graft particles
2. Infection
3. Fibrous encapsulation
Postoperative regimen:
1. Antibiotic: Amoxicillin 500mg tid for 7 days or clindamycin (in penicillin-allergic patients)
2. Pain medications: With or without codeine
3. Chlorhexidine mouth rinse

J. Longer healing period is required, prior to implant placement, compared with regular extraction socket healing:
- Invasive and technique-sensitive procedure
- Need to place the patients on a postoperative antibiotic regimen (development of antibiotic resistance)
- Additional cost
- Soft tissue dehiscence defects frequently observed in bone grafted sites compared with nongrafted sites

Case 4

Ridge Split and Osteotome Ridge Expansion Techniques

Case 4A

CASE STORY
A 53-year-old female was referred from her prosthodontist for a consultation for dental implant placement and restoration in her upper right edentulous area (Figures 1 and 2). The patient's chief complaint was the inability to properly masticate food due to the loss of multiple posterior teeth.

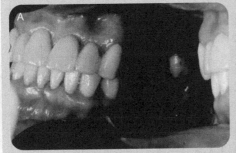
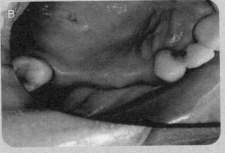
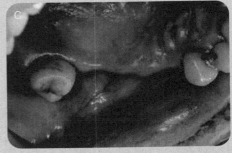

Figure 1: Preoperative clinical presentation of maxillary right quadrant. (A) Buccal view; (B), occlusal view; (C) palatal view.

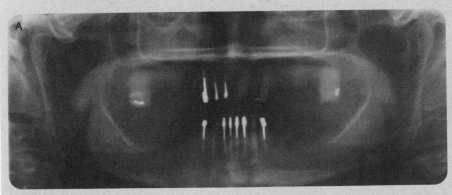
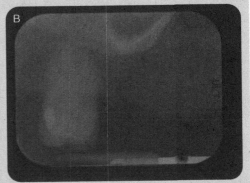

Figure 2: Preoperative radiographs. (A) panoramic radiograph; (B) periapical radiograph.

LEARNING GOALS AND OBJECTIVES

■ To identify the indications and rationales for the ridge split procedure

■ To understand the surgical technique for ridge split with or without simultaneous implant placement

■ To understand the presurgical and postsurgical considerations

Medical History

The patient's medical history was not significant. The patient was not taking any medications and denied having any allergies.

Review of Systems

• Vital signs
  ○ Blood pressure: 128/76 mm Hg
  ○ Pulse rate: 68 beats/minute
  ○ Respiration: 14 breaths/minute

Social History

The patient did not smoke cigarettes but occasionally drank alcohol during social events. The patient denied ever having used recreational drugs. The patient brushed twice a day and flossed at least once a day.

Extraoral Examination

No significant findings were present.

Intraoral Examination

• Oral cancer screening was negative. Soft tissues including buccal mucosa, hard and soft palate, floor of the mouth, and tongue all appeared normal.

• There was an adequate amount of attached keratinized gingiva present on all of the remaining teeth.

• The patient had excellent oral hygiene with minimal amounts of plaque accumulation and localized mild gingival inflammation.

• A full periodontal charting was completed (Figure 3).

• There was some mild clinical attachment loss with no probing depths >3 mm, no tooth mobility, and no furcation involvement.

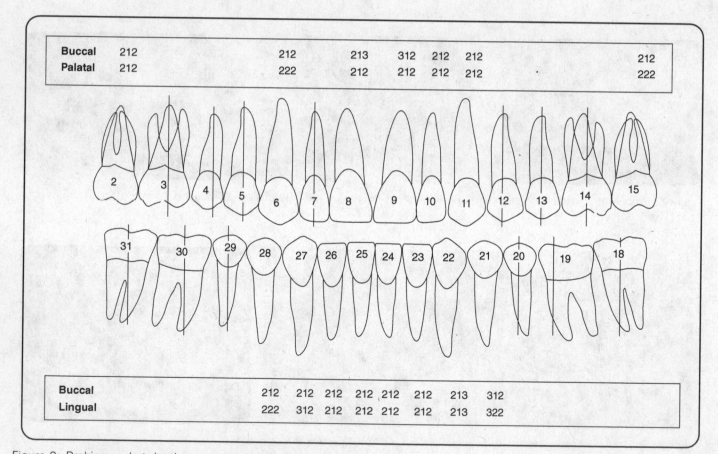

Buccal	212			212	213	312	212	212				212
Palatal	212			222	212	212	212	212				222

Buccal	212	212	212	212	212	212	213	312
Lingual	222	312	212	212	212	212	213	322

Figure 3: Probing pocket depth measurements during initial visit.

- The patient was partially edentulous and was missing teeth #1, 3, 4, 5, 7, 12, 13, 14, 16, 17, 18, 19, 20, 29, 30, 31, and 32. All the remaining teeth were temporized.
- A Seibert class I defect was present on maxillary right quadrant.

Occlusion

The patient had Angle's class I canine occlusion. The patient was wearing maxillary and mandibular removable partial dentures for posterior occlusal support. No occlusal interferences and fremitus were detected.

Radiographic Examination

There was no evidence of periapical radiolucencies and pathologic lesions (Figure 2). With respect to edentulous sites #3, #4 and #5, preoperative computed tomography (CT) scan revealed mainly an insufficient horizontal ridge dimension for implant placement, although site #3 also exhibited slight bone loss in vertical dimension (Figure 4).

Diagnosis

A diagnosis of localized chronic mild periodontitis was given based on the clinical and radiographic examinations.

Treatment Plan

Based on the periodontal and prosthodontic evaluation, guided bone regeneration (GBR) using a split ridge technique was recommended for edentulous sites #3, 4, and 5. After 6 months, a postoperative CT scan will be taken to evaluate the amount of bone generated. If adequate amount of bone is present, three implants at sites #3, 4, and 5 will be placed. Each implant will be restored with single unit crown 4–6 months after implant placement. Soft tissue manipulation will be done to ensure adequate amount of attached keratinized gingival around each implant.

Treatment

The patient was encouraged to continue practicing good oral hygiene. A wax-up of the edentulous sites #3, 4, and 5 was done by the prosthodontist to outline the ideal implant position and angulation.

Ridge Split Procedure

One day preoperatively, the patient was given a 6-day regimen of Medrol Dosepak (methylprednisolone with a start of 24 mg /day, tapering by 4 mg/day over 6 days per package instructions) to reduce the anticipated swelling and inflammation associated with the surgery. After achieving local anesthesia, a palatal-crestal incision was made from mesial of #2 to distal of #6 with intrasulcular incisions around #2 and #6. No vertical incisions were made. Full-thickness flap was raised using periosteal elevators to expose the native bone. Clinically, there was in general about a 2- to 3-mm ridge width present at the crest at edentulous sites #3, 4, and 5 (Figure 5A). To preserve as much crestal bone as possible, a ridge split was initiated by using a sharp #15 blade. Specifically, the midcrestal bone was first scored using the #15 blade to delineate the line of the split. Then it was used as a "chisel" in combination with a mallet to start the split. As shown in Figure 5B, the #15 blade was inserted apically to about 6–7 mm between the buccal and palatal plates. Caution was taken to avoid breaking the sinus floor while splitting the ridge. A chisel was then used to continue the split to push the two cortical plates buccally and palatally (Figure 5C). Figure 5D shows the ridge after the split. To widen and maintain the split at the crest of the ridge, surgical screws were used to push the buccal cortical plate buccally, resulting in about a 3- to 4-mm crestal split between the two cortical plates (Figure 5E). A few tenting screws were then inserted through the buccal cortical plate to maintain the space for augmenting bone on the buccal aspect of the resorbed ridge (Figure 5F). A mixture of freeze-dried bone allograft (FDBA) and Bio-Oss was packed on the buccal aspect of the ridge defect as well as between the two split cortical plates. A bioresorbable collagen barrier membrane was used to cover the bone grafting material (Figure 5G). The buccal flap was advanced coronally to allow for tension-free primary closure. The surgical site was then sutured with a few horizontal mattress and multiple single-interrupted sutures (Figures 5H and I). Hemostasis was achieved, and postoperative instructions and an ice pack were given to the patient. Amoxicillin (500 mg tid for 7 days), chlorhexidine 0.12% mouthwash (bid for 7 days), and ibuprofen (800 mg every 6 hours as needed) were prescribed.

Sutures were removed 2 weeks postoperatively, and the soft tissues at the surgical site were healing well with no signs of infection (Figure 5J). Two months postoperatively, the surgical site appeared healthy, and clinically there was evidence of augmentation at sites #3, 4, and 5 (Figure 5K). The area was temporized with a fixed provisional prosthesis.

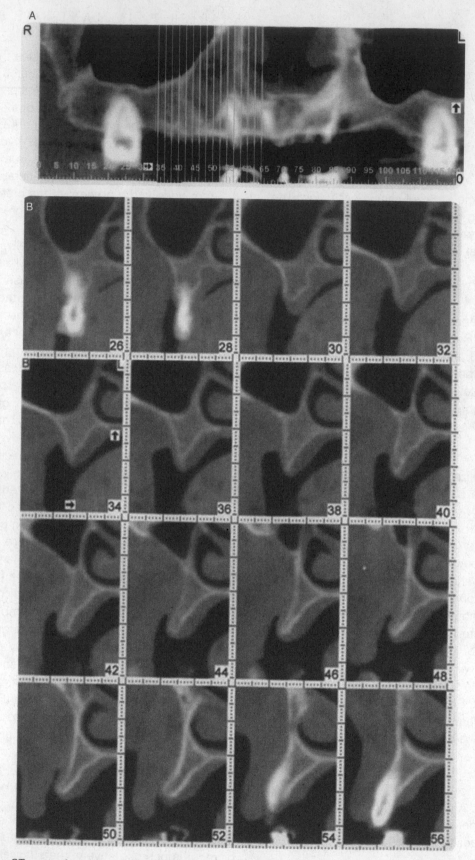

Figure 4: Preoperative CT scan of maxillary right quadrant. (A) Panoramic view; (B) lateral slice cross-sectional view for edentulous sites #3, 4, and 5.

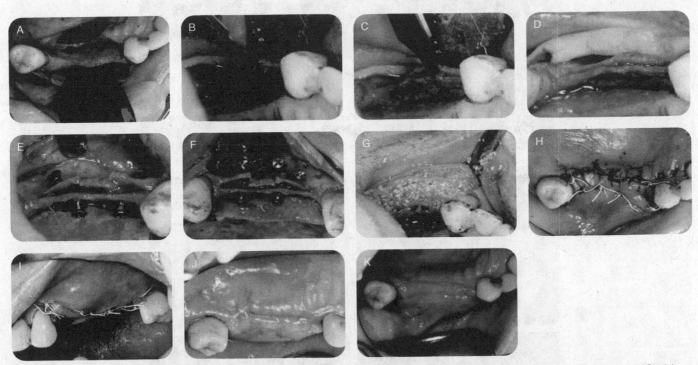

Figure 5: Ridge split at sites #3, 4, and 5. (A) Residual native bone prior to ridge split; (B) ridge split using #15 blade; (C) ridge split using chisel; (D) ridge after the split; (E) surgical screws used to increase and maintain the split between buccal and palatal plates; (F) tenting screws used on the buccal aspect of the ridge to maintain space for buccal ridge augmentation; (G) bone grafting materials and barrier membrane in place; (H) occlusal view of primary closure of the surgical site; (I) buccal view of primary closure of the surgical site; (J) 2-week postoperatively at surgical site; (K) 2-month postoperatively at surgical site.

A CT scan was taken 6 months postoperatively with the patient wearing the radiographic stent indicating the proposed ideal implant position. The CT scan showed a tremendous amount of bony augmentation, on average 5 mm, on the buccal aspect of the previously resorbed alveolar ridge (Figure 6).

Clinically, there was a significant amount of bone regenerated at the ridge split area 6 months after ridge augmentation (Figures 7A and B). Three Straumann tissue level implants 4.1 × 10 RN, 4.1 × 10 RN, and 4.8 × 10 WN were placed at sites #3, 4, and #5, respectively (Figures 7C–F).

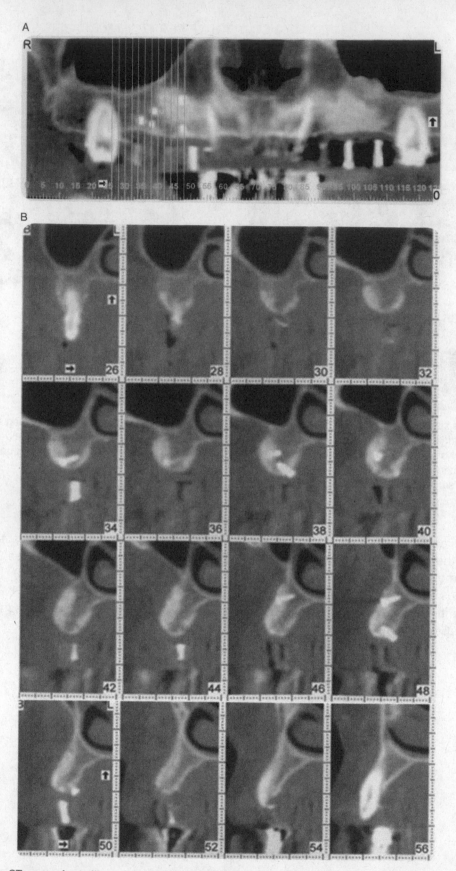

Figure 6: Postoperative CT scan of maxillary right quadrant. (A) Panoramic view; (B) lateral slice cross-sectional view for edentulous sites #3, 4, and 5.

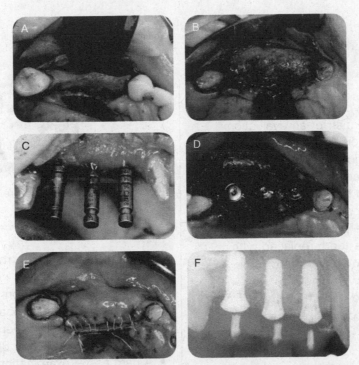

Figure 7: Ridge augmented site and implant placement. (A) Preaugmented alveolar ridge; (B) alveolar ridge 6 months after augmentation; (C) implant guide pins showing the implant position at sites #3, 4, and 5; (D) implant placement in alveolar ridge; (E) occlusal view of primary closure of the surgical site; (F) periapical radiograph showing implant placement in alveolar ridge.

Case 4B

CASE STORY

The patient was a 48-year-old female who was referred by the prosthodontist for an evaluation for an implant placement on #9; she had had the tooth extracted 2 years ago. There was an existing ridge deformity and the referring clinician had been worried there was not sufficient bone in the buccolingual direction for an implant placement. The patient's chief complaint was to have the tooth replaced with an implant and a single crown and restore the maxillary anterior sextant with single ceramo-metal crowns. Figures 1 to 4 illustrate the clinical situation at the first periodontal examination.

LEARNING GOALS AND OBJECTIVES

- To identify the indications and rationale for osteotome ridge expansion
- To understand the surgical technique for ridge expansion with or without simultaneous implant placement
- To understand the presurgical and postsurgical considerations

Medical History

The patient was healthy and received a medical examination every year. She did not take medications and did not report any allergies or any medical problems.

Review of Systems

- Vital signs
  - Blood pressure: 125/75 mm Hg
  - Pulse rate: 60 beats/minute (regular)

Social History

The patient did not drink alcohol; she did not smoke and denied ever having used recreational drugs.

Extraoral Examination

No significant findings were noted. The patient had no masses or swelling and the temporomandibular joints were within normal limits.

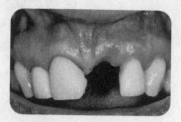

Figure 8: Preoperative picture.

Intraoral Examination

- The soft tissues of the mouth appeared normal. The oral cancer screen was negative.
- The gingival examination in the maxillary anterior sextant revealed a thick and flat periodontium with localized mild marginal erythema, rolled margins, and blunted papillae (Figure 8).
- A hard tissue examination had been completed by the prosthodontist; who had found enough sound tooth structure available for the prosthetic restoration of teeth #7, 8, 10, and 11.
- A periodontal examination was completed by the periodontist and all probing depths were within normal limits of 2–3 mm and clinical attachment level <2 mm with no bleeding on probing.
- The edentulous ridge on site #9 had a ridge deformity in the buccolingual direction (Seibert class 1).

Occlusion

The canine and molar relationships were Angle class 1. There was posterior group function in lateral excursion, anterior guidance in protrusion, and 1 mm of overbite with 2 mm of overjet in the anterior sextant. No fremitus or interferences were detected.

Radiographic Examination

There was no evidence of periapical radiolucencies, horizontal or vertical bone loss, and the lamina dura was visible and continuous (Figure 9).

Treatment Plan

Periodontal, prosthodontic, and endodontic evaluations were performed to assess the restorability of the teeth. The multidisciplinary team deemed the teeth restorable with ceramometal crowns and without endodontic treatment for teeth #7, 8, and 10, a ridge augmentation procedure for the edentulous area of #9

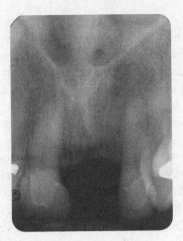

Figure 9: Radiograph.

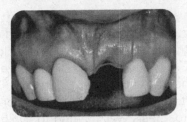

Figure 10: The incision design.

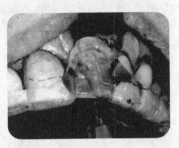

Figure 11: The full-thickness flap reflection with the surgical guide in place and the 2-mm twist drill in the correct prosthetic position.

followed by a single-tooth replacement for #9, with an implant-retained ceramometal crown.

Treatment

The patient received oral hygiene instructions and a prophylaxis. A wax-up of the anterior sextant was done by the prosthodontist as well as a fabrication of a surgical guide.

Preoperative Consultation

The medical history was reviewed. Clinical and radiographic examinations were performed. The amount of remaining native bone was determined by bone sounding after local infiltration of anesthesia in the edentulous area of #9. Alternatively, a CT scan could have been taken to determine more accurately the existing bone dimensions. It was determined that the existing buccolingual dimension of the edentulous ridge was approximately 4 mm in width and sufficient to place a 4-mm implant fixture with a simultaneous ridge augmentation procedure or ridge expansion. A consent form addressing benefits and risks associated with the procedure was reviewed with the patient. Preoperative prescriptions were delivered to the patient: ibuprofen 600 mg (every 4–6 hours as needed for pain), Peridex 0.12% (bid), and amoxicillin 500 mg (tid for 7 days starting the night prior to procedure).

Ridge Expansion Procedure

Anesthesia of the maxillary anterior sextant was achieved by a local infiltration with lidocaine 2% (epinephrine 1/100,000). A surgical incision was made on the palatal-crestal edentulous ridge of #9 with a vertical releasing incision on the mesiobuccal line angle of #10 and a vertical releasing incision preserving the papillae along the frenum on the mesiobuccal line angle of edentulous #9 (see outline in Figure 10).

A full-thickness flap elevation was done to expose the crestal bone, and the surgical guide was placed to determined the optimum prosthetic implant position, which guided the initial 2-mm twist drill to final length for the initial implant osteotomy (Figure 11).

After the initial osteotomy of 2 mm, the remaining bony wall from the buccal was about 1 mm and the palatal aspect about 1.5 mm in thickness; because the desired implant fixture was 4 mm in diameter, two drilling sequences for the final osteotomy needed to be performed; however, if performed, the risk of a full dehiscence or complete destruction of any of the remaining bony walls was evident. Thus a 2.5-mm tapered osteotome was inserted into the 2-mm osteotomy and tapped to final length (Figure 12A). Although there was a fenestration on the apical extent on the buccal side due to the normal ridge concavity, the coronal bony wall remained intact. A 3-mm tapered osteotome was then inserted and tapped to final length, followed by a 3.5-mm osteotome, also tapped to final length (Figure 12B). A 4.2-mm diameter by 10-mm tapered implant fixture was then placed into the expanded osteotomy to a 35 Ncm torque with primary stability (Figure 13A). An FDBA was placed on the buccal aspect to cover the existing fenestration and to augment the remaining buccal bone (Figure 13B). A resorbable cross-linked bovine collagen membrane was placed over the bone graft (Figure 13C). A tension-free flap was repositioned and secured in placed with sutures obtaining primary closure (Figure 13D). A radiograph was taken to verify the position of the implant fixture (Figure 14). Full clearance in the area of #9 of the transitional removable prosthesis was created to avoid any pressure on the surgical site.

Postoperative instructions including oral hygiene were delivered, and an ice pack was placed against the patient's lip.

The patient was seen for a postoperative consultation at 14 days for suture removal, and then after 1, 3, and 6 months (Figure 15). After 6 months of healing and osseointegration time, implant was exposed in a stage 2 procedure using an apically repositioned flap procedure where implant stability was tested and a healing abutment was placed (Figure 16).

After 4 weeks, the healing abutment was replaced by a final prosthetic ceramic abutment on implant #9 torqued at 35 Ncm, and adjacent #7, 8, and 10 were prepared for a final single-unit crown restoration (Figure 17). Two weeks later, the final restorations on these teeth were delivered and the final restorations for all mandibular anterior teeth completed (Figure 18).

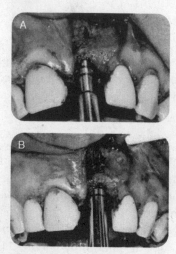

Figure 12 (A, B): The sequential osteotome expansion.

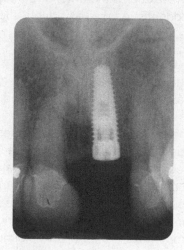

Figures 14: Postoperative radiograph.

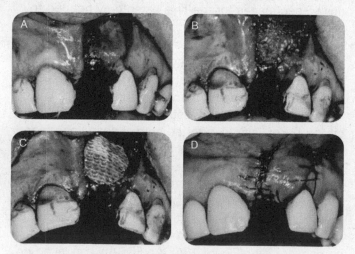

Figures 13 (A–D): Steps followed after the osteotome expansion was completed: implant placement (A), FDBA placement (B), collagen membrane adapted (C), and primary closure and suturing (D).

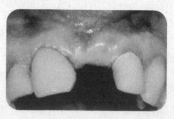

Figure 15: Healing response 6 months postoperatively.

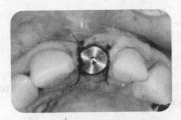

Figure 16: Implant exposure and healing abutment by means of an apically repositioned flap.

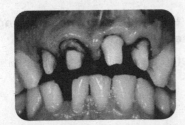

Figure 17: Placement of a full ceramic aesthetic abutment on implant #9 and final preparation of teeth #7, 8, and 10.

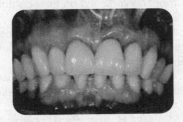

Figure 18: Final delivery of permanent restorations and the completion of the case.

Discussion

A clinician can choose from a variety of treatment modalities to provide dental implant therapy for alveolar ridge deformities. With respect to the cases presented here, the choices for treatment may include a GBR procedure and a subsequent implant placement or implant placement with simultaneous bone grafting of the remaining bony walls or implant surfaces, among others. Ultimately, the choice of treatment relies on the amount of native bone remaining as well as the clinical expertise of the clinician. In case 4A, a ridge split technique was performed without simultaneous implant placement due to a considerable amount of buccal concavity at the edentulous site and the amount of bone remaining on the crest of the alveolar ridge (2–3 mm), which was insufficient to obtain implant stability. A ridge split technique was used in conjunction with a bone graft expecting the native bone to provide containment and stability of the bone grafting material a well as to supply osteogenic cells needed for bone regeneration

(see question B for advantages on ridge split procedure).

In contrast, in case 4B the remaining amount of native bone was sufficient to provide the primary stability of the implant; in this case the osteotome expansion allowed the preservation of the buccal and palatal native bone that otherwise would have been drilled away if a standard implant placement protocol was followed. Although the bone expansion allowed for the preservation of the native bone, the remaining buccal wall was thinner than the suggested 1.5–2 mm outlined in the literature; thus the need of bone graft material to increase the buccal bone width was evident.

When discussing the specifics of each approach, one could argue the use of different instrumentation to achieve the desired goal; for instance, in case 4A, a #15 blade was used as a chisel in conjunction with a light tapping with a mallet to initiate the split and to preserve as much bone as possible. Alternatively, one could have used bone chisels, piezo surgical tips, or a bone saw. However, it is necessary to keep in mind that the thinner the bone-cutting instrument, the better preservation of the native bone is attained. In case 4B, the initial 2-mm twist drill was used to initiate the osteotomy followed by a sequential use of the osteotome; conversely, one could have considered the use of bone expanders that come in a shape of slightly tapered threaded, and noncutting drilling bits and in different diameters that attach to a handpiece or to a hand ratchet. One could argue that the tapping of the osteotome at the time of the expansion could be more traumatic for the patient and the bone itself than with the use of the expanding bits; although the according to the literature, both are equally successful. In either case the direction of the osteotome or expanding bits is critical because the implant will follow the direction of the expanded osteotomy.

Like other guided bone regeneration surgeries, the success of a ridge split or expansion procedures depends on the medical status of the patient for an optimal host response, the availability of osteogenic cells from the surgical site, the vascularity of the surgical site, the stability and the turnover rate of the bone graft materials, the epithelial exclusion through a barrier membrane, and the soft tissue management to achieve primary closure. Factors that would lead to less favorable results are infection, absence of primary closure, sloughing of flap edges with soft tissue dehiscence, loss of bone graft materials, and lack of implant stability if implants are simultaneously placed [1,2].

Self-Study Questions

A. What is the purpose of doing ridge split and osteotome ridge expansion, and when should one consider a staged approach or simultaneous placement of a dental implant?

B. What are the advantages and indications for doing ridge split or ridge expansion?

C. What are the disadvantages, limitations, and complications associated with ridge split and ridge expansion?

D. Describe Seibert's classification system for alveolar ridge defect.

E. How are ridge split and osteotome ridge expansions performed?

F. What are the criteria needed for doing ridge split and osteotome ridge expansion?

Answers located at the end of the chapter.

ACKNOWLEDGMENT
Special thanks to Dr. Jacob Pourati for his contribution to this chapter.

References

1. Coatoam GW, Mariotti A. The segmental ridge-split procedure. J Periodontol 2003;74:757–770.
2. Machtei EE. The effect of membrane exposure on the outcome of regenerative procedures in humans: a meta-analysis. J Periodontol 2001;72:512–516.
3. Donos N, Mardas N, et al. Clinical outcomes of implants following lateral bone augmentation: systematic assessment of available options (barrier membranes, bone grafts, split osteotomy) [review]. J Clin Periodontol 2008;35(8 Suppl):173–202.
4. Tonetti MS, Hämmerle CH; European Workshop on Periodontology Group C. Advances in bone augmentation to enable dental implant placement: Consensus Report of the Sixth European Workshop on Periodontology. J Clin Periodontol 2008;35(8 Suppl):168–172.
5. Flanagan D. Labyrinthine concussion and positional vertigo after osteotome site preparation. Implant Dent 2004;13:129–132.
6. Kaplan DM, Attal U, et al. Bilateral benign paroxysmal positional vertigo following a tooth implantation. J Laryngol Otol 2003;117:312–313.
7. Peñarrocha M, Pérez H, et al. Benign paroxysmal positional vertigo as a complication of osteotome expansion of the maxillary alveolar ridge. J Oral Maxillofac Surg 2001;59:106–107.
8. Seibert JS. Reconstruction of deformed, partially edentulous ridges, using full thickness onlay grafts. Part I. Technique and wound healing. Compend Contin Educ Dent 1983;4:437–453.
9. Rambla-Ferrer J, Peñarrocha-Diago M, et al. Analysis of the use of expansion osteotomes for the creation of implant beds. Technical contributions and review of the literature. Med Oral Patol Oral Cir Bucal 2006;11:E267–271.

TAKE-HOME POINTS

A. Both ridge split and osteotome ridge expansion procedures are surgical approaches used to augment atrophic edentulous alveolar ridges to generate adequate amount of bone for implant placement (see previous chapters for discussion on other types of bone grafting procedures).

A ridge split is usually performed over a larger span of the edentulous area rather than a single-tooth site. In ridge split, implants can either be placed concomitant with the procedure or at a later time, depending on the size of the ridge defect, the presence of implant primary stability, and the appropriateness of the anticipated implant angulation.

In an osteotome ridge expansion, an implant is usually placed simultaneously with ridge expansion because the implant is needed to maintain the expansion. In both cases the bone is subject to fractures or microfractures; the traumatic events will initiate a bone healing response and the preservation of as much native bone as possible will aid in the osteoprogenitor cells availability for the regeneration of the defect and the added bone graft material.

B. Among the factors for a predictable ridge split procedure for alveolar ridge augmentation is the concept that the bone grafting material is placed in a well-contained, "four-wall" defect between the two cortical bony plates. This four-wall defect will also provide sufficient number of osteogenic cells needed for bone regeneration [3,4].

Ridge split and ridge expansion techniques allow simultaneous implant placement in an atrophic alveolar ridge that otherwise would not have been possible. Note that ridge expansion technique is almost always done with simultaneous implant placement.

Unlike onlay bone grafting procedures, ridge split and ridge expansion procedures do not require a second surgical site to harvest a block of autogenous bone. Hence these procedures reduce the morbidities associated with bone harvesting.

Comparing this technique with a procedure when an implant is placed over a thin shell of cortical plate or a bony dehiscence that require additional bone grafting, ridge split and ridge expansion techniques are more advantageous because a minimal amount of bone is lost during the procedures. Often times, a lesser amount of bone grafting materials is required during simultaneous implant placement.

C. Performing a ridge split or ridge expansion procedure can produce a traumatic event in the bone, and thus depending on the surgical experience of the clinician and the nature of the patient's bone quality, splitting or expanding the alveolar ridge may sometimes result in unintentional fracture or displacement of cortical plate(s), which may lead to bone necrosis of the displaced segment. In certain areas of the mandible where the cortical bone is denser with lower plasticity and the alveolar ridge is too thin, usually <3 mm, a ridge split procedure represents a higher risk and may not be recommended. In addition, tapping on the alveolar ridge using a surgical mallet may be unpleasant for patients. An uncontrolled force applied during these procedures could also damage anatomic structures such as nerves, arteries, and facial spaces, among others, so caution must be exercised and therefore site and case selection are important. Typically an osteotome ridge expansion is not recommended in the mandible, so alternative expansion techniques should be considered like the use of expansion bits as outlined in the discussion. Although chisels could be used for a mandibular ridge split, when addressing a surgical site in the mandible one should also consider alternative instrumentation.

Other side effects that patients may develop as a result of these procedures and that have been reported in the literature include postoperative nausea, vomiting, and dizziness. In more serious situations, patients may develop benign paroxysmal positional vertigo and labyrinthine concussion due to traumatic percussion from tapping [5–7]. These complications are self-limiting and usually last for several days to a week. Finally, local paresthesia, transitional or permanent, could occur due to the nature of the instrumentation and the damage to nerves that are in close proximity to the surgical site.

D. Seibert's classification of alveolar ridge defect [8]:
- Class I defect: Buccolingual loss of tissue with normal ridge height in apico-coronal dimension
- Class II defect: Apico-coronal loss of tissue with normal ridge width in buccolingual dimension
- Class III defect: Combined buccolingual and apico-coronal loss of tissue resulting in loss of normal ridge height and width

E. *Ridge split:* The operator should make a soft tissue incision slightly palatal or lingual to midcrest where the ridge will be split. After raising a full-thickness flap and removing all the soft tissue tags, the operator will determine the extent of alveolar ridge defect. Should the defect qualify for ridge split, the procedure can then be started. First, use a sharp chisel or a #5 blade to score a line along the crest of the alveolar ridge. The score line should come no closer than 2mm from the adjacent teeth [1]. Deepen the entire score line to about 3mm by using a surgical mallet to gently tap on the flat end of the chisel. Continue deepening the entire score line until desired depth has been reached. Alternatively, the score line can be made by using piezo surgical tips. Piezosurgery offers ease in making the initial score line; however, about 1mm of crestal bone will be lost when using piezo surgery because the piezo surgical cutting tips is itself about 1mm in thickness. Depending on the preference of the clinician, bony vertical releases at the two ends of the crestal bony incision/split line can then be made. Gently separate the two cortical plates of the split ridge as much as possible by twisting the chisel while preventing the fracture of the bony plates to maintain bone vitality. If the surgical site allows for the simultaneous placement of the implant, prepare the implant osteotomy utilizing the drilling sequence that best fit the split to the desired diameter and length. However If only bone grafting procedure is desired, place the bone grafting material between the two cortical plates. In some situations surgical screws can be used in a buccopalatal/lingual direction to maintain the space created between the two cortical plates. A membrane barrier may be used prior to the closure of the flaps. It is crucial to achieve tension-free primary closure to ensure optimal bone grafting results.

Ridge expansion with osteotomes: Ridge expansion is usually performed in conjunction with implant placement and is similar to performing osteotome sinus elevation [9]. After a full-thickness flap elevation is achieved, a surgical guide is used to determine the optimal position of the implant fixture; then a 2-mm twist drill is used to final length to obtain the initial implant osteotomy.

After the initial osteotomy of 2mm, it is necessary to determine the amount of residual buccal and palatal bone remaining and the diameter of the desired implant fixture, accounting for an optimal buccal and palatal bone width of 1.5–2mm prior to the final insertion of the implant. Insert and tap into final length a 2.5-mm osteotome, remove and repeat procedure with the 3-mm osteotome; continue with the same sequence until the final diameter of the desired implant fixture minus 0.5mm has been achieved. Place implant and ensure primary stability. If any of the remaining bony walls are less than 1.5–2mm in width, place a bone graft material on the bony surface, cover it with a barrier membrane, and ensure tension-free primary flap closure or proceed with a stage I implant.

F. Ridge split:
- It can be done for individual in the mandible or maxilla.
- A minimum of 3mm of existing bone is needed
- Usually performed in large edentulous areas but it can be done for single-tooth edentulous sites for as long as the split is kept at 2mm from the adjacent teeth
- Beware of the limitations outlined in question C
  Ridge expansion:
- It can be done for individual or multiple implant sites
- A minimum of 4mm of existing native bone is needed
- Limited to maxillary sites when utilizing osteotomes. However if performing an expansion in mandibular edentulous sites, consider the used of expansion bits instead of osteotomes as previously described
- Beware of the limitations outlined in question C

8

Dental Implants

Clinical Cases in Periodontics, First Edition. Nadeem Karimbux.
© 2012 John Wiley & Sons, Inc. Published 2012 by John Wiley & Sons, Inc.

Case 1

Conventional Implant Placement

CASE STORY

A 38-year-old Caucasian male presented with a chief compliant of: "I need a cleaning and also I have a tooth missing." The patient had not had a teeth cleaning in 3 years (Figure 1), and tooth #19 had been extracted elsewhere 18 months ago (Figure 2) due to extensive caries (Figure 3). The patient claimed to brush his teeth two to three times daily. He flossed once a day but denies use of any mouth rinse.

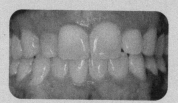

Figure 1: Preoperative frontal view.

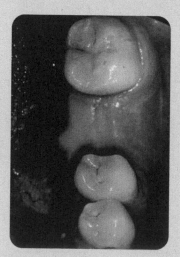

Figure 2: Missing mandibular first molar area.

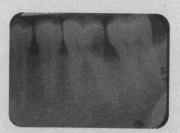

Figure 3: Tooth #19 was extracted due to large distal caries.

LEARNING GOALS AND OBJECTIVES

- To understand the indications of implant treatment
- To interpret radiographic examinations for implant surgical planning
- To understand the sequence of conventional implant therapy

Medical History

The patient was prehypertensive but had no other significant medical problems and no known allergies. Occasionally the patient took diphenhydramine hydrochloride (Benadryl) for seasonal allergy.

Review of Systems

- Vital signs
  - Blood pressure: 138/86 mm Hg
  - Pulse rate: 67 beats/minute (regular)

Social History

The patient was a social drinker (three to four glasses per weekend). Currently he did not smoke, but he had a history of social smoking for 1 year during college.

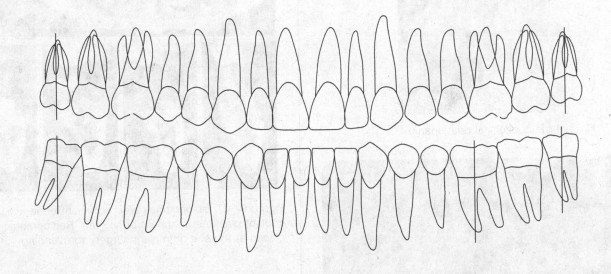

Buccal	323	323	323	313	323	323	222	212	212	213	322	213	224	323
Palatal	333	323	323	323	323	223	212	212	212	222	323	323	313	322

Buccal	322	323	223	324	323	223	222	233	313	323	313	323	323
Lingual	223	323	312	313	213	212	212	212	313	323	312	223	322

Figure 4: Probing pocket depth measurements.

Extraoral Examination

No significant findings were noted. The patient had no masses or swelling and the temporomandibular joint was within normal limits (Figure 4).

Intraoral Examination

- There was no lymphadenopathy and oral cancer screen was negative.
- There was an adequate band of attached gingiva. Stippling was present.
- A hard tissue and soft tissue examination was completed (Figures 4–6).

Occlusion

The patient presented normal molar relationship and no interference in excursive movements (Figure 7).

Radiographic Examination

There were no caries or significant crestal bone loss seen on examination of the bite-wing radiographs (Figure 8).

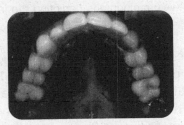

Figure 5: Occlusal view of the maxillary arch.

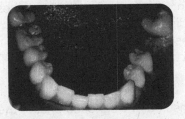

Figure 6: Occlusal view of the mandibular arch.

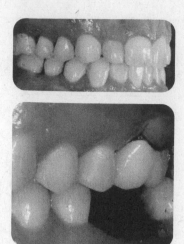

Figure 7: Normal molar occlusal relationship.

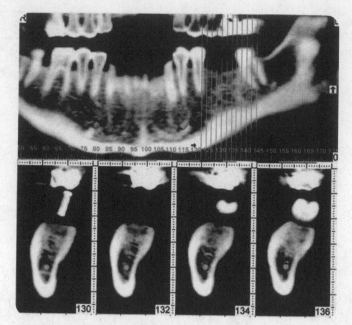

Figure 9: CT radiographs reveal sufficient bone available for implant placement without bone graft. Radiographic guide is placed at the site of implant surgery for planning.

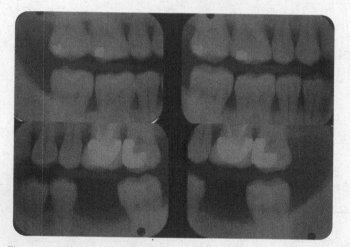

Figure 8: Bite-wing radiographs depicting the interproximal bone levels.

A computer tomographic (CT) image (Figure 9) revealed the presence of available bone >15 mm in height and sufficient width for wide diameter implant placement. Therefore no bone graft was necessary for implant placement (Figure 9).

Diagnosis

The patient had partial edentulism and was diagnosed as American Dental Association type I due to gingivitis.

Treatment Plan

The treatment plan for this patient includes an initial phase of scaling with polishing and implant-supported porcelain fused to metal (PFM) crown for the area of #19.

Treatment

After the consult and diagnostic phase, the patient received initial therapy of scaling and polishing. The patient was able to maintain good oral hygiene in follow-up visits. Study models of maxillary and mandibular arch were fabricated to evaluate adequate spacing of area #19. The mesiodistal space of missing molar #19 area was compatible with the contralateral molar. A radiographic template was fabricated before sending the patient for CT evaluation. The CT revealed adequate quantity of bone and healing of extraction site with normal pattern of trabeculation.

The patient refused the alternative treatment option of a three-unit fixed partial denture #18-X-20 because the virgin abutment teeth would require preparation. A step-by-step description of implant therapy was discussed including possible complications. A consent form was obtained prior to the procedure.

On the day of the procedure, the patient's blood pressure was measured, and it was in a similar range of hypertensive level as the initial visit. Local infiltration anesthesia was given in the surgical area with lidocaine 2% (epinephrine 1:100,000). A full-thickness flap was raised after midcrestal incision. A surgical template was used to guide sequential drilling with copious irrigation to prepare the site for implant placement (Figure 10). One-stage implant of 4.8 × 10 mm and a wide neck platform for prosthesis connection was placed (Figure 11). The implant was clinically stable and a short healing abutment was screwed in (Figures 12 and 13). A periapical radiograph

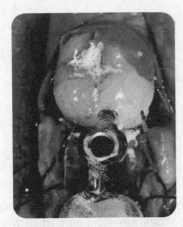

Figure 10: A surgical template was used to guide angulations of drills.

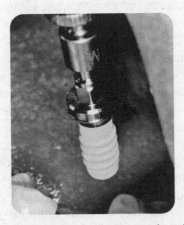

Figure 11: A wide diameter implant was placed in the molar region.

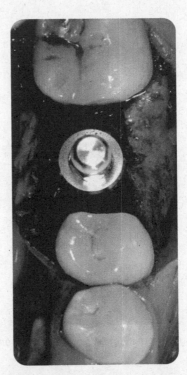

Figure 12: Implant placed in the molar area with appropriate angulation and distance from adjacent teeth.

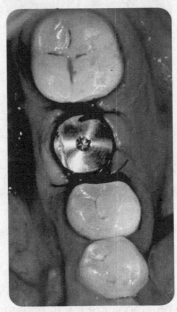

Figure 13: A short healing abutment placed and sutured for primary closure.

confirmed appropriate implant angulation and a safe distance from the inferior alveolar nerve. Flaps were sutured for primary closure. Minimum bleeding was observed before the patient left. Postoperative instructions were given. The patient received prescriptions for pain medication and an oral rinse.

One week later, sutures were removed and soft tissue was healing normally. Minimum postoperative discomfort was reported.

The prosthetic phase of the case was initiated 2 months after the surgery. An impression coping was attached for closed final impression using polyether. An appropriate shade was selected for porcelain fabrication. The favorable implant position allowed for selection of a prefabricated straight abutment (Figure 14).

Four weeks after the final impression, final implant-supported PFM was cemented (Figure 15). A periapical radiograph was taken as a baseline for future reference. Oral hygiene instruction was reinforced

and the patient was scheduled for recall visit every 6 months.

Discussion

Implant-supported restorations have become routine treatment in dental practice with predictable outcome

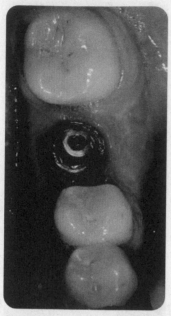

Figure 14: A straight prefabricated final abutment was used for restoration.

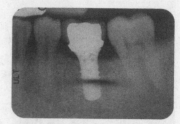

Figure 16: Postoperative periapical radiograph.

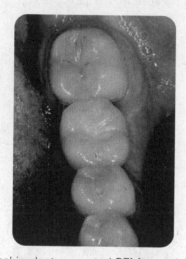

Figure 15: Final implant-supported PFM was delivered.

and a high success rate [1]. However, the prevention aspect should be emphasized with patients so loss of tooth due to caries or periodontal disease may be minimized. Effective oral home care including fluoride with periodic professional visits is crucial for appropriate prevention and early detection of oral disease.

The initial therapy of oral prophylaxis and compliance of oral home care is an important factor before considering implant therapy [2]. Once the

implant option is chosen, study models and radiographic images are used as part of the planning. The planning should be done with the final outcome in mind. Various radiographic examinations may be prescribed such as conventional two-dimensional (2D) panoramic or computer tomography, which has the advantage of three-dimensional analysis of anatomic structures with minimum distortion [3]. When the radiographic template has the appropriate angulation, the same device may be used as a surgical template. If incorrect angulation is detected in the radiograph, appropriate modification should be made before the surgery.

In radiographic analysis, important anatomic structures should be identified. Ideally in the maxilla, implants should not penetrate the maxillary sinus space. In the mandible, the apex of implants should be 2 mm away from the inferior alveolar nerve or the mental foramen. Convergence of roots should be also be evaluated, especially in patients with a history of orthodontic treatment to avoid damaging root structure during implant placement. Implant diameter is selected to give appropriate support and emergence profile for the size of the crown. However, there should be a space of approximately 2 mm from implant to root surface [4].

Once the implant is placed, a certain period of time is necessary for healing and osseointegration. Branemark originally suggested a healing time of 4 months for the mandible and 6 months for the maxilla [5]. Recent advances in bone biology and implant designing have allowed a shortening of the waiting time from implant placement and final delivery of crown with predictable results [6]. In limited cases, it is also possible to extract the tooth, place the implant, and restore it all in the same day [7].

After final delivery of the restoration, the patient should be in strict recall protocol for professional oral hygiene and radiographic reevaluation.

Self-Study Questions

A. Is there any age limitation to place a dental implant?

B. What kind of radiographs could be ordered for an implant case planning?

C. What are the advantages and disadvantages of implant treatment compared with conventional fixed-partial denture (FPD)?

D. What is the difference between the one-stage and two-stage implant approach?

E. What are the possible postoperative complications in the short and long term?

Answers located at the end of the chapter.

References

1. Adell R, Eriksson B, et al. Long-term follow-up study of osseointegrated implants in the treatment of totally edentulous jaws. Int J Oral Maxillofac Implants 1990;5:347–e59.
2. Wennström JL, Ekestubbe A, et al. Oral rehabilitation with implant-supported fixed partial dentures in periodontitis-susceptible subjects. A 5-year prospective study. J Clin Periodontol 2004;31:713–724.
3. Harris D, Buser D, et al; European Association for Osseointegration. E.A.O. guidelines for the use of diagnostic imaging in implant dentistry. A consensus workshop organized by the European Association for Osseointegration in Trinity College Dublin. Clin Oral Implants Res 2002;13:566–570.
4. Buser D, Martin W, et al. Optimizing esthetics for implant restorations in the anterior maxilla: anatomic and surgical considerations. Int J Oral Maxillofac Implants 2004;19:43–61.
5. Branemark PI, Hansson BO, et al. Osseointegrated implants in the treatment of the edentulous jaw. Experience from a 10-year period. Scand J Plast Reconstr Surg Suppl 1977;16:1–132.
6. Bornstein MM, Schmid B, et al. Early loading of non-submerged titanium implants with a sandblasted and acid-etched surface. 5-year results of a prospective study in partially edentulous patients. Clin Oral Implants Res 2005;16:631–638.
7. Misch CE, Hahn J, et al. Workshop guidelines on immediate loading in implant dentistry. Immediate Function Consensus Conference. J Oral Implantol 2004;30:283–288.
8. Op Heij DG, Opdebeeck H, et al. Age as compromising factor for implant insertion. Periodontol 2000 2003;33:172–184.
9. Park SH, Wang HL. Implant reversible complications: classification and treatments. Implant Dent 2005;14:211–220.

TAKE-HOME POINTS

A. There is no upper age limit for implant placement as long as the patient fulfills the prerequisites for general surgery. However, an implant placed in a young patient may work as an ankylosed structure and interfere with the growth of facial bones [8]. In general, growth spurt occurs at the age of 12 years for girls and 14 for boys. However, the craniofacial/skeletal growth may continue further, and individual variation could be up to 6 years of difference. Therefore the chronological age is not sufficient to estimate growth cessation. A more reliable test would be superimposing tracings of cephalometric radiographs taken at least 6 months apart and determining the growth cessation.

B. Bite-wing, periapical, and panoramic radiographs are the most common radiographic techniques in the dental setting. Bite wing is not appropriate for implant planning because it only shows a limited range of the crestal bone area. A periapical radiograph may be used in limited cases, but it may fail to show anatomic sites such as the maxillary sinus and inferior alveolar nerve. Panoramic radiograph has the advantage of showing a large area, but it has greater distortion than a periapical radiograph. Because it is a superimposed 2D image, bone width cannot be determined. The CT scan is the ideal radiograph for planning since it is a three-dimensional image with minimum distortion. CT images can also be applied to software to fabricate computer-generated surgical templates.

C. The greatest advantage of a dental implant is that the preparation of neighboring teeth is avoided. The physiological stimulation to the alveolar bone through the dental implant also prevents further bone loss. In cases where distal abutment is absent, a dental implant may be the only alternative to deliver a fixed prosthesis option. However, treatment length for an implant may be longer compared with conventional FPD, and patients may reject the idea of having surgical intervention, especially when it requires the additional steps of bone grafting.

D. Traditionally, implants were designed to be closed with the soft tissue at the time of implant placement. After a period of healing, implants would be uncovered by placing a healing abutment at the second stage. This two-stage approach would require a second surgical intervention and further waiting time for soft tissue maturation.

Other implants are designed with a longer neck; therefore soft tissue would be adapted around it instead of covering the implant at the time of placement. This one-stage approach eliminates the necessity of a second surgical intervention to expose the implant. Two-stage designed implants can be used as one-stage approach by inserting a healing abutment at the time of implant placement.

E. Some of the intraoperative surgical-related complications are as follows [9]:
- Damage of adjacent teeth
- Lack of primary stability
- Hemorrhage
- Nerve injury
- Penetration of sinus floor
- Fracture of mandible

Careful planning and knowledge of anatomy are important to avoid these types of complications. Minor complications such as a small perforation of sinus floor may not require removal of implants, and antibiotics and a decongestant may help to avoid complications. Complications such as nerve injury and fracture of the mandible require immediate removal of implant, and further treatment should be considered.

These are the postoperative surgical-related complications:
- Incision line opening
- Prolonged pain

- Fistula and abscess
- Peri-implantitis

Even if sutures are loosen earlier that expected, it may not require resuturing. If pain persists longer than usual period, the dentist should suspect overheating during drilling preparation or carefully evaluate for possible anatomlc injuries. Abscess and fistula may occur when cover screws become loose. Debridement of implant surface in conjunction with an antibiotic may be necessary in case of infection; even implant removal may be indicated in more advanced peri-implantitis.

Case 2

Immediate Implant Placement

CASE STORY
A 24-year-old Caucasian female presented with a chief compliant of: "My front tooth is changing color." The patient noted discoloration following traumatic injury as a child. This tooth was later treated endodontically, and the patient had been told in subsequent visits that the tooth had a fair prognosis. There had never been any swelling or pain associated with the change in color. The patient claimed to brush her teeth three times a day and to visit her dentist regularly (Figure 1).

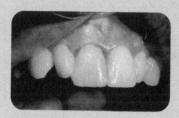

Figure 1: Preoperative presentation. Tooth #8 is discolored.

LEARNING GOALS AND OBJECTIVES
■ To be able to decide when and where an extraction and immediate Implant placement can be planned
■ To understand the advantages/disadvantages of immediate implant placement
■ To understand the possible complications and outcomes of immediate implant placement

Medical History
There were no significant medical problems; however, the patient reported an allergy to penicillin. She had no known medical illnesses and exercised regularly. On questioning the patient stated that she took no medications except for birth control pills.

Review of Systems
• Vital signs
  ○ Blood pressure: 118/75 mm Hg
  ○ Pulse rate: 76 beats/minute (regular)
  ○ Respiration: 15 breaths/minute

Social History
The patient did not drink alcohol and did not smoke (B).

Extraoral Examination
No significant findings were noted. The patient had no masses or swelling, and the temporomandibular joint was within normal limits.

Intraoral Examination
• The soft tissues of the intraoral mucosa, gingiva, palate, and tongue appeared normal.
• The gingival examination revealed a normal gingival architecture including the gingival margins and interdental papillae.
• Moderate mobility was noticed on tooth # 8 with an enamel fracture line extending to the gingival margin.
• Mild tenderness to apical percussion was noted.

Occlusion
The patient demonstrated class I occlusion with slight drifting of the two central incisors buccal and

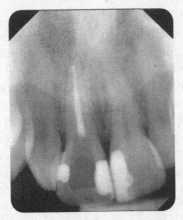

Figure 2: A periapical radiograph of the maxillary anteriors.

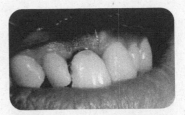

Figure 3: Preoperative view of tooth #8.

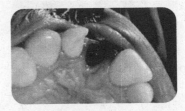

Figure 4: View following the extraction.

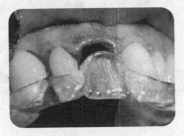

Figure 5: The surgical guide.

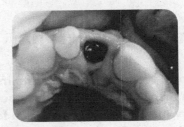

Figure 6: Implant placed.

downward. The interincisal relationship showed an overbite with no occlusal discrepancies or interferences (C).

Radiographic Examination

A single periapical film was ordered. On radiographic examination it was determined that tooth #8 had endodontic treatment and loss of the tooth structure of the crown. No periapical radiolucency was seen (Figure 2).

Diagnosis

After reviewing the history and completing the clinical and radiographic examination, a differential diagnosis was generated.

Treatment Plan

The treatment plan is extraction of tooth #8 followed by immediate implant insertion (D) and a temporary crown. Following the osseointegration period, a permanent crown can be fabricated (E).

Treatment

Anesthesia was achieved via infiltration buccal and lingual for the purpose of hemostasis and analgesia. Tooth #8 was extracted atraumatically. During the extraction the crown separated from the root, due to a horizontal tooth fracture (Figure 3). The root was retrieved using small elevators and periotomes to preserve the integrity of the extraction socket walls (Figure 4). Following the extraction the socket was examined and showed no granulation tissue. Using the consecutive drills the implant osteotomy was completed utilizing the surgical stent as a guide (Figure 5). The osteotomy was planned to be approximately

2 mm beyond the apical portion of the extraction socket and 2–3 mm subgingivally (Figure 6). The implant was torqued to 35 Ncm and a periapical film was taken that showed a good position of the implant in relationship to the neighboring teeth and good clearance from the incisive foramen and the floor of the nasal sinuses (Figure 7). A temporary abutment was placed and restored with a provisional crown (Figure 8). Incisal occlusion was adjusted to avoid excessive forces on the implant crown, and the patient was advised to avoid biting on hard objects. Postoperative instructions were given. The patient tolerated the procedure very well. She was alert with no signs of distress upon dismissal (F).

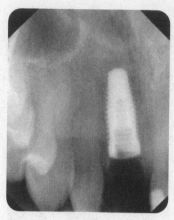

Figure 7: Postoperative radiograph.

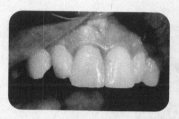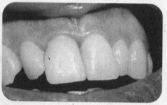

Figure 8: Preoperative and postoperative view of tooth #8.

Discussion

In this case the patient was conscious about abnormal changes that took place in her dentition following trauma. Early diagnosis and treatment will impact the treatment outcome. If no treatment was rendered, an infection could eventually develop that would alter the treatment plan. Antibiotics would have to be prescribed followed by a follow-up visit to determine the best treatment options based on the extent of the infection and the amount of remaining bone to host an implant with or without the need for bone augmentation. Another treatment option would be an extraction followed by the fabrication of a fixed or removable prosthesis.

The initial stability of the immediate implant placement is crucial for the survival afterward of the implant. This can only be accomplished by placement of the implant beyond the apical portion of the extraction socket and torqued as recommended by the implant manufacturer. The atraumatic extraction will aid in the preservation of the bone to host the implant. Finally, the placement of the implant and the provisional crown subgingivally will help preserve the interdental papillae for the best aesthetic results.

Self-Study Questions

A. List the local reasons why patients might present with discolored teeth. What questions in a dental history might help you begin to form a differential diagnosis?

B. What effects can smoking have on dental implants?

C. Can occlusal discrepancies and parafunctional habits be responsible for tooth fracture?

D. What are the factors to consider when recommending immediate implants?

E. What are other treatment options should be considered in this case?

F. What are the possible complications associated with immediate implant placement in the anterior region?

Answers located at the end of the chapter.

References

1. Chung EM, Sung EC. Dental management of chemoradiation patients. J Calif Dent Assoc 2006;34:735–742.
2. Kidd EA, Joyston-Bechal S, et al. Staining of residual caries under freshly-packed amalgam restorations exposed amalgam to tea/chlorhexidine in vitro. Int Dent J 1990;40:219–224.
3. Billings RJ, Berkowitz RJ, et al. Teeth. Pediatrics 2004;113:1120–1127.
4. Doyle SL, Hodges JS, et al. Factors affecting outcomes for single implants and endodontic restorations. J Endod 2007;33:399–402.
5. Proceedings of the Fourth International Team for Implantology (ITI) Consensus Conference. Int J Oral Maxillofac Implants 2009;(24 Suppl): 39–65.
6. Udoye CI, Jafarzadeh H. Cracked tooth syndrome: characteristics and distribution among adults in a Nigerian teaching hospital. J Endod 2009;35:334–336.
7. Cohen S, Berman LH, et al. A demographic analysis of vertical root fractures J Endod 2006;32:1160–1163.
8. Thompson BA, Blount BW, et al. Treatment approaches to bruxism. Am Fam Physician 1994;49:1617–1622.
9. De Rouck T, Collys K, et al. Single-tooth replacement in the anterior maxilla by means of immediate implantation and provisionalization: a review. Int J Oral Maxillofac Implants 2008;23:897–904.
10. Kan JY, Rungcharassaeng K, et al. Immediate placement and provisionalization of maxillary anterior single implants: 1-year prospective study Int J Oral Maxillofac Implants 2003;18:31–39.
11. Casado PL, Donner M, et al. Immediate dental implant failure associated with nasopalatine duct cyst. Implant Dent 2008;17:169–175.
12. Casap N, Zeltser C, et al. Immediate placement of dental implants into debrided infected dentoalveolar sockets. J Oral Maxillofac Surg 2007;65:384–392.
13. Artzi Z, Nemcovsky CE, et al. Displacement of the incisive foramen in conjunction with implant placement in the anterior maxilla without jeopardizing vitality of nasopalatine nerve and vessels: a novel surgical approach. Clin Oral Implants Res 2000;11:505–510.

TAKE-HOME POINTS

A.

- **Foods/drinks:** Coffee, tea, colas, wines, and certain fruits and vegetables (e.g., apples and potatoes) can stain teeth.
- **Tobacco use:** Smoking or chewing tobacco can stain teeth.
- **Bor dental hygiene:** Inadequate brushing and flossing to remove plaque and stain-producing substances like coffee and tobacco can cause tooth discoloration.
- **Disease:** Treatments for certain conditions can also affect tooth color. For example, head and neck radiation and chemotherapy can cause teeth discoloration [1]. In addition, certain infections in pregnant mothers can cause tooth discoloration in the infant by affecting enamel development.
- **Medications:** The antibiotics tetracycline and doxycycline are known to discolor teeth when given to children whose teeth are still developing (<8 years of age). Mouth rinses and washes containing chlorhexidine and cetylpyridinium chloride can also stain teeth. Antihistamines (like Benadryl), antipsychotic drugs, and drugs for high blood pressure also cause teeth discoloration.
- **Dental materials:** Amalgam restorations can stain teeth a gray-black color [2].
- **Age:** As people age, the outer layer of enamel gets worn away revealing the natural yellow color of dentin.
- **Genetics:** Some people have naturally brighter or thicker enamel than others.
- **Environment:** Excessive fluoride either from environmental sources (naturally high fluoride levels in water) or from excessive use (fluoride applications, rinses, toothpaste, and fluoride supplements taken by mouth) can cause teeth discoloration [3].
- **Trauma:** For example, damage from a fall can disturb enamel formation in young children whose teeth are still developing. Trauma can also cause discoloration to adult teeth due to internal bleeding.

B. There is an increased risk of peri-implantitis in smokers compared with nonsmokers. Studies have shown survival rate of implants in smokers is 73% [4]. The deleterious effects includes impaired wound healing, reduced collagen production, impaired fibroblast function, reduced peripheral circulation, and compromised function of the neutrophils and macrophages. Heavy smokers are not good candidates for dental implants; light to medium smokers should be informed of the increased risk of peri-implantitis and implant failure [5].

C. Porcelain fracture associated with an implant-supported, metal ceramic crown, or fixed partial denture occurs at a higher rate than in tooth-supported restorations, according to the literature [6]. There is a significantly higher risk of porcelain fracture in patients with bruxism habits when the patient has no protective occlusal device. In addition, parafunctional habits have resulted in vertical loss of the peri-implant bone [7,8].

D. Immediate anterior implants should be considered in cases where the configuration of the extraction is still intact and no pathology exists. The implant length should be selected 3 mm longer than the extraction socket so it will integrate into the bone beyond the apical portion for primary stability. Subcrestal placement should be considered for anticipation of bone remodeling following the placement of the prosthesis. A bone graft should be considered to fill in the gap between the walls of the extraction socket and the implant body with the use of a membrane [9,10].

E. A fixed or removable prosthesis can be considered; however, advantages and disadvantages of each option should be discussed with the patient.

F.
- Infection can occur due to possible preexisting pathology into the socket [11,12]
- Nerve damage to the incisive foramen [13]
- Iatrogenic damage to neighboring teeth
- Interproximal bone loss followed by loss of the interdental papillae
- Primary wound closure

Case 3

Sinus Lift and Immediate Implant Placement

CASE STORY

A 43-year-old female was referred by an endodontist, who had suggested placing an implant after sinus grafting due to the fracture of tooth #3. The patient presented with pain upon biting hard materials, with no other symptoms. Tooth #3 exhibited a mobility of 1, and there was moderate pain upon percussion. A tooth fracture was suspected, and extraction, bone graft, sinus graft, and implant placement was recommended. The patient will need to go back to Korea once her husband finished his work in the United States, so the treatment needed to be finished in 8 months. In addition, the patient preferred not to have multiple surgeries done. Therefore, a crestal approach using an internal sinus lift (using the Crestal Window Technique) with immediate implant placement was recommended (Figure 1).

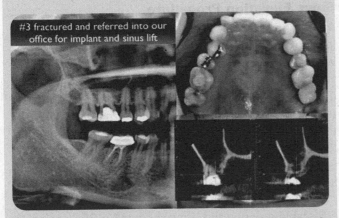

#3 fractured and referred into our office for implant and sinus lift

Figure 1: Initial clinical examination: Preoperative #3 tooth fracture after endodontic attempt. Slightly thickened maxillary sinus membrane due to irritation from tooth #3.

LEARNING GOALS AND OBJECTIVES

- To learn how to perform a sinus lift from a molar extraction socket
- To learn how to place an immediate dental implant at the time of the extraction/sinus lift
- To understand the decision-making process for doing a sinus lift/extraction and immediate implant placement in one visit
- To discuss the indications/contraindications for a sinus lift/extraction/immediate placement

Medical History

The patient was in good health, and her last physical checkup had been within 6 months.

Review of Systems

- Vital signs
  - Blood pressure: 107/65 mm Hg
  - Pulse rate: 60 beats/minute (regular)

Social History

The patient did not drink alcohol or smoke.

Extraoral Examination

No significant findings were noted. The patient had no masses or swelling, and no trismus. No palpable lymphadenopathy was observed, and the temporomandibular joints were within normal limits (Figure 2).

Intraoral Examination

- The soft tissues of the mouth including the tongue appeared normal. The oral cancer screening was negative.

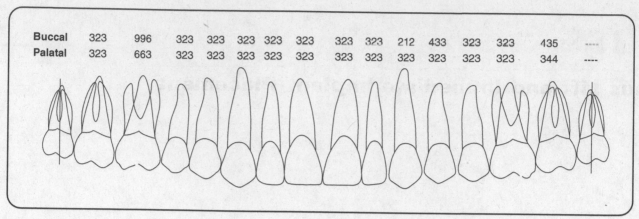

Buccal	323	996	323	323	323	323	323	323	323	212	433	323	323	435	----
Palatal	323	663	323	323	323	323	323	323	323	323	323	323	323	344	----

Figure 2: Probing pocket depth measurements.

- The gingival examination revealed a generalized mild marginal erythema.
- A hard tissue examination was completed by referring endodontist
- The patient had moderate pain upon biting (tooth #3) and a tooth fracture was suspected (Figure 1).

Occlusion

Canine guidance, deep bite, and a mild Curve of Spee. Opposing occlusion were natural teeth.

Radiographic Examination

A digital panoramic radiograph (Figure 1) showed a temporary filling material in the pulp chamber of #3. The computed tomography (CT) scan showed mild inflammation of the sinus membrane. There was 4-m initial bone height from crestal bone to sinus floor (Figure 1).

Treatment

The patient received oral hygiene instructions and a prophylaxis. She was premedicated with amoxicillin 500 mg tid, metronidazole 500 mg tid, and Sudafed 30 mg.

Preoperative Consultation

The medical history was reviewed. The consent form addressing benefits and risks associated with the procedure was reviewed with the patient. The patient was seeking a fixed restoration so implant was recommended. Because the sinus floor was only 5 mm from the crestal bone, a sinus grafting procedure was recommended. However, due to the limited time available, the patient asked if the restoration could be placed within 1 year (Figure 3).

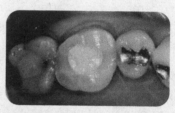

Figure 3: Preoperative image, prior to extraction.

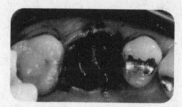

Figure 4: After extraction, note preservation of buccal plate.

Sinus Elevation Procedure

A posterior superior alveolar (PSA) nerve block and local infiltrations were achieved with Septocaine 4% with epinephrine 1:100,000. An atraumatic extraction was done on tooth #3 preserving the buccal plate (Figure 4). A blunt-ended Glick instrument was used to probe around the socket to get a mental three-dimensional "view" of the socket and to ensure there were no major dehiscence or fenestrations. Several methods could be used to achieve the internal sinus lift. In this case a pointed trephine was used to mark the location of the implant (Figure 5). The adjustable stopper and bone ejector (ASBE) trephine is use to set the stopper 1 mm short of the sinus floor (Figure 6). This ensures that the sharp teeth of the ASBE trephine do not penetrate the Schneiderian

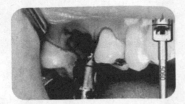

Figure 5: Pointed trephine to mark implant location precisely.

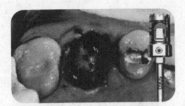

Figure 6: ASBE trephine to go 1 mm below estimated sinus floor.

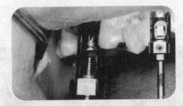

Figure 7: Slow speed is used with ASBE trephine.

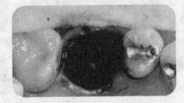

Figure 8: After ASBE trephine.

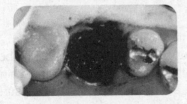

Figure 9: Bone core removed.

membrane. Slow speed is recommended to induce fracture of the bone core (Figure 7). Location and trephine should be verified again to ensure that the implant is placed in the center of the extraction socket (Figure 8). The bone core should be removed after use of the elevator to fracture it off the sinus floor (Figure 9). A flat-ended diamond drill is used to grind away the

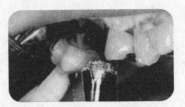

Figure 10: Flat diamond bur to expose sinus membrane.

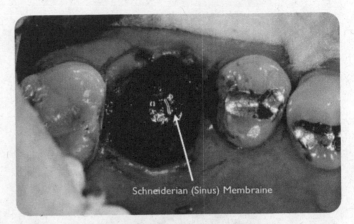

Schneiderian (Sinus) Membraine

Figure 11: Sinus membrane exposed.

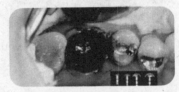

Figure 12: Series of mushroom elevators used to detach and elevate sinus membrane.

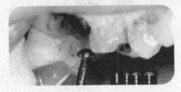

Figure 13: Mushroom elevators are also used to make crestal window larger by pulling sinus floor away from membrane.

sinus floor without perforating the Schneiderian membrane (Figure 10). Cold saline should be used to clean the socket visualizing the Schneiderian membrane. The cold temperature reduces blood flow to the socket, therefore improving visibility to the crestal window (Figure 11). A series of mushroom elevators are used to elevate the sinus membrane (Figure 12) as well as to pry away bony tips from the sinus floor, thus further enlarging the crestal window (Figure 13). A Cobra instrument is used to further

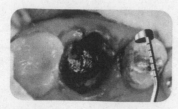

Figure 14: Cobra instrument is used to further elevate the sinus membrane.

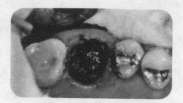

Figure 15: Movement of sinus membrane is verified to check if membrane perforation occurred.

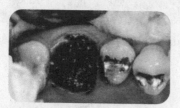

Figure 16: FDB bone graft is introduced to sinus window as well to socket.

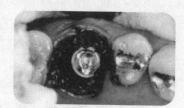

Figure 17: Implant, MEGAGEN Rescue 6.5 × 10 mm is placed slowly.

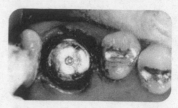

Figure 18: An 8-03 healing abutment is placed to seal the socket retaining bone graft material.

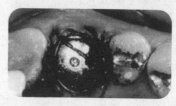

Figure 19: A 4-0 gut suture is used to further tighten and seal the socket to prevent loss of blood clot and bone graft materials.

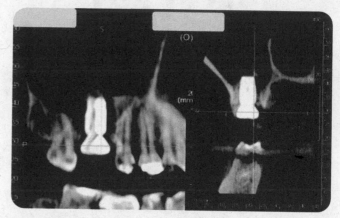

Figure 20: Postoperative CT scan showing bone graft intact under the Schneiderian membrane.

elevate the sinus membrane (Figure 14), but this step can usually be skipped if the sinus membrane is thick (white color). The patient is asked to breath in and out via nose to verify that membrane is not torn (Figure 15). An intact membrane moves up and down versus a perforated membrane where expelled air can be detected [1]. Then 1.5 ml of bone graft (freeze-dried bone allograft [FDBA]) is packed into the sinus and around the socket (Figure 16). A wide diameter implant (Megagen Rescue Implant 6.5 × 10 mm) was inserted slowly with good initial stability >20 Ncm (Figure 17). If poor initial stability is achieved, then a greater diameter implant insertion is recommended [2] (e.g., 7.0 mm or 7.5 mm). A super-wide diameter healing abutment is used to seal the socket (Figure 18) to retain the bone graft material and to achieve primary closure. Simple interrupted sutures or continuous locking sutures are recommended with 4-0 gut chromic to further tighten and seal the socket (Figure 19). A postoperative radiograph should be taken to verify that bone graft material is well retained below the Schneiderian membrane (Figure 20).

Discussion

As mentioned earlier, most crestal approaches are "blind techniques" [3]. In contrast, this technique is not a blind technique. It is especially useful in extraction of multirooted teeth because elevation of sinus can be achieved via socket without laying any flap [4].

The average buccal lingual dimension of molar tooth is 11 mm. Therefore, the crestal approach can be done with a 5- to 6-mm window via septum of the molar socket. A trephine is used to cut septal bone 1 mm below the sinus wall. Slow speed <30 rpm and a twist of ASBE trephine when reaching close to the sinus floor are recommended to aid in fracture of the septal bone away from the sinus floor. Slow speed increases friction between the bone core and inner side of the ASBE trephine, thus inducing fracture of bone. The ASBE trephine has an inner shank that can be used to expel bone core from the trephine. If the septal bone does not come out with the ASBE trephine and stays intact like in this case (Figure 8), induction of septal fracture is done with a narrow Luxator or thin elevator. After removal of this bone core, flat diamond drill is used. The flat diamond drill has a large surface area at the tip of the bur; thus it puts a low amount of pressure onto the Schneiderian membrane (P = F/A) [4]. As emphasized earlier, this technique is *not* a blind technique, and manual elevation is done with mini instruments with the aid of magnification (loupe).

In contrast to the conventional recommendation of the two-stage approach when the initial bone height is <5 mm, this unique technique shortens treatment time by 6–8 months and reduces the multiple number of surgeries for our patients [5] (Table 1). No flap is raised; therefore patients do really well postoperatively without any pain, swelling, nor bruising [3]. Case selection is critical in these cases. Clinicians need to select cases that have low initial bone height (1–5 mm) with wide buccal lingual bone (>9 mm) [4]. If there are periapical lesions, or fracture of buccal bone during extractions two-stage approaches are recommended (bone graft first, then sinus and implant later). Clinicians should strive for primary stability and not overtorque the implant. Also, care should be taken not to displace the implant into the sinus.

The initial stability is achieved with very minimal bone to implant contact. Therefore, once in a while (<10%), the implant might lose stability as the bone

heals. Therefore, a monthly checkup is recommended. A dental #5 explorer is used on the screw hole of the healing abutment and a light shake is done to determine the stability of an implant. If any mobility is suspected (usually in the first month after surgery), the implant is rotated out counterclockwise, and a larger implant by 1 mm in diameter is placed after degranulating the osteotomy site. The same healing abutment is placed back. This procedure usually takes <3 minutes, and there is no associated postoperative discomfort. This ensures that the implant will integrate well.

The use of super-large healing abutments (8–10 mm in diameter) can help achieve primary closure in large extraction socket without raising any flap. If a small gap <2 mm is still present, suturing with 4-0 chromic gut will close it. If >2 mm of gap is present, collagen tape can be used around this gap, or semilunar coronally positioned flap can be elevated to close the gaps. This super-large healing abutment prepares the gingival for a good emergence profile for molar restoration.

Table 1: Comparison of Crestal Window Technique to Conventional Two-Stage Approach*

Timeline	Conventional Two-Stage Approach	Crestal Window Technique Right After Extraction
First surgery (4–6 months)	Extraction and ridge preservation	Extraction, sinus grafting, implant placement, ridge preservation, and one-stage surgery (healing abutment
Second surgery (4–6 months)	Sinus grafting	Already done on first surgery
Third surgery (4–6 months)	Implant placement	Already done on first surgery
Fourth surgery (3 weeks)	Second-stage surgery	Already done on first surgery

*This technique shortens treatment time by threefold and reduces multiple number of surgeries to patients. Thus this is a less traumatic approach for patients needing an implant in the pneumatized posterior maxilla.

Self-Study Questions

A. What are the advantages of using the internal sinus lift (in this case the Crestal Window Technique) in an extraction socket?

B. What speed is recommended when using ASBE trephine and why?

C. Which bone (wall) is the most important bone to preserve in an extraction?

D. If good initial stability of an implant is not achieved, which protocol should be followed?

E. What is recommended postoperative follow-up with the Crestal Window Technique in an extraction socket?

F. If the gap between the super-large healing abutment and the gum still exists, what are three techniques discussed that can be used to achieve good primary closure?

G. What are two clinical advantages of using a super-large healing abutment?

H. What are the contraindications to performing a sinus lift/extraction/immediate implant placement? How do you manage complications (torn membrane, no primary stability, etc.)?

Answers located at the end of the chapter.

References

1. Soltan M, Smiler DG. Antral membrane balloon elevation. J Oral Implantol 2005;31:85–90.
2. Torelli S, Bercy P. Incidence and primary prevention of complications related to the placement of dental implants. Rev Belge Med Dent (1984);2001;56:35–61.
3. Chen L, Cha J. An 8-year retrospective study: 1,100 patients receiving 1,557 implants using the minimally invasive hydraulic sinus condensing technique. J Periodontol 2005;76:482–491.
4. Lee S. Crestal sinus lift: a minimally invasive and systematic approach to sinus grafting. J Implant Adv Clin Dent 2009;1:7588.
5. Bruschi GB, Scipioni A, et al. Localize management of the sinus floor with simultaneous implant placement: a clinical report. Int J Oral Maxillofac Implants 1998;13:219–226.
6. Lindhe J, Lang NP et al. Clinical Periodontology and Implant Dentistry. 5th ed. Oxford, UK: Wiley-Blackwell, 2008.
7. Yamashita M, Horita S, et al. Minimally invasive alveolar ridge preservation/augmentation procedure (open barrier membrane technique). Paper presented at: American Academy of Periodontology 96th Annual Meeting; 2010; Honolulu, HI.

TAKE-HOME POINTS

A. The Crestal Window Technique is a minimally invasive procedure, and the clinician is able to lift sinus in predictable manner because it is not a blind technique. There is no flap elevation in an extraction socket, resulting in less postoperative pain and swelling. In addition, sinus lift, socket grafting, implant placement, and the one-stage approach are all done in one visit, reducing treatment time by threefold compared with conventional techniques (Table 1).

B. Slow speed <30 rpm is recommended for ASBE trephine. Slow speed increases the friction between the bone core and the trephine, increasing chances of bone core fracture from the sinus floor. Slow speed eliminates the need to use irrigation (to reduce bone heating); thus patient comfort is increased and visibility is also improved compared with high speed, which requires irrigation (1000 rpm).

C. The buccal plate is made of bundle bone [6]. It is the weakest bone in an extraction socket. Therefore, preservation of buccal bone is important key in immediate implant placement. No elevator should be used directly on buccal bone, and care should be taken not to fracture this thin bone.

D. If the stability of an implant is <10 Ncm, then a larger size (0.5 mm larger diameter) implant should be placed to increase initial stability. Any micromovement of an implant will not integrate with bone and will be surrounded by granulation tissues [2]. However, if buccal bone is thin and the distance from buccal plate to implant is <2 mm, a larger diameter implant should not be placed. Instead, a two-stage approach with healing cap is recommended, or the open membrane technique should be used to cover the socket [7].

E. Initial stability decreases as bone remodels, and it is weakest during the third week. Therefore, the first month check-up of these implants is crucial to check mobility. Remember that initial stability in this technique is achieved by only thin cortical bone of the sinus floor. If any movement of an implant is suspected, it should be removed by counterclockwise rotation and replaced with a larger implant by 1 mm diameter.

F. Semilunar coronally repositioned flap (Figures 21 and 22)
1. Apply CollaTape around the healing abutment
2. Suture with 4–0 chromic gut if gap is <2 mm

G. Super-large healing abutment (8–10 mm in diameter) is useful in sealing the extraction site. This technique preserves the zone of keratinized tissue and reduces patient morbidity. It also molds tissue to achieve an excellent emergence profile for molar restorations.

H. The contraindications for performing a sinus lift/extraction/immediate implant placement are sinus pathology, lack of buccal bone or palatal bone, and the presence of pus in a socket.

A small torn sinus membrane (<4 mm) can be patched with collagen membrane if access is

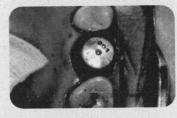

Figure 21: Palatal flap is opened even with a super-wide diameter healing abutment.

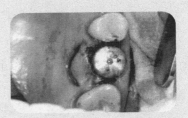

Figure 22: Semilunar coronally positioned flap used to close the palatal gap.

possible. If not, lateral window can be performed to have better access to the torn membrane, and it can be patched with collagen membrane. If the tear is >7 mm, the procedure should be avoided and retried in 3 months.

In case of lack of initial stability (spinner), a larger implant can be used to achieve better initial stability. If larger implant cannot be used, the implant should be submerged, and an "open membrane technique" should be used with nonresorbable membrane. If the implant rocks mesial-distally or buccal-lingually, just bone grafting (socket preservation) should be used.

9

Preventive Periodontal Therapy

Clinical Cases in Periodontics, First Edition. Nadeem Karimbux.
© 2012 John Wiley & Sons, Inc. Published 2012 by John Wiley & Sons, Inc.

Case 1

Plaque Removal

CASE STORY
A 55-year-old Caucasian male, a plumber by trade, presented with a chief complaint of: "I know that my teeth are bad, and I want them fixed" (Figures 1 and 2).

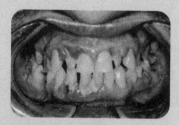

Figure 1: Initial examination presentation.

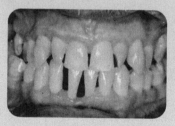

Figure 2: One year following plaque control instruction and scaling and root planing.

LEARNING GOALS AND OBJECTIVES
- To understand that the behavioral motivation of a patient, to be consistent and thorough with biofilm removal, is of paramount importance in successful dental therapy, and that no matter how thorough scaling and root planing therapy is done, it is the *daily* removal of biofilm by the patient that sustains the professional therapy
- To know that the removal of the etiologic agents can lead to healing with repair of the periodontium and sometimes even to regeneration
- To learn various techniques of behavioral motivation and of plaque removal

Medical History
The patient had no significant past medical problems, nor were there any known allergies other than the severe periodontal infection. He reported no present medical illnesses and stated that he was taking no medications. He had not had a general physical examination for several years.

Dental History
Over the past several years, the patient had noticed blood on his toothbrush and in his saliva whenever he brushed his teeth, and he stated that he had bad breath. The patient claimed to brush his teeth only once a week because he did not like the taste of blood. He did not use dental floss or any other means of interproximal plaque control. He used mouthwash occasionally. His most recent visit to the dentist had been 12 years ago for "some fillings."

Review of Systems

- Vital signs
  - Blood pressure: 120/65
  - Pulse rate: 72 beats/minute (regular)
  - Respiration: 15 breaths/minute

Social History

The patient did not drink alcohol. He had smoked cigarettes since he was age 23 and currently smoked a half a pack (10 cigarettes) daily.

Extraoral Examination

No significant findings were noted. The patient had no masses or swelling, and the temporomandibular joint was within normal limits (Figure 3).

Intraoral Examination

- Plaque control techniques were observed and were inadequate for complete plaque removal.
- The soft tissues of the mouth with the exception of the gingiva appeared normal.
- The gingival examination revealed severe marginal erythema, with rolled margins and edematous, bulbous, and spongy papillae (Figure 1).
- A dental examination revealed cervical and interproximal smooth surface caries.

Occlusion

There were no occlusal discrepancies or interferences. There were no parafunctional problems, and there was no significant attrition.

Radiographic Examination

A complete mouth series of periapical radiographs revealed calculus, caries, defective restorations, evidence of from 25% to 85% angular bone loss, a loss of crestal-septal density, and a root tip with root canal therapy #29. (See Figure 4 for the patient's mandibular anterior periapical radiographs pretreatment and Figure 5 showing 1 year post-treatment.)

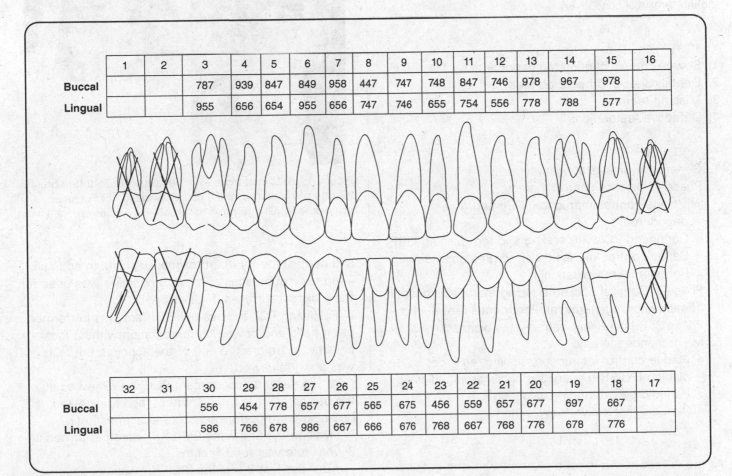

	1	2	3	4	5	6	7	8	9	10	11	12	13	14	15	16
Buccal			787	939	847	849	958	447	747	748	847	746	978	967	978	
Lingual			955	656	654	955	656	747	746	655	754	556	778	788	577	

	32	31	30	29	28	27	26	25	24	23	22	21	20	19	18	17
Buccal			556	454	778	657	677	565	675	456	559	657	677	697	667	
Lingual			586	766	678	986	667	666	676	768	667	768	776	678	776	

Figure 3: Probing pocket depth measurements.

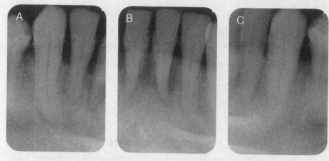

Figure 4: (A–C) Periapical preoperative radiographs depicting the interproximal bone levels.

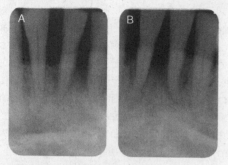

Figure 5: (A,B) Periapical postoperative radiographs depicting the interproximal bone levels.

Diagnosis

1. Severe chronic generalized periodontitis
2. Dental caries and fractured teeth
3. Missing teeth
4. Defective restorations

Treatment Plan

1. General physical examination
2. Phase 1: Disease control therapy:
   - Plaque control instruction (PCI) and gross debridement
   - Continued PCI with scaling and root planing (SRP)
   - Caries control, extraction of nontreatable teeth
   - Periodontal reevaluation
3. Phase 2: Surgical pocket-reducing therapy as needed (resective or regenerative): Periodontal reevaluation
4. Phase 3: Restorative treatment (as planned)
5. Maintenance therapy:
   - Plaque control Instruction, scaling, and root planing (PCISRP) every 3 months or as indicated
   - Periodic periodontal reevaluation
   - Periodic restorative reevaluation

Treatment

At the outset of the initial treatment visit, the patient was instructed in an intrasulcular technique of brushing

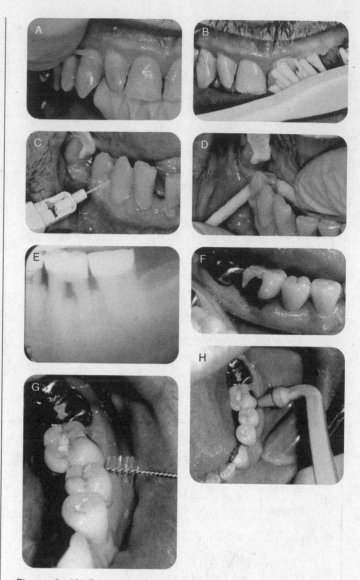

Figure 6: (A) Dental tape; (B) intrasulcular multi-tufted brush; (C) interproximal brush; (D) gauze bandage. (E) Furcation involvement; (G) interproximal brush; (H) rubber tip.

and dental tape for interproximal cleaning. In addition, interproximal brushes and gauze bandage was used for the proximal surfaces (Figures 6A–D).

Following PCI, a gross debridement was performed using hand and power instrumentation without local anesthetic. Before the end of the appointment PCI was again reviewed.

At the second appointment PCI was reviewed at the beginning of the appointment, and scaling and polishing were performed using local anesthetic.

Hygiene therapy visits (PCISRP) were performed at 2-week intervals for 3 months.

After the first 3 months, PCISRP was continued at 5-week intervals. After 1 year of treatment the patient had achieved excellence in home care techniques and consistency. There was a significant resolution of the inflammation and reduced pocketing (Figure 2).

Postoperative radiographs of the mandibular anterior teeth at 1 year revealed apparent bone fill associated with tooth #24 (Figure 5).

Discussion

Because periodontitis is a plaque-induced inflammatory disease initiated by the periodontal pathogens in the plaque [1] and plaque adheres to the tooth surface, the treatment of periodontitis involves three factors:

1. That the patient be *motivated* to perform daily home care techniques
2. That the patient *kows and per forms appropriate* techniques to remove the plaque
3. That the patient is able to *access* the tooth to perform the correct techniques

The theory of plaque removal from teeth is a basic principle of physics: "Two objects cannot occupy the same place at the same time and the object of the greater mass will displace the object of the lesser mass." Plaque removal is a displacement process, not an abrasive process. Thus scrubbing one's teeth is not only unnecessary but might be harmful. If the toothbrush bristles are moving across a tooth in the cervical third, abrasion of the teeth or gingiva might occur (especially if toothpaste is used), and the bristles will not enter into the gingival crevice.

The techniques shown to the patient were an intrasulcular technique of brushing, the "stationary jiggle technique," which is a modification of the Bass technique [2]. This technique involves using a multi-tufted nylon toothbrush with bristle diameters of 0.007. The brush head is angled slightly toward the gingival crevice (approximately 70°). The brush head is placed approximately at the middle of the clinical crown and pressure is applied against the tooth to place the bristle tips into the gingival sulcus and to maintain them in the gingival third of the tooth "stationary" on the tooth surface. The handle of the brush is moved in a *short* back-and-forth (vibratory) motion for 3–4 seconds without the bristle tips moving on the tooth (no scrubbing). This technique is repeated in the same location three times, each time removing the bristles from the tooth and replacing them. We recommended that the patient begin on the facial aspect of the most posterior tooth in any quadrant and move anteriorly overlapping the bristle placement, once crossing the midline then moving posteriorly and ending on the facial aspect of the most posterior tooth in the opposite quadrant. The patient then will continue on the lingual surfaces of the teeth in a like manner until ending back at the beginning point. The opposite arch is cleaned in the same manner. Most people brush randomly and by rote. With a power brush, the same technique is used *without moving the handle*.

For interproximal plaque control we recommended dental tape, a rubber tip, and interproximal brushes. The technique we instructed for the dental tape was to anchor the tape on the ring finger, to use the index finger and thumb to wrap the tape in a "C" fashion around the tooth, and to use a buccolingual-apicoocclusal movement of the tape with firm lateral pressure against the tooth surface, similar to the method people use to dry their back with a towel following a bath or shower. The tape is placed subgingivally until the base of the sulcus is reached. There should be *no* apical pressure against the epithelial attachment, only lateral pressure against the proximal surface of the tooth and the line angles. All mesial and distal surfaces are to be cleaned in this fashion.

We recommended a rubber tip be used from the facial to the lingual and vice versa for interproximal pockets that cannot be accessed by the dental tape, where there are subgingival tooth concavities, where the papilla are edematous, or where pockets exceed 4 mm. The rubber tip is also effective when used to displace plaque from furcations. The interproximal brush is effective supragingivally and when there are tooth concavities or class 2 or 3 furcation involvements (see Chapter 4).

Other interproximal plaque control devices include bridge threaders to carry the dental tape interproximally where contacts are not open. Balsa wood triangular interdental devices, which simulate a rubber tip, are difficult to use. Two-inch-wide by 10-inch-long moist gauze bandage strips are recommended to clean the proximal surfaces of teeth next to edentulous areas.

Other brush-type devices are single tufted brushes to enter into furcations and end-tuft brushes to remove plaque on the distal of posterior teeth next to an edentulous area, especially if there are furcations exposed (Figure 6A–H).

Self-Study Questions

A. When in a treatment plan should plaque control therapy (P ISRP be instituted?

B. How frequently should patients clean (brush, floss, etc.) their teeth?

C. Why is it recommended to concentrate on brushing and flossing (taping) techniques, and what is the concern about "random" brushing?

D. Why use an intrasulcular technique, and what is the advantage of dental tape?

E. Why is an angle of the toothbrush bristles to the tooth of 70° recommended over the classic 45°?

F. Why place the toothbrush bristles on the clinical crown of the tooth and into the gingival crevice and not half on the tooth and half on the gingiva?

G. How often should plaque control instruction (P I) be done and why?

H. Why do P I at the outset of the appointment and not following the debridement?

I. How can smoking mask the signs of gingival inflammation and mislead the clinician and patient?

J. How is it possible to achieve regeneration from excellent plaque removal by a patient and comprehensive root debridement (root planing)?

K. Why were all of the pockets not resolved?

L. What questions should be asked in cases where the gingivitis or periodontitis do not resolve?

Answers located at the end of the chapter.

References

1. Haffajee AD, Socransky SS. Microbiology of periodontal diseases: introduction. Periodontol 2000. 2005;38:9–12.
2. Bass CC. The optimum characteristics of dental floss for personal oral hygiene. Dent Items Interest 1948;70:921–934.
3. Rosenberg ES, Evian CI, Listgarten MA. The composition of the subgingival microbiota after periodontal therapy. J Periodontol 1981;52:435–441.
4. Bergström J, Preber H. The influence of cigarette smoking on the development of experimental gingivitis. J Periodontal Res 1986;21:668–676.
5. Bergström J, Floderus-Myrhed B. Co-twin control study of the relationship between smoking and some periodontal disease factors. Community Dent Oral Epidemiol 1983;11:113–116.
6. Preber H, Bergström J. Occurrence of gingival bleeding in smoker and non-smoker patients. Acta Odontol Scand 1985;43:315–320.
7. Bergström J. Cigarette smoking as risk factor in chronic periodontal disease. Community Dent Oral Epidemiol 1989;17:245–247.
8. Bergström J. Oral hygiene compliance and gingivitis expression in cigarette smokers. Scand J Dent Res 1990;98:497–503.
9. Johnson GK, Hill M. Cigarette smoking and the periodontal patient [review]. J Periodontol 2004;75:196–209.
10. Papapanou PN. Periodontal diseases: epidemiology [review]. Ann Periodontol 1996;1:1–36.
11. Tonetti MS. Cigarette smoking and periodontal diseases: etiology and management of disease [review]. Ann Periodontol. 1998;3:88–101.
12. Stambaugh RV, Dragoo M, et al. The limits of subgingival scaling. Int J Periodontics Restorative Dent 1981;1:30–41.

TAKE-HOME POINTS

A. Plaque control therapy should be the *first* on the definitive treatment plan sequence following these steps:

- Any medical consultations that need to be done where treatment could negatively affect the patient's health.
- All dental consultations have been done that might affect whether or not a tooth should be retained.
- Any emergency therapy that is needed to eliminate pain, acute infection, and replace an avulsed tooth in the aesthetic zone.
- Any emergency caries control to prevent an irreversible pulpitis.
- Any emergency extraction of an extremely mobile and nontreatable tooth.

B. Because plaque generally matures in 1–3 days, the ideal habit for a patient to remove all plaque (biofilm) from all tooth surfaces to preserve health is once daily. This said, however, it depends on the patient's susceptibility to dental caries and/or periodontal infections (gingivitis and periodontitis). Clearly if the patient has a high caries rate, shows significant gingival inflammation, and/or exhibits evidence of attachment loss caused by present or past periodontitis, thorough plaque removal should be done twice a day.

If the patient has malposed teeth where there is a high likelihood for food to collect, if they exhibit oral malodor or "feel" their teeth are not clean, the removal of food debris and plaque is indicated more than once daily.

C. Plaque is generally invisible to patients and to us when we are cleaning our teeth. Subgingival plaque is always invisible even if erythrosine plaque-disclosing preparations are used. Even with them, it is virtually impossible to see interproximally and to see the lingual surfaces of most teeth. In fact, the disclosing preparations used by the patient to detect for unremoved plaque show the surfaces of the teeth most easily cleaned and not the hard-to-clean surfaces. Cleaning plaque from teeth is like trying to paint a wall without missing any area when we are blindfolded. Like painting a wall, once the techniques are learned, they are not difficult; however, unlike painting a wall, we cannot see plaque that is missed with our techniques. Thus brushing and flossing techniques need to be done with concentration. That means thinking as one is doing plaque removal techniques: "Do I feel the toothbrush bristles in the gum crevice? Am I keeping the toothbrush bristle tips stationary on the tooth at the gum crevice and not scrubbing? Am I overlapping strokes so as not to miss an area? Am I adapting the dental tape to the tooth surface and moving it up and down (apically occlusally) and not sawing it into the gum? Am I using adequate pressure with the dental tape horizontally against the tooth?" Not concentrating on techniques can lead to a rote repetitive situation where plaque can remain on the teeth following home care, which might cause caries, gingival inflammation, attachment loss, and perhaps abrade the gingiva or the teeth.

D. In 1948, C.C. Bass [2], a physician from Louisiana, wrote in the *Louisiana Medical Journal* that it was bacterial toxin collecting under the gum that created the gingival inflammation, which was the cause of gingivitis and periodontitis. He advocated a brushing technique that used a soft multi-tufted nylon toothbrush and an intrasulcular technique of brushing. Prior to that and for many years thereafter, the brushing technique that was advocated was a Stillman's or Charter's (sweeping technique or fones (scrubbing technique). The Stillman's and Charter's techniques recommended an extra-hard natural bristle toothbrush be used.

Dental tape is wider than dental floss. Although it is made of the type of filaments as dental floss, there are a greater number of them. The benefit of dental tape over dental floss is that dental tape covers a greater surface area of the tooth, and there is increased frictional grip to the tooth with dental tape rather than dental floss. The frictional grip is important because it helps prevent the tape from slipping into the gingival crevice with force that could cause damage to the epithelial attachment. There has been a misconception that dental tape is thicker and more difficult to bring through the contact area between the teeth. On the contrary, dental tape is made with the same diameter filament as dental floss of the same manufacturer, and actually most dental tape shreds less than dental floss.

E. An angle of 70° of the toothbrush bristles to the tooth will access *all* gingival crevices, whereas a 45° angle many times does not allow the toothbrush bristles to access the gingival crevice on the lingual of the mandibular posterior teeth, which is a very common area for gingival/periodontal infection. That said, it is not recommended to explain any "angle" to a patient because many people do not remember or never studied geometry and do not understand angle dimensions. In addition some might be confused with whether it is the inside or outside angle of the bristles to the tooth. An intrasulcular technique of brushing is a technique whereby the patient can "feel" the bristles enter into the gum crevice.

Our suggestion is to recommend that the patient angle the brush bristle tips toward the gum crevice and place the bristles about in the middle of the tooth (clinical crown of the tooth) and press the bristles into the tooth until they "feel" the toothbrush bristles *enter into* the gum crevice. Then if using a hand (nonpower) brush, move the handle in short strokes back and forth with enough pressure to maintain the bristles tips at the gum crevice stationary and connected with the tooth. This technique avoids scrubbing and toothbrush abrasion of the gingiva and the tooth. We have named it the "stationary jiggle" technique. It differs only slightly from the Bass technique in that it avoids talking about a 45° angle, and it suggests that the bristles be entirely on the tooth and not half on the tooth and half on the gingiva. The reasons for not using the statement of half on the tooth and half on the gingiva is because dental biofilm, which can cause caries or periodontal disease, resides on the tooth, and thus we do not want to confuse the patient that the gums must be deplaqued for gum health. Along the same lines, many people believe they need to "exercise" or "stimulate" their gingiva to make it healthy.

Brushing the gingiva can be more harmful than good and can lead to gingival recession in a thin periodontal biotype or ulceration of the gingiva due to epithelial and connective tissue abrasion.

F. Plaque/biofilm resides on the tooth in quantities that can cause infection because the tooth is an unchanging surface. Placing the toothbrush bristles on the gingiva can lead to abrasion of the gingiva, might be uncomfortable, and does not remove plaque that will cause disease. It also is confusing to patients because they think the brush is "stimulating the gingiva" and thereby providing health. This is a nonproven theory, and the detriment of brushing the gingiva far outweighs any possible advantage.

G. The need for PCI depends on the patient's abilities with a toothbrush, dental tape (floss), and other recommended plaque removal aids. From a physical therapy viewpoint, it is imperative that a patient demonstrate brushing and flossing (taping) techniques at the outset of their initial comprehensive examination. Many times we find that a patient who seemingly has excellent plaque control and who shows no signs of gingival inflammation is scrubbing the teeth and is likely in time to cause cervical abrasion and gingival recession. Part of a comprehensive examination is knowing the patient's dental hygiene techniques. We cannot rely on the patient to describe it to us any more than a golf coach can rely on a client's description of how the golf club is swung.

PCI should be done at each visit for hygiene therapy regardless of whether the visit is a periodic maintenance appointment or part of initial phase therapy including scaling and root planning [3] and regardless of how much plaque we can see because we cannot visualize subgingival and interproximal plaque. It should be done at the inception of the visit and if necessary repeated at the end. It should be done *before* local anesthesia is used (topical or injectable) because all the intrasulcular brushing techniques rely on the patient's proprioception, which will be lost following anesthesia. If the patient's plaque control is unacceptable and the patient is being seen for a visit for other than hygiene therapy, PCI should be instituted at the outset of that appointment and before local anesthesia is administered.

The answer to "why" is that for a patient with natural teeth or with implants, the key to oral and general health is controlling the biofilm on the tooth or implant. This must be primarily done by the patient because plaque can mature in as little as 24 hours, and it is the patient's responsibility to achieve and preserve dental health and our responsibility to be their coaches and assist them in removing what cannot be removed with a brush, dental tape (floss), and other aids for plaque removal.

H. Most individuals have always been told that one does the most important things first. Reviewing hygiene therapy at the end of the appointment connotes to the patient that it is *less* important than the hygiene therapy (scaling, root planing, or polishing) that we do as professionals. The lasting effect of what we do depends on the patient's home care.
1. At the end of the appointment following our professional therapy, the patient is tired and ready to leave. The attention span then is likely to be short at the end of an appointment.
2. If, when doing PCI at the outset of therapy, the patient has difficulty manipulating the dental tape (floss) or toothbrush, there is the end of the appointment to review the techniques again.

I. Smoking appears to reduce the clinical signs of inflammation with plaque accumulation [4].
1. Clinical studies show that smokers exhibit less inflammation than nonsmokers [5–8].
2. Although the signs if inflammation appear less in smokers than in nonsmokers, the preponderance of studies show that smoking is a major risk factor for periodontitis and that periodontitis is more prevalent and more severe in smokers than nonsmokers [9–11].

J. Periodontal regeneration (see Chapter 4) can occur when the conditions for healing are present. Regeneration can occur in these situations:
1. The tooth is thoroughly debrided of biofilm, calculus, and has been thoroughly root planed to remove bacterial toxins.

2. There is an adequate blood supply.
3. The defect is narrow and generally has three walls and one tooth surface.
4. There is an adequate surface area of periodontal ligament exposed inside the infrabony defect.
5. The patient is performing an excellent level of supra- and subgingival plaque control.
6. The patient is systemically healthy and a nonsmoker.

K. The most likely answer is that not all of the calculus was completely removed from the tooth surface. Stambaugh and Dragoo [12] stated that it was unlikely in pockets ≥5 mm to do complete root debridement and calculus removal. In addition, most of the infrabony osseous defects were not narrow with three walls and one tooth surface.

L. The first thing is to determine the etiology:
1. **Are the patients concordant with their home care and do they use the correct techniques?** If the patients are not consistent with brushing and taping (flossing), then continue to explain that they have disease and only they can eliminate it with thorough and consistent plaque removal. If the patient is consistent, however, on observing the techniques and plaque is not being removed, work on techniques and emphasize the need to concentrate on techniques and not to do them by rote.
2. **Are there any systemic factors preventing normal healing?** Assess when the patient last had a general physical examination. If it has been >2 years or if there is a suspected systemic problem and it has not been diagnosed, consult with the patient's physician.
3. **Does the patient use tobacco products?** If so and the patient wishes to eliminate the tobacco habit, offer a tobacco cessation program or refer the person to their physician or to an ongoing tobacco cessation program.
4. **Is there detectable subgingival calculus?** If so, redo the scaling and root planing.
5. **Are there pockets that cannot be accessed for complete daily plaque control?** If so, explain pocket-reducing surgical therapy and initiate therapy or refer the patient to a periodontist for diagnosis and therapy.

Never give up and write off a patient as noncompliant and never compliant. Sometimes it takes years; however, most patients eventually see the value in correct and consistent plaque control techniques. When we remain silent when there is inadequate plaque control, nobody will benefit. The patient's dental health will deteriorate, the work we do for the patient will deteriorate, and our self-esteem will also deteriorate. If we continue the mantra of emphasizing excellence in home care, we have done all that is possible to assure that our patients will receive the best treatment we can provide.

INDEX

Note: Page numbers in *italics* indicate figures.

Clinical Cases in Periodontics, First Edition. Nadeem Karimbux.
© 2012 John Wiley & Sons, Inc. Published 2012 by John Wiley & Sons, Inc.

Printed in the United States
by Bookmasters

Printed in the United States
By Bookmasters